Editor

Claudio Barigozzi
Via Celoria 10
Milan
Italy

W0042609

AMS Subject Classifications (1980): 92 XX

ISBN-13:978-3-540-10279-3   e-ISBN-13:978-3-642-93161-1
DOI: 10.1007/978-3-642-93161-1

2141/3140-543210

FOREWORD

The idea of organizing a symposium on mathematical models in biology came to some colleagues, members of the Accademia dei Lincei, in order to point out the importance of mathematics not only for supplying instruments for the elaboration and the evaluation of experimental data, but also for discussing the possibility of developing mathematical formulations of biological problems. This appeared particularly appropriate for genetics, where mathematical models have been of historical importance.

When the organizing work had started, it became clear to us that the classic studies of Vito Volterra (who was also a Member of the Academy and its President from 1923 to 1926) might be considered a further reason to have the meeting in Rome at the Accademia dei Lincei; thus the meeting is dedicated to his memory.

Biology, in its manifold aspects proved to be a difficult object for an exhaustive approach; thus it became necessary for practical reasons to make a choice of problems. Therefore not all branches of biology have been represented.

The proceedings of the symposium, as a whole, assume a knowledge of mathematics on the part of the reader; however the problem of teaching mathematics to biologists was the subject of a round table discussion, not recorded in these proceedings. On this were brought up some basic points to be recommended to teachers on an international basis, and a statement was prepared for circulation.

The Organizing Committee

Lecture Notes in Biomathematics

Vol. 1: P. Waltman, Deterministic Threshold Models in the Theory of Epidemic 101 pages. 1974.

Vol. 2: Mathematical Problems in Biology, Victoria Conference 1973. Edited by P den Driessche. VI, 280 pages. 1974.

Vol. 3: D. Ludwig, Stochastic Population Theories. VI, 108 pages. 1974.

Vol. 4: Physics and Mathematics of the Nervous System. Edited by M. Conrad, W. tinger, and M. Dal Cin. XI, 584 pages. 1974.

Vol. 5: Mathematical Analysis of Decision Problems in Ecology. Proceedings 1 Edited by A. Charnes and W. R. Lynn. VIII, 421 pages. 1975.

Vol. 6: H. T. Banks, Modeling and Control in the Biomedical Sciences. V, 114 pages. 19

Vol. 7: M. C. Mackey, Ion Transport through Biological Membranes, An Integr Theoretical Approach. IX, 240 pages. 1975.

Vol. 8: C. DeLisi, Antigen Antibody Interactions. IV, 142 pages. 1976.

Vol. 9: N. Dubin, A Stochastic Model for Immunological Feedback in Carcinogenn Analysis and Approximations. XIII, 163 pages. 1976.

Vol. 10: J. J. Tyson, The Belousov-Zhabotinskii Reaktion. IX, 128 pages. 1976.

Vol. 11: Mathematical Models in Medicine. Workshop 1976. Edited by J. Berger, W. I ler, R. Repges, and P. Tautu. XII, 281 pages. 1976.

Vol. 12: A. V. Holden, Models of the Stochastic Activity of Neurones. VII, 368 pages. 19

Vol. 13: Mathematical Models in Biological Discovery. Edited by D. L. Solomone C. Walter. VI, 240 pages. 1977.

Vol. 14: L. M. Ricciardi, Diffusion Processes and Related Topics in Biology. VI, 200 pa 1977.

Vol. 15: Th. Nagylaki, Selection in One- and Two-Locus Systems. VIII, 208 pages. 19

Vol. 16: G. Sampath, S. K. Srinivasan, Stochastic Models for Spike Trains of Si Neurons. VIII, 188 pages. 1977.

Vol. 17: T. Maruyama, Stochastic Problems in Population Genetics. VIII, 245 pages. 19

Vol. 18: Mathematics and the Life Sciences. Proceedings 1975. Edited by D. E. Mattho VII, 385 pages. 1977.

Vol. 19: Measuring Selection in Natural Populations. Edited by F. B. Christiansene T. M. Fenchel. XXXI, 564 pages. 1977.

Vol. 20: J. M. Cushing, Integrodifferential Equations and Delay Models in Popula Dynamics. VI, 196 pages. 1977.

Vol. 21: Theoretical Approaches to Complex Systems. Proceedings 1977. Editeo R. Heim and G. Palm. VI, 244 pages. 1978.

Vol. 22: F. M. Scudo and J. R. Ziegler, The Golden Age of Theoretical Ecology: 1923–19 XII, 490 pages. 1978.

Vol. 23: Geometrical Probability and Biological Structures: Buffon's 200th Annivers Proceedings 1977. Edited by R. E. Miles and J. Serra. XII, 338 pages. 1977

Vol. 24: F. L. Bookstein, The Measurement of Biological Shape and Shape Chan VIII, 191 pages. 1978.

Vol. 25: P. Yodzis, Competition for Space and the Structure of Ecological Communin VI, 191 pages. 1978.

Lecture Notes in Biomathematics

Managing Editor: S. Levin

39

Vito Volterra Symposium on Mathematical Models in Biology

Proceedings of a Conference
Held at the Centro Linceo Interdisciplinare,
Accademia Nazionale dei Lincei, Rome
December 17 – 21, 1979

Edited by Claudio Barigozzi

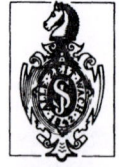

Springer-Verlag
Berlin Heidelberg New York 1980

TABLE OF CONTENTS

TOPIC I   MODELS OF NATURAL SELECTION   1

R. C. Lewontin:
Models of Natural Selection   3

M. Nei:
Stochastic Theory of Population Genetics and Evolution . .   17

A. Robertson:
Natural Selection and Continuous Variation   48

S. A. Levin:
Some Models for the Evolution of Adaptive Traits   56

J. Maynard Smith:
Evolutionary Game Theory   73

G. Malécot:
Variability and Permanence in Molecular Genetics   82

A. Piazza:
Evolution in Human Populations: Data and Models   98

C. Matessi and S.D. Jayakar:
Models of Density- and Frequency- Dependent Selection for
the Exploitation of Resources. II. Coevolution of Species
in Competition 133

F. B. Christiansen and V. Loeschke:
Intraspecific Competition and Evolution 151

L. R. Ginzburg:
Ecological Implications of Natural Selection 171

TOPIC II   PROBLEMS IN POPULATION BIOLOGY AND RELATED
           DISCIPLINES 185

L. Cavalli-Sforza:
Areas of Overlap of Population Genetics with Related
Disciplines 187

L. B. Slobodkin:
Completeness and Craft Standards in Ecological Theory . . . 195

C. Matessi:
A Theoretical Approach to the Dynamics of Single
Populations 222

L. M. Ricciardi:
Stochastic Equations in Neurobiology and Population
Biology 248

K. Dietz:
Models for Vector-Borne Parasitic Diseases 264

R. M. Anderson:
The Dynamics and Control of Direct Life Cycle
Helminth Parasites 278

B. Cvjetanović:
Epidemiologic Models of Bacterial Diseases 323

E.G. Knox:
Strategic Planning Models for Rubella Vaccination
Programmes 329

J. Wyman:
The Cybernetics of Biological Macromolecules 338

J. D. Murray:
A Pattern Formation Mechanism and its Application
to Mammalian Coat Markings 360

A. M. Liquori and A. Tripiciano:
Cell Growth as an Autocatalytic Relaxation Process 400

A. Borsellino:
Vito Volterra and Contemporary Mathematical Biology 410

TOPIC I

Models of Natural Selection

Models of Natural Selection

R.C. Lewontin

Museum of Comparative Zoology

Harvard University

Cambridge, Massachusetts 02138 USA

Introduction

Darwin's theory of evolution by natural selection has had such an immense success in
explaining the historical changes that have occurred in life on earth that it has come
to be regarded by many people as the model for the dynamics of all historical processes.
"Evolutionary change" has become identified as identical with "change by natural selection," although there exist, in fact, two quite different modes of explanation for
the evolution of systems in time. In the variational mode, which is characteristic of
Darwinism, there is variation among the individual units comprising the whole system.
The system changes in time by a change in the proportions of the different kinds of
units, as a consequence of the differential survival and reproduction of the units.
It is interesting that the only natural system known with certainty to evolve by this
variational-selectional mode is the biological diversity of species.

The alternative mode of evolutionary change, exemplified by cosmological evolution, is
transformational. In this case the objects whose history is in question all undergo
the same transformation of state as a result of some mechanism of internal individual
development and is a direct consequence of their current state. The cosmos does not
evolve by the differential reproduction and survival of stars of different luminosities
and masses. Rather, each star undergoes the same transformations of state from its
first condensation, through the main sequence, to the red giant and finally white dwarf.
In biology, the example is the development of the embryo from egg to adult as a consequence of an internal ontogenetic program interacting with and incorporating the external milieu. The population of newly formed eggs becomes a population of adults by
the transformation of every individual in ontogeny.

It is important to understand that different domains of phenomena evolve by different
modes. The transformational mode, which is clearly the correct description for gal-
axies and embryos, is not correct for species. It was Darwin's triumph that he introduced the variational mode to our understanding, and so solved the problem which could
not be solved by Lamarck's transformationism. But the issue between variational and
transformational theories remains open in other spheres. For example, in immunology,
instructional (transformational) and selective theories remain as alternatives about
which there is much controversy. While transformational theories have been the domi-

nant ones in anthropology and political economy for a long time as explanations of
short-term historical changes, there has been a recent flowering of Darwinian theories
of long-term cultural evolution using natural selection either metaphorically or literally as the mechanism of human history. It is clear that many of these theories
assume that the variational mode is the only possibility for an evolutionary process,
or at least this is the only one they consider. So, for example, the recent very interesting fusion of genetic and cultural transmission by Cavalli-Sforza and Feldman
considers culture to be the aggregate of individual properties which are, in turn,
transmitted at different rates from individuals or groups of individuals in one generation to individuals in the next. The entire dynamic is the consequence of differential rates of transmission, survival, and reproduction of different cultural variants.
We must constantly bear in mind that such variational models are not the only, and
perhaps even not the most common, mode of historical change.

Phenotype and Genotype

A complete model of natural selection entails both genotypic and phenotypic descriptions of organisms. Obviously it is the phenotype of an organism that is most directly
concerned with the fertility and survival of the individual. Indeed fertility and
survival are part of the phenotype itself. Yet, at the same time, evolution by natural selection means a change in the frequency of genotypes. The change of a population from one generation to another can only be adequately modeled by passing back
and forth between phenotypic and genotypic descriptions as illustrated in Figure 1.

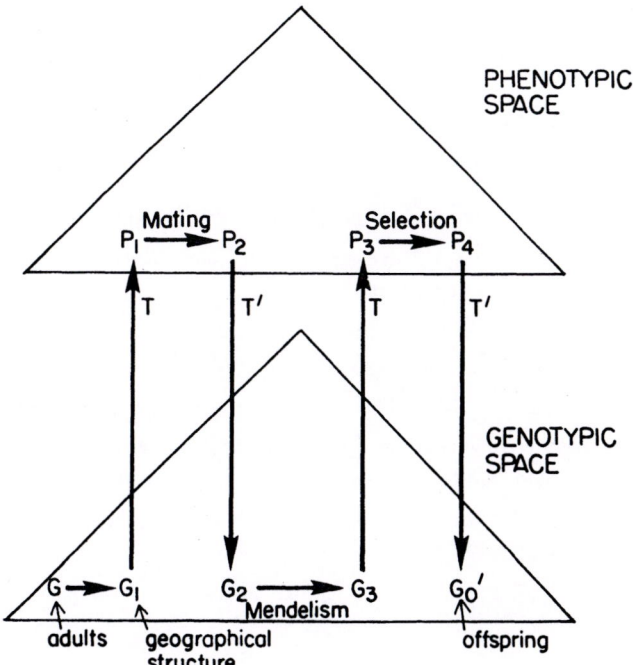

Figure 1.

We may begin in some generation with a population of adult genotypes G_0. There is some set of rules that describes how these genotypes are arranged in space and according to their degree of genetic relationship so as to make a pool of potential mates, G_1. But the actual processes of forming mating pairs depend upon assortative mating by phenotype so we must move from the genotypic space into the phenotypic space by the epigenetic laws, T, that govern the transformation of gene into developed organism in interaction with the environment. This set of laws of development is completely unknown at the moment. We do not know how to predict the distribution of phenotypes that will result from an array of genotypes developing in a set of environments, except in a few cases of simple one-locus traits. For the vast majority of genes and phenotypes concerned with size, shape, metabolic rates, behavior, etc., this is terra incognita. Given that we can predict the phenotypes P_1, then the laws of assortative mating would allow us to give the distribution of mated pairs P_2. But the consequences of mating are genotypes so we must again pass to the genotypic space. To do this requires the inverse epigenetic transformation, T´, that would allow the prediction of the distribution of genotypes given the distribution of phenotypes. Again, we are totally unable to make this transformation except for trivially simple characters that bear a one-to-one relationship with genotype. If the genotypic distribution among mating individuals, G_2, is known, then the laws of Mendel, the phenomena of cytogenetics and of recombination will predict the distribution of offspring genotypes at the moment of conception, G_3. There remains a last step, selection, to connect this distribution at conception to the new adult generation. But such selection depends upon the phenotypes of the organisms, so once again the epigenetic transformation T must be invoked to carry the genotypic distribution back into the phenotypic space. From the phenotypes P_3 before selection, the selected phenotypes P_4 can be derived. This final phenotypic array must then be converted by T´ into the selected genotypic distribution that constitutes the starting point for the next generation.

In order to create a model of genetic change from generation to generation, we see that the laws of correspondence between genotype and phenotype must be known, and they are invoked at several places in the cycle. Yet we do not know these laws. How have models of selection been constructed? There have been two traditions of modeling selection, one that has operated entirely in the phenotypic space and one entirely in the genotypic space. The phenotypic models are those of the biometrical geneticists, largely concerned with artificial selection of complex continuously varying traits in domesticated animals and plants. For such traits, the observations are of phenotypic values only, and no inference is possible to specific genotypes at specific Mendelian loci. The characteristic mathematical model of artificial selection of such traits is

$$(1) \qquad \Delta P = i \ h^2$$

where $\underline{P}$ is the phenotypic mean of the population, $\underline{i}$ is the difference between the mean phenotype of the selected parents and the mean phenotype of the entire population before selection, and $\underline{h}^2$ is the heritability in the narrow sense.

Genotypic models of selection are constructed by what we may call "Mendelian" population geneticists concerned with natural selection of polymorphisms in natural populations. While observations must be, by their nature, of phenotypes, an immediate inference is made about genotypic classes, and the models that are constructed are framed in terms of gene frequencies. The classical mathematical model of selection in Mendelian population genetics is

$$(2) \qquad \Delta q_i = \sum_j \frac{q_i q_j (\bar{W}_i - \bar{W}_j)}{\bar{W}}$$

where q_i is the frequency of the ith allele at some locus, $\bar{W}_i$ is the mean fitness of the ith allele, and $\bar{W}$ is the mean fitness of the population. $\bar{W}$ is itself defined in terms of allelic frequencies and the fitness of diploid genotypes, W_{ij}:

$$\bar{W} = \sum q_i \bar{W}_i = \sum q_i q_j W_{ij}.$$

Thus we have two parallel theoretical structures of evolutionary genetics, one operating apparently entirely in the phenotypic space and one in the space of genotypes with no reference to the laws of epigenetic transformation. But this is a pure illusion. In fact, both equations (1) and (2) contain both genetic and phenotypic information concealed in them in the disguise of constants. The biometrical equation contains h^2, the heritability which is the ratio of the additive genetic variance, σ_A^2, to the total phenotypic variance, σ_P^2. However, σ_A^2 and σ_P^2 are not constants. They depend upon allelic frequencies at the various loci influencing the trait, and these allelic frequencies are themselves changing during the course of selection. A total description of the course of evolution would then be a pair of simultaneous equations of the form

$$(3) \qquad \Delta P = i h^2$$

$$(4) \qquad \Delta h^2 = f(q)$$

coupled to each other by an epigenetic function relating gene frequencies to phenotype:

$$(5) \qquad P = e(q).$$

In like manner, the apparently purely genotypic equation (2) contains hidden phenotypic relations in the expression for the mean fitness, $\bar{W}$. The fitnesses of the genotype W_{AA}, W_{Aa}, etc. are not constants but, in general, depend upon the composition of the population. If the largest individuals in the population survive best, for example, then the probability of survival of different genotypes will change progressively as the population distribution moves to higher means. Thus, a full description of selection for Mendelian systems is necessarily the set of equations

$$(6) \qquad \Delta q_i = \frac{q_i \, \Sigma \, q_j (\bar{W}_i - \bar{W}_j)}{\bar{W}}$$

$$(7) \qquad \Delta W_{ij} = f(P)$$

coupled by the epigenetic laws

$$(8) \qquad P = e(q).$$

In fact, both biometrical and Mendelian systems need the same information. In biometrical selection models, the problem of missing information is met by abandoning any attempt at long-range prediction. Each generation or every few generations h^2 is remeasured in the population, so that an empirical evolution of this quantity is established. In other words, h^2 is treated at any moment as if it were a constant, but the value of the constant is continually readjusted to accord with the changing reality. Mendelian geneticists deal with the problem by pretending that constant fitnesses are the most common case and putting "frequency-dependent selection" in the category of special cases of secondary interest, by carefully choosing for actual experimental study those cases that most nearly conform to the constant fitness model, and when faced with fitnesses that are, in fact, changing, by reassessing them every generation just as the biometrical geneticists do. In the end, long-term prediction of evolutionary change under selection will depend upon solutions to the problems of developmental genetics, so that the epigenetic transformations can be built into evolutionary models.

Does Natural Selection Optimize Fitness?

An alternate form of equation (2) is

$$(9) \qquad \Delta q_i = \frac{q_i(1-q_i)}{2\,\bar{W}} \frac{d\bar{W}}{dq_i} = \frac{q_i(1-q_i)}{2} \frac{d \ln \bar{W}}{dq_i}.$$

This form has a great deal of intuitive appeal because it separates genetic variance

$q_i(1-q_i)$ from the derivative of a potential function

$$\frac{d \ln \bar{W}}{dq_i}$$

where $\ln \bar{W}$ plays the role of potential in physics. It can then be stated that the change in gene frequency will be large at intermediate gene frequencies where the variance term $q(1-q)$ is large, and small near gene fixation. Moreover, since there is a potential function involved, selection can be described according to a maximization (or minimization) principle. The principle in the case of equation (9) is that gene frequencies change in such a way as to maximize the mean fitness of the population $\bar{W}$.

The search for a Hamiltonian in biology has been strongly influenced by the history of physics. Mathematical biologists, especially, analogize their work to mathematical physics, and the power of extremal principles in physics, such as Fermat's Principle of Least Action, or the minimization of potential energy, has provided a model for what theoretical biologists have hoped to accomplish. Ernst Mach spoke for physics of the 19th century and biology of the 20th when he wrote about science that:

> It has as its highest and most coveted aim the solution of the
> problem of condensing all natural phenomena which have been observed
> and are still to be observed into one simple principle, that allows
> the computation of past, and more especially, of future processes
> from present ones. . . . Amid the more or less general laws which
> mark the achievements of physical science during the course of the
> last centuries, the principle of least action is perhaps that which,
> as regards form and content, may claim to come nearest to that
> ideal final aim of theoretical research.

While equation (9) seems to fulfill the hope of finding a maximization in principle in evolutionary theory, this is illusory. In fact, neither the maximization of fitness nor the simple relation between the speed of selection and heterozygosity, $q(1-q)$, is realized in fact. Only in the case of a single locus with constant genotypic fitnesses is equation (9) an adequate representation of selection. In all other cases there is neither a necessary maximization of fitness (it may even be minimized!) nor does selection operate most rapidly at intermediate allele frequencies. Several cases illustrate the problems.

1. Two loci without linkage.

Let us consider two loci each with two alleles simultaneously under selection, and ignore for the moment the complication of linkage by assuming that at every moment the loci are in linkage equilibrium with each other (although that will not generally be true). Then letting p and r represent the allele frequencies at the two loci, we have

$$(10a) \qquad \frac{dp}{dt} = \frac{1}{2} p(1-p) \frac{d\bar{W}}{dp}$$

(10b) $\qquad \dfrac{dr}{dt} = \dfrac{1}{2} r(1-r) \dfrac{d\bar{W}}{dr}$

as the time continuous analogue of equation (9). Combining (10a) and (10b) together to get rid of the time dimensions will give us a single differential equation describing the trajectory of allele frequencies in relation to each other as the population evolves along the fitness surface:

(11) $\qquad r(1-r) \dfrac{d\bar{W}}{dr}\, dp = p(1-p) \dfrac{d\bar{W}}{dp}\, dr\ .$

But the equation that describes a trajectory that maximizes the rate of increase of $\bar{W}$ is simply

(12) $\qquad \dfrac{d\bar{W}}{dr}\, dp = \dfrac{d\bar{W}}{dp}\, dr\ ,$

and the rate of change of fitness along such a maximum path would be given by

(13) $\qquad \dfrac{d\bar{W}}{dC} = \sqrt{(\dfrac{d\bar{W}}{dp})^2 + (\dfrac{d\bar{W}}{dr})^2}\ .$

The discrepancy between (11) and (12) means that Fermat's principle does not hold for gene frequency change under selection even though $\bar{W}$ is eventually maximized. The population takes an "indirect" path through the gene frequency space rather than the path of steepest ascent of $\bar{W}$ that is demanded by a least action principle. This discrepancy is present even though we assume the simplest model of constant genotypic fitnesses.

2. "Frequency dependent" fitness.

If the genotypic fitnesses, W_{ij}, are not constant but change as some function of the frequencies of the genotypes in the population, then Δq is some complicated function of the allele frequencies which will be different in each case. Formally, however, we can always represent the change in gene frequencies as:

(14) $\qquad \Delta q = f(q) = \dfrac{q(1-q)}{\bar{U}} (\bar{U}_1 - \bar{U}_2)$

which looks like the standard equation for Δq because I have arbitrarily factored out the term $q(1-q)/2\bar{U}$ and arbitrarily written what is left in parentheses as the difference in mean allelic fitnesses. There is nothing to prevent me from doing this operation mathematically, but the function that is left in the parentheses may be a complicated expression with no obvious meaning. It certainly will not, in general, be of the form $d\bar{U}/dq$. Having written the expression for Δq in the form of (14), I now give the illusion that selection depends upon the heterozygosity $q(1-q)$, but because of the form of $\bar{U}_1-\bar{U}_2$ this may be false. For example, in a constant fitness model with no dominance and the fitness of aa = 1-s

(15) $\Delta q = \dfrac{-q(1-q)s}{2\bar{W}}$.

But now suppose s is a function of frequency and in particular has the relationship of the general form

(16) $s = \dfrac{K}{q(1-q+K)}$

at least for q not too close to 0 or 1. Then

(17) $\Delta q = \underline{K}$!

That is, the change in gene frequency is independent of q and is uniform across the whole range of allelic frequencies. Indeed, if the frequency dependence of s is made even more concave than in (16), the effect of selection may grow greater as allelic frequencies depart more and more from intermediate values. The segregation of a term for heterozygosity as determining the rate of evolution is, in general, uninformative. Moreover, since equation (16) no longer can be written, in general, in the form of (9), it is no longer the case that $\bar{W}$ is eventually maximized, even by an indirect path. There is no general rule at all for the eventual value of mean fitness when there is frequency dependent selection.

3. The complication of linkage.

If we return to the problem of two or more loci taking into account now the actual linkage relations, then assuming constant genotypic fitnesses the equation for the change of a gametic type, A_iB_j, can be written as:

(18) $\Delta g_{ij} = \dfrac{g_{ij}(1-g_{ij})}{2\bar{W}} \dfrac{d\bar{W}}{dg_{ij}} + R(W,g,r)$

where $R(W,g,r)$ is a function of the fitnesses of various multiple heterozygotes, $\underline{W}$, the gametic frequencies, $\underline{g}$, and the recombination fractions among the loci, $\underline{r}$. Again, such an operation does not, in general, maximize $\bar{W}$, and it is easy to produce cases in which $\bar{W}$ decreases as selection progresses.

In general, then, the kinetics of gene frequency change cannot, except under very special circumstances, be described as the product of the heterozygosity and the gradient in fitness. The attempt to analyze the selection process into two simple components, the amount of heterozygosity and the force of selection, is an attempt to force a general principle on natural selection, where none has been found.

What is Fitness?

What is meant in population genetics by fitness? In fact, the development of this concept has a curious form. Population geneticists begin with the simplest biological model of natural selection that assumes differential viability of immature stages. These differential probabilities of survival are then called "fitness" because in this simplified model only survival probabilities are assumed to differ among the genotypes. From the differential viability model, it is trivial to construct a mathematical expression for the change of gene frequency. It is simply an expression of (2),

$$(19) \qquad \Delta q = \frac{q(1-q)[q(W_{aa}-W_{Aa}) - p(W_{AA}-W_{Aa})]}{p^2 W_{AA} + 2pqW_{Aa} + q^2 W_{aa}}$$

where the $\underline{W}$'s are the viabilities of the genotypes. This expression is then taken as the general model for selection and is used in actual cases of gene frequency change when the actual biological situation is not known. Successive values of $\underline{q}$ are observed, and from these values one estimates the $\underline{W}$'s. That is, an equation originally designed as a deductive tool for predicting changes in gene frequency from a particular biological situation is used as an inductive device to make statements about fitness from observed changes in gene frequency. In the process the $\underline{W}$'s become tautological rather than causal. They are simply the value of $\underline{W}$ that will fit the observed value of $\underline{q}$. If, for example, it is not differential viability, but differential fertility, that is the cause of gene frequency change, because fertility is a property of couples rather than individual genotypes, equation (19) is inappropriate as a deductive causal equation. In place of the three $\underline{W}$'s of genotypes, we must build a model containing all nine pairwise fertilities. If, in ignorance, equation (19) is used to infer genotypic fitnesses, values of the three $\underline{W}$'s will be produced, as they must be, but these are totally artificial and have nothing to do with the actual situation. Moreover, the three $\underline{W}$'s will be found to be frequency dependent in this case, although, in fact, the fertilities are fixed properties of the pairs. Equation (19) always yields values for the $\underline{W}$'s which are instantaneous genotypic fitnesses, by definition, and they are, in some sense, the fitnesses of the genotypes, but only at that instant. Thus, "frequency dependent fitness" is really a reification of a mathematical artifact that comes from using an inappropriate deductive model to define fitness.

There is a second, deeper problem in using equation (19) inductively. How do we know that selection is going on at all? In any real population gene frequencies will change because of random events, and some family lines will go extinct while others increase. In probability theory there is a well known result called "the extinction of family names," that eventually every family except one in a population will go extinct by

chance. Does it then follow that the families that increase over some particular period have higher fitnesses than those that decrease? In what sense are the Bianchi
more fit than the Sforze? In an a posteriori sense the genotypes that increase are
more fit, and, if the change in gene frequency is used, it will be impossible to distinguish between random increase of genotypes and a selective increase where selection
coefficients have some random variation from generation to generation. This indistin-
guishability is the direct consequence of the tautological nature of inferred fitnesses.

To resolve the problem we must return to the a priori concept of fitness as causing
gene frequency change. But we cannot estimate such fitnesses from the changes. They
must be deduced from physiological, morphological, and behavioral information about
the phenotypes that have developed from the genotypes. The fitness of a genotype must
be defined as the expectation of the reproductive rate over some fixed set of environments. Moreover, even the concept of the fitness of a genotype should be abandoned
and replaced by the separate biological properties of viability and fertility. A single fitness of a genotype does not exist except in the special case of constant viability selection, or special fertility relations where the fertilities of couples are
the products of the fertilities of the individuals. For all other models of natural
selection, when they are built up from the biological description, no simple genotypic
fitnesses will appear, except in a formal mathematical sense that will require them to
be reevaluated every generation. "Fitness" is indeed a tautology, as Darwin's critics
claimed. Viabilities, fecundities, and mating propensities are the real dynamic forces
of natural selection which must enter into the kinetic models.

The Dialectics of Selection

The simple models of natural selection, even those that take specific components of
the life cycle into account, make apparent separation between the cause of change,
genetic variance in fitness, and the consequence which is the genetic change itself.
However, the situation is more complicated. The genetic changes that occur as a consequence of fitness variation are themselves causes of fitness variation. Natural
selection is like a fire that consumes its own fuel, genetic variation in fitness.
But a fire does not burn wood; it burns the hot gases that are produced from the wood
by the action of the fire itself. So selection is both the creator and consumer of
the conditions for its existence. I will give three examples briefly.

1. Selection occurs at different levels of the genome.
Figure 2 shows the genetic changes that occur in a population when several loci are
segregating and influencing a trait for which there is an intermediate selective optimum [2]. There are five loci, each with two alleles. Figure 2A shows the change
in allelic frequency at the five loci under conditions of very loose linkage among

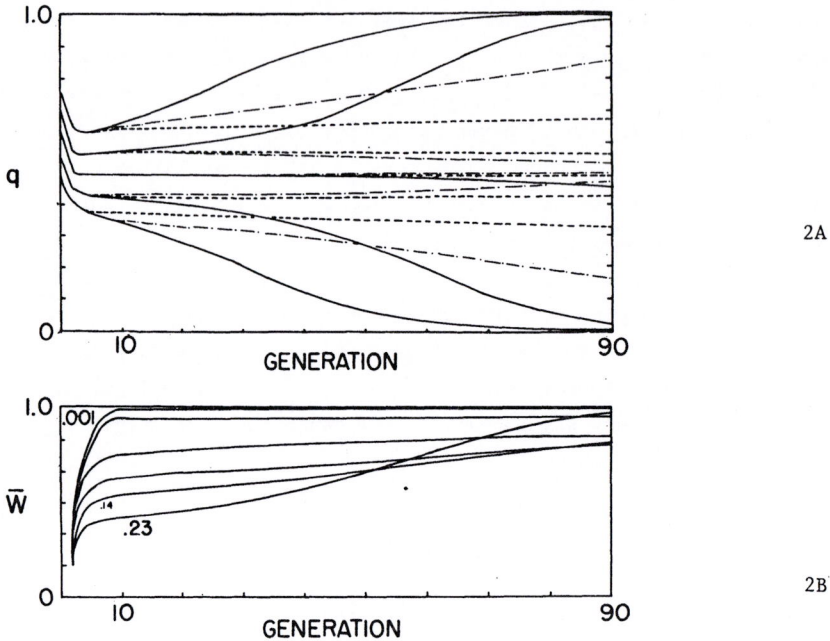

Figure 2.

them (solid line), when they have intermediate linkage (dashes and dots), and when they are tightly linked (dashes). Figure 2B shows the changes in mean fitness, $\bar{W}$, of the population under the various amounts of recombination. When there is loose linkage ($R = .23$) allele frequencies change rather rapidly, two loci going toward fixation at $q = 1.0$ and two at $q = 0.0$ with the fifth locus changing slowly. These changes in allele frequency result in a slow but steady increase in mean fitness, $\bar{W}$. In contrast, for tight linkage ($R = .01$), the allele frequencies remain virtually constant at intermediate values, yet the mean fitness, $\bar{W}$, rises very dramatically at once and nearly reaches its maximum possible value after only 10 generations. This remarkable change despite a constancy of allele frequency is a result of the buildup of linked complementary gametic types, for example AbCdE and aBcDE, and a removal of others. This creation of super-genes, without changing allele frequencies, is a consequence of natural selection operating on linked loci. Once the super-genes are created, they are kept in the population in quasi-equilibrium by the selection. Moreover, the building of the super-gene occurs by a crystallization process in which alleles at two neighboring loci form a small super-gene early in selection, and this unit drives the loci on either side of it also to become highly correlated with it. This process of the spread of the super-gene along the chromosome until only two complementary gametes exist in the population can be more easily seen in models involving more loci [1]. Thus, selection has actually built up the genetic structure on which it continues to operate.

2. Selection creates genetic variance on the fitness scale.

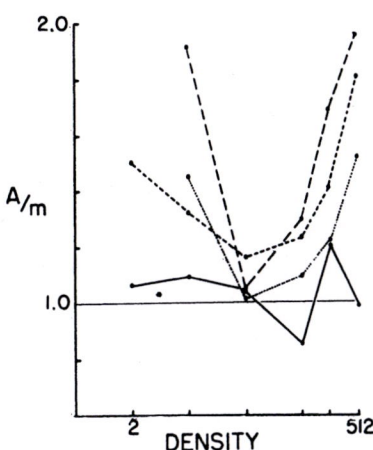

Figure 3.

Figure 3 shows the relative viability of larvae of a wild type A and a mutant m in
Drosophila busckii at different densities and in different proportions [4]. The solid
line gives the relative viability A/m when the two genotypes are tested separately in
pure culture. They are essentially equivalent to each other in viability. The other
lines show the relative viability realized when there is competition between the genotypes in the same culture with 75% A (long dashes), 50% A (short dashes), and 25% A
(dots). Especially at higher densities, the greater the relative frequency of A, the
greater its viability. Suppose a population of type m is invaded by a few type A by
migration or mutation. There will be virtually no fitness differential at this mixture. However, as A grows in frequency, its relative viability grows greater and
greater so that fitness variance is actually being created by the selection process,
quite apart from the purely statistical effect on variance of changing q. This is a
classical case of "frequency dependent fitness."

Another example of the same creation of variance by selection is in the work of Rendel
[5] on canalized characters. Ordinarily there is no phenotypic variance for the number of scutellar bristles in Drosophila. All flies have four bristles. By disturbing
the system of developmental buffering, Rendel revealed that there was genetic variation
at loci influencing the trait and that this variation could be selected. After selection had operated for some period, variation in scutellar bristle number appeared even

in the absence of the disturbance of buffering. Now selection could operate on the
character even under normal genetic and environmental conditions. Selection had created phenotypic variance on which to operate further, where none had existed before.

3. <u>Selection</u> <u>is</u> <u>an</u> <u>historical</u> <u>process</u>.

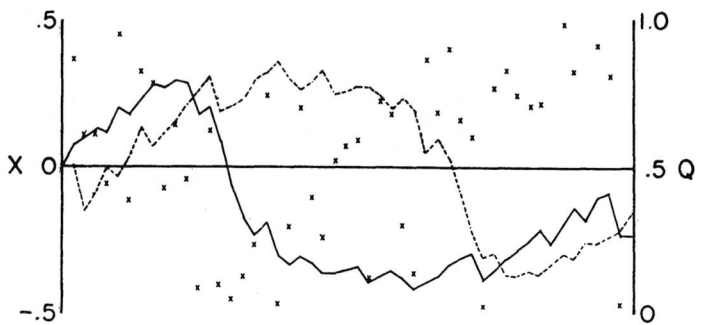

<u>Figure</u> <u>4</u>.

Figure 4 shows the outcome of a simple exercise with random members [3]. We assume
a locus with two alleles and no dominance. A selection coefficient <u>s</u> is assigned each
generation to the allele <u>a</u>, by choosing a number from a uniform distribution between
−0.5 and +0.5. The successive selection coefficients are shown by the crosses. The
resulting trajectory of gene frequency change in this randomly varying environment is
then plotted as the solid line. Whenever the selection coefficient is above 0, the
gene frequency increases, while it decreases for negative values of <u>s</u>. Although 60%
of the values of <u>s</u> were positive, the gene frequency was below .5 for 75% of its history, and the mean value of <u>q</u> was .38. This is because the negative selective values
were concentrated in a nearly uninterrupted sequence during early and middle generations, so that the later positive selection could not compensate. The <u>order</u> of environments plays an important role in a continuous historical process like selection. The
fact is even more strikingly seen in the history given by the broken line in Figure 4.
In this case exactly the same environments were encountered by the population <u>in</u> <u>ex-</u>
<u>actly</u> <u>the</u> <u>same</u> <u>sequence</u> <u>except</u> <u>that</u> <u>the</u> <u>entire</u> <u>environmental</u> <u>sequence</u> <u>was</u> <u>taken</u> <u>in</u>
<u>reverse</u> <u>order</u>. Now we see that the gene frequency is <u>above</u> .5 about 60% of .the time
with a mean q = .57 and a much larger variance of gene frequency. A totally different
population history was generated from exactly the same set of environments but taken
in reverse order. In fact, no set of statistics about the environment can distinguish
these two cases. All moments of the environmental distribution are identical obviously,

as is the serial autocorrelation of the environment. What is different between the
environments is that up to any given moment, t, the past histories have been different,
and, therefore, the state of the population at that moment is different. Since the
size of Δq at each moment depends upon the present value of q, then two populations
that have had different past histories will also have different futures. Moreover,
at any instant, one cannot interchange past and future. In this sense, the evolutionary history of a population is like the developmental transformation of an organism.
The final outcome of an historical process depends uniquely on the historical order
in which events occur. The future contains the past.

References

[1] Franklin, I. and R.C. Lewontin. 1970. Is the gene the unit of selection?
     Genetics 65: 707-734.

[2] Lewontin, R.C. 1964. The interaction of selection and linkage. II. Optimum
     models. Genetics 50: 757-782.

[3] Lewontin, R.C. 1966. Is nature probable or capricious? BioScience 16: 25-27.

[4] Lewontin, R.C. and Y. Matsuo. 1963. Interaction of genotypes determining via-
     bility in Drosophila busckii. Proc.Nat.Acad.Sci.U.S. 49: 270-278.

[5] Rendel, J.M. 1959. Canalization of the scute phenotype of Drosophila. Evolution
     13: 425-439.

STOCHASTIC THEORY OF POPULATION GENETICS AND EVOLUTION

Masatoshi Nei
Center for Demographic and Population Genetics
University of Texas at Houston, Houston, Texas   77025

INTRODUCTION

The stochastic theory in population genetics has a long history.   In
his 1922 paper Fisher first studied the effect of genetic drift on the
genetic variability of a random mating population, introducing a new
concept of stochastic change of gene frequencies. He reached the conclusion that the rate of change of genetic variability due to genetic
drift is extremely small in a large population.   This study affected
his view as well as his followers on the role of genetic drift in evolution. Some of his followers (e.g. Ford 1975) still maintain the view
that virtually all characters of an organism are the product of natural
selection and genetic drift is unimportant except in an extremely small
population.   Fisher himself, however, was aware of the importance of
the stochastic factor in evolution at least in the initial process of
gene frequency increase.   In fact, it was Fisher (1922, 1930) and Haldane
(1927) who showed that genetic drift will eliminate a majority of advantageous mutations in a few generations after they occur and only a small
proportion of them will be fixed in the population.
     Sewall Wright's view on the role of genetic drift in evolution is
considerably different from that of the Fisherian school.   In his 1931
paper he developed a number of mathematical models to treat this factor
and presented a general formula for the gene frequency distribution under
the joint effects of selection, mutation, migration, and genetic drift.
Because of his early studies on the coat color variation in guinea pigs,
he was convinced that each locus has many multiple alleles and there is
strong gene interaction among different loci in determining a phenotypic
character.   He thought that in general there is no selective advantage
or disadvantage for a specific allele but a particular combination of
alleles at different loci produces advantage or disadvantage to a given
individual.   It was this idea that led him to propose his so-called shifting balance theory of evolution.   In this theory he conceived a multi-

dimensional surface of fitness determined by many loci and regarded evolution as a process of a population moving from one adaptive peak on this surface to another higher adaptive peak. In this process the population has to go through a valley between the two peaks and this passage of a valley is facilitated by genetic drift if a large population is subdivided into many subpopulations. In this theory most loci are assumed to be polymorphic at any moment of the time, and attainment of a higher adaptive peak is accomplished by gene frequency shifts at many loci rather than by complete substitution of genes at any particular loci (Wright 1931, 1971). Recently Wright (1978) stated that some data on protein polymorphism support this theory.

Recent studies on evolutionary change of proteins and nucleic acids (DNA and RNA) have made it clear that stochastic factors are even more important in evolution than Wright thought. Zuckerkandl and Pauling (1965) have shown that the evolutionary change of proteins is similar to the process of radioactive decay. Indeed, Fitch and Margoliash (1967) and Langley and Fitch (1974) have shown that this change can be described roughly by the Poisson process, which is one of the simplest stochastic processes. This type of observation led Kimura (1968) to propose the hypothesis that the majority of gene substitutions at structural loci are due to random fixation of neutral or nearly neutral mutations and a majority of the protein polymorphisms observed in the present natural populations simply represent a transient state of gene substitution by random genetic drift. This hypothesis generated a great controversy among evolutionary biologists who were educated under the influence of neo-Darwinism or the synthetic theory of evolution.

Kimura's mutation-drift hypothesis is intended to explain the evolution at the molecular level. At the morphological level natural selection must play an important role, since the morphology of an organism is well adapted to the environment in which the organism is placed. However, some parts of morphological variation in populations do not appear to be directly related to the adaptability of organisms, and the mutation-drift hypothesis possibly applies even to morphological evolution to some extent (Nei 1975).

At any rate, the importance of stochastic factors in evolution has been firmly established at least at the molecular level. However, this does not mean that the two major evolutionary theories based on stochastic factors, i.e. the neutral mutation theory and shifting balance theory, are proven to be correct. To see the validity of these theories, careful studies are required. In the past several years I have been studying the applicability of the neutral mutation theory to protein polymorphism data in collaboration with my colleagues. In this study we have collected gene frequency data from all species in which a large number of protein loci have been examined and tested the agreement of various statistical quantities with the values predicted from the neutral theory (Nei et al. 1976 a,b, 1978; Fuerst et al. 1977; Chakraborty et al. 1978, 1980). We have also studied various mathematical properties of the neutral theory and its alternatives (Nei et al. 1975, 1976a; Li and Nei 1975, 1977; Nei and Li 1975, 1976, 1980; Nei and Tateno 1975; Nei and Yokoyama 1976; Li 1976, 1977, 1978, 1979 a,b; Nei 1976, 1978; Chakraborty and Nei 1976, 1977; Maruyama and Nei, unpublished).

The purpose of this paper is threefold. First, a summary of the results of our theoretical and statistical studies on protein polymorphism will be presented. A general discussion about the mechanism of protein polymorphism will also be given. Second, the applicability of the shifting balance theory to protein polymorphism data will be discussed. Third, the role of stochastic factors in morphological evolution will be examined.

PROTEIN POLYMORPHISM

Neutral Mutation Theory

Let me first discuss the properties of the neutral theory, since this theory has been misunderstood by many authors. (1) Kimura's neutral theory refers only to molecular variation and evolution and does not apply to morphological evolution. (2) It is concerned with the behavior of a "majority" of the genes that are incorporated into the population during evolution and allows the existence of a small proportion of advantageous or overdominant mutations. (3) It is assumed that the majority of fresh mutations are deleterious but they are quickly eliminated from the population and thus contribute little to the genetic variation or gene substitution in a population. This large fraction of deleterious mutations occurs because most of new mutations disturb the function of the protein encoded (Kimura and Ohta 1973). (4) Neutral genes are not functionless genes but generally of vital importance to the organism. At any locus a pair of alleles are called neutral if they are functionally equivalent and thus equally important to the survival of the organism. In population genetics, however, the definition of neutrality of a gene depends on whether the behavior of the gene in a population is dictated by genetic drift or not relative to the other allele. Suppose that there are two alleles at a locus, and let s be the selective advantage of one

allele to the other. Then, if $Ns \leq 1$, the pair of alleles are called
neutral, where N is the effective population size (Kimura 1968; Li 1978).
Therefore, a mutant gene, which is advantageous in a large population,
may become neutral in small populations. (5) The rate of gene substitution for neutral genes is equal to the mutation rate, v, (Kimura 1968),
whereas the average heterozygosity per locus is $4Nv/(1 + 4Nv)$ (Kimura
and Crow 1964). This latter statement is true only for the infinite
allele model but this model seems to be quite realistic even for electrophoretic data (Li 1976; Fuerst and Ferrell 1980; Ramshaw et al. 1980).
For more detailed properties of the neutral theory, see Nei (1975) and
Kimura (1979a).

It is clear from the above properties that the validity of the neutral theory should be tested by examining many loci; demonstration of
selection at one or two loci does not refute the neutral theory. Namely,
the test should be statistical. It should also be noted that since the
protein polymorphism and molecular evolution represents two different
aspects of the same phenomenon as emphasized by Kimura and Ohta (1971),
any reasonable theory must be able to explain both polymorphism and evolution with the same population parameters. With these understandings,
we have initiated a statistical study of protein polymorphism and examined the neutral theory as a null hypothesis. In this test we tried
to eliminate subjective judgements as far as possible.

In the neutral theory, the level of heterozygosity in an equilibrium population depends on the value of $4Nv$, as mentioned earlier. In
practice, however, it is very difficult to estimate the $4Nv$ value in any
particular population. In our test, therefore, we avoided this problem,
and used the relationship among various quantities. For example, the
theoretical mean and variance of heterozygosity for neutral genes are
given by

$$H = M/(1 + M) \tag{1}$$

and

$$V = \frac{2M}{(1 + M)^2 (2 + M)(3 + M)}, \tag{2}$$

respectively, where $M = 4Nv$. The relationship between these two quantities is given by the solid line in Figure 1. Therefore, we can test
the null hypothesis of neutral mutations by examining whether the observed mean and variance follow this relationship or not (Nei 1975;
Nei et al. 1976b; Fuerst et al. 1977). (If formulae (1) and (2) are
to be applied to data from a large number of different protein loci in

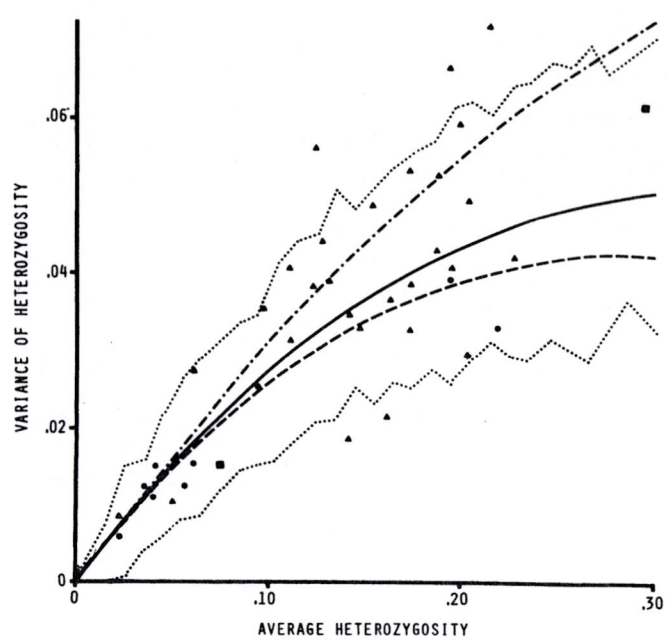

Figure 1. Relationships between the estimates of average heterozygosities ($\hat{H}$) and the interlocus variances of heterozygosity ($\hat{v}$) for invertebrate species. Thirty-four species and five differentiated subspecies were used.
———— : theoretical relationship for the infinite allele model.
— — — : theoretical relationship for the stepwise mutation model.
—•—•— : theoretical relationship for the infinite allele model with varying mutation rate (coefficient of variation of mutation rate = 1.0).
••••• : 95% significance intervals obtained by computer simulation.
▲ Drosophila; ■ non-Drosophila insects; ● non-insect invertebrates

a population, the variation in mutation rate among loci should be taken into account; Nei et al. 1976a.) We have examined similar relationships for various quantities, i.e. the relationship between average heterozygosity and proportion of polymorphic loci (Fuerst et al. 1977), the relationship between the mean and variance of genetic distance (Chakraborty et al. 1978), the relationship between gene identity and correlation of heterozygosity (Chakraborty et al. 1978), the relationship between subunit molecular weight of protein and heterozygosity (Nei et al. 1978), the distribution of allele frequencies (Chakraborty et al. 1980), and others. In this test we used more than 130 species in which 20 or more protein loci have been examined. They included various organisms from invertebrates to vertebrates. Our general conclusion is that most data on protein polymorphism can be accounted for by the neutral theory but in a significant proportion of species there is an excess of rare alleles. In this paper I shall present only a few of the results obtained from these studies.

Figure 1 shows the theoretical and observed relationships between the mean and variance of heterozygosity in 34 species and 5 differentiated subspecies of invertebrates. It is clear that the agreement between theory and data is satisfactory in most species. A similar study was conducted for 95 species and one subspecies of vertebrates, but the agreement was again satisfactory. Therefore, this test could not reject the null hypothesis of neutral mutations (Fuerst et al. 1977).

Figure 2 shows the theoretical and observed distributions of single-locus heterozygosity. The theoretical distribution was obtained by computer simulation under the assumption of $4Nv = 0.1$. It is noted that

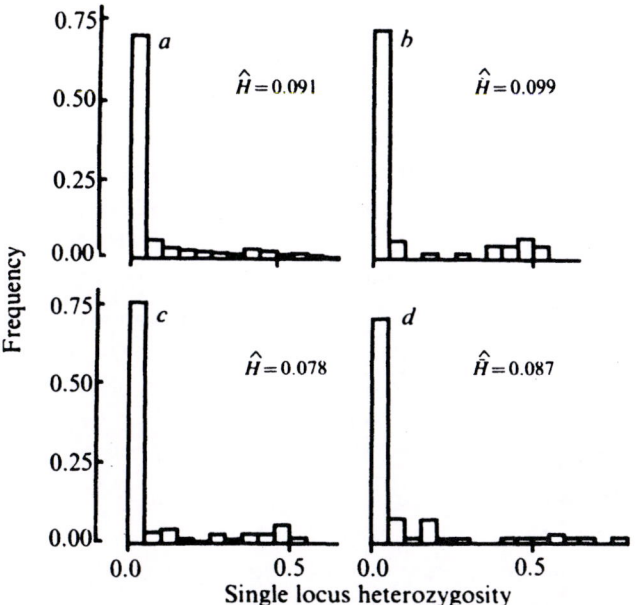

Figure 2. Distributions of single-locus heterozygosities for b, man (Caucasian); c, the house mouse (*Mus musculus*) and d, the *Drosophila mulleri* species group. The theoretical distribution (a) was obtained by computer simulation with the infinite allele model. $\hat{H}$ stands for the average heterozygosity. The distribution for the stepwise mutation model is almost identical with that for the infinite allele model when $\hat{H} = 0.09$.

although $4Nv$ is the same for all loci, the single-locus heterozygosity varies greatly among loci and this variation is purely due to random genetic drift. Therefore, a single observation of single-locus hetero-zygosity is a very poor estimate of mean heterozygosity $H = M/(1 + M)$ = 0.091. Figure 2, b-d, show the observed distributions of single-locus heterozygosity for three different species in which the average hetero-zygosity was close to the expected value of $H = 0.09$. It is clear that the agreement between theory and data is again quite satisfactory. Actually we have studied the agreement for all the species examined by using the Kolmogorov-Smirnoff test (Fuerst et al. 1977). The results obtained indicated that the agreement was satisfactory in a majority of species.

The final example I would like to show is the distribution of allele frequencies in a population. The theoretical and observed distributions of allele frequencies for 4 different species are presented in Figure 3. The theoretical distribution was obtained by using Nei et al.'s (1976b) formula for the allele frequency distribution for the case of varying mutation rate, i.e.,

$$\Phi(x) = \frac{\overline{M}(1 - x)^{-1} x^{-1}}{[1 - \overline{M} \log_e (1 - x)]^2} , \tag{3}$$

where $\Phi(x)dx$ represents the expected number of alleles whose frequency in the population is between x and $x + dx$ and $\overline{M}$ is the mean of M for all loci. Figure 3 shows that in all species the distribution is U-shaped and in view of the relatively small number of loci examined the agreement between theory and data is quite satisfactory except in the Japanese macaque. Indeed, statistical tests did not show any signifi-cant discrepancy in the three species. In the Japanese macaque, how-ever, the number of rare alleles was excessive compared with the theo-retical number. Similar tests for 138 populations (mostly species or subspecies) have shown that in all the species examined the distribu-tion is U-shaped and the agreement between theory and data are generally satisfactory but in about a quarter of the populations there was an ex-cess of rare alleles. Particularly in the *D. willistoni* group species the excess of rare alleles was conspicuous, as noted earlier by Ohta (1975) and Latter (1975). (In some populations there was a deficiency of rare alleles as in the case of *Taricha rivularis*, though the defi-ciency was not statistically significant.) Nevertheless, the excess of rare alleles does not create much problem for the neutral theory, since whenever there is a bottleneck in population size the excess is

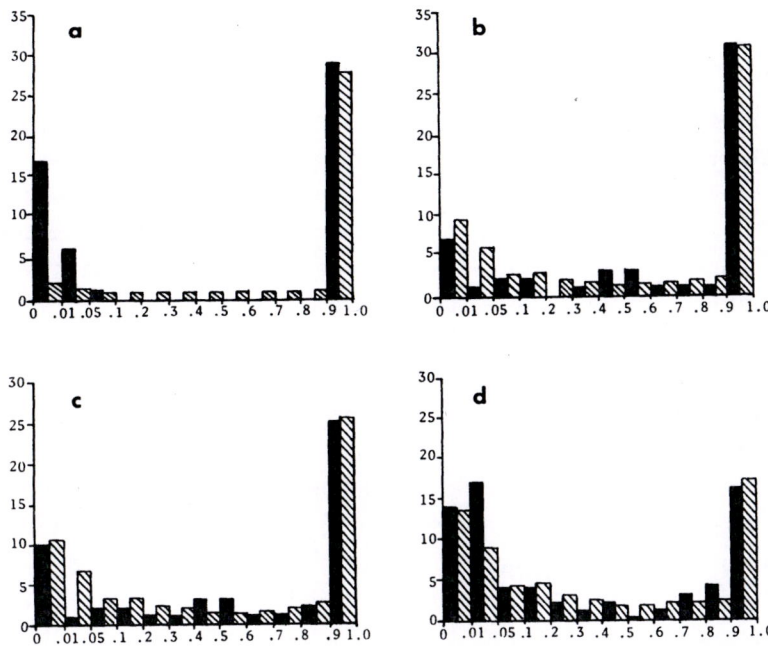

Figure 3.   Observed and expected distributions of allele frequencies
in four species representing different average heterozygosity values:
(a) Japanese macaque (20 loci, average heterozygosity $\bar{H} = 0.018$, $n = 1976$),
(b) *Taricha rivularis* (37 loci, $\bar{H} = 0.077$, $n = 784$), (c) *Zoarces viviparus*
(32 loci, $\bar{H} = 0.102$, $n = 757$), and (d) *Drosophila heteroneura* (25 loci,
$\bar{H} = 0.162$, $n = 605$).   The observed distributions are represented by
solid columns, whereas the expected distributions by slashed columns.
The abscissa gives allele frequency classes and the ordinate the number
of alleles.

expected to occur (Nei 1976; Chakraborty et al. 1980).   We shall discuss
the bottleneck effect on protein variation in more detail later.

In this connection it should be noted that overdominant selection
is expected to increase the number of intermediate frequency alleles
(Li 1978), and thus the distribution tends to be W-shaped.   In practice,
however, no such distribution was observed in any species.

Alternative Theories

There are a large number of ways natural selection can operate at
a genetic locus, but they can be classified into two categories from
the viewpoint of maintenance of polymorphism, i.e., diversity-enhancing

(or retaining) selection and diversity-reducing selection. The former category includes any type of selection that increases the genetic variability of an equilibrium population compared with that for neutral mutations. Typical of this category is overdominant selection, but any type of selection that produces a stable equilibrium of gene frequencies in an infinite population without the aid of mutation and migration may be included. The latter category includes selection against deleterious mutations and selection for advantageous mutations that will eventually be fixed in the population. Recently, Lewontin et al. (1978) studied the likelihood of stable equilibria for multiple alleles under overdominant selection and concluded that overdominant selection is unlikely to maintain many alleles at a locus. However, they did not consider the effect of mutation. If they had considered mutation, they would have reached a different conclusion. To make the overdominance model realistic, we must consider selection, mutation, and random genetic drift simultaneously (Wright 1949; Watterson 1977; Li 1978).

Before going into the discussion of alternative theories, I would like to emphasize that in the study of molecular evolution there are two observations that cannot be disputed. One is the rate of amino acid substitution in proteins that is *approximately* constant per year and the same for many groups of organisms (Wilson et al. 1977). The other is the average heterozygosity studied by electrophoresis in a large number of organisms. If we consider only those organisms in which 20 or more protein loci are studied, the average heterozygosity ranges from 0 to 0.3 in vertebrates and invertebrates (Fuerst et al. 1977). Any realistic evolutionary theory must be able to explain these two observations with the same set of population parameters. In this type of study it is convenient to translate the rate of amino acid substitution into the rate of gene substitution detectable by electrophoresis. According to Kimura and Ohta (1971) and Nei (1975), this rate is roughly 10^{-7} per gene per year. It is noted that the rate of gene substitution per year is constant but the rate per generation is not. In Drosophila there are about 10 generations in a year, so that the rate of gene substitution per generation is about 10^{-8} per gene, whereas in human lineages it is about 2×10^{-6} per gene under the assumption that one generation corresponds to 20 years.

In the past several years our Houston group (Ranajit Chakraborty, Paul Fuerst, Wen-Hsiung Li, Takeo Maruyama, and myself) have studied various quantities expected under diversity-enhancing and diversity-reducing selections. Since space limitation does not allow me to present all the results obtained by these works, I would like to discuss only one aspect, i.e., the level of heterozygosity in relation to gene substitution. It should be noted that the level of heterozygosity is affected drastically by the bottleneck effect even in the absence of selection (Nei et al. 1975; Chakraborty and Nei 1977). Therefore, I shall first discuss this effect.

Bottleneck effect: As mentioned earlier, the expected heterozygosity for neutral genes is given by (1). In the neutral theory, the v value in (1) may be estimated by the rate of gene substitution, since the latter is equal to the mutation rate. Thus, in Drosophila the mutation rate under the null hypothesis of neutral mutation is estimated to be 10^{-8}, whereas in man it is 2×10^{-6}. In *Drosophila willistoni* Ayala (1972) estimated the effective population size to be at least 10^9. If we assume $N = 10^9$, then the expected heterozygosity for this organism is 0.976. The observed average heterozygosity has been reported to be 0.176 (Ayala 1972). Therefore, there is a great discrepancy between theory and data. The current human population on earth is about 4×10^9, and the effective size would be about 10^9. Therefore, the expected heterozygosity will be nearly 100 percent. Yet the observed heterozygosity is about 0.1 (Nei and Roychoudhury 1974). Indeed, whenever a rough estimate of effective population size is obtainable, the observed heterozygosity is almost always lower than the expected. (Soulé (1976) argued that in a substantial number of species the observed heterozygosity is higher than the expected, but in these species he used unrealistically small effective size. For example, the effective size he used for *Thomomys bottae* was 10^{2-3} (Soulé, personal communication.) It should be noted that the N in (1) refers to the entire species rather than to a local population (Kimura and Maruyama 1971).) However, these discrepancies do not pose any serious problem to the neutral theory. This is because the effective size to be used in (1) is not that of the current populations but that of the past populations. The size of a population in nature almost always fluctuates from time to time, and when population size fluctuates, the effective size is known to be close to the minimum size (Wright 1938). Furthermore, if a population goes through a bottleneck, the level of heterozygosity is reduced drastically and takes a long time — more than $4N/(1 + 4Nv)$ generations — before the original level is restored (Nei et al. 1975). In Drosophila the time required could often be more than 10 million generations. If we note that the last glaciation ended only about 10,000 years ago and at the time of glaciation the population size was apparently much smaller than the present size in many organisms, the observed heterozygosity is indeed expected to be smaller than the theoretical value based on the current population size.

Overdominant selection: Let us now consider overdominant selection, which has been favored by many selectionists. The mathematical model for overdominant selection has not been well developed, but in recent years some progress has been made. Let A_i be the ith allele existing in a population. We assume that the fitness of heterozygote $A_i A_j$ is 1 irrespective of i and j and denote the fitness of homozygote $A_i A_i$ by $1 - s_i$. Using the infinite allele model, we have studied the expected heterozygosity and other quantities for the case where s_i is constant (s) and the case where it varies with allele according to an exponential distribution. The result for the latter case is nearly the same as that for the first case if the mean of s_i is equal to s. Therefore, we consider only the first case here.

When $4Ns$ and $4Nv$ are sufficiently large, the expected hetero-zygosity for overdominant alleles is given by

$$H = 1 - \frac{\Gamma(1 + B)\,_1F_1(2,2 + B,S)}{\Gamma(2 + B)\,_1F_1(1,1 + B,S)} \, ,$$

where $B = 4N(v + s)$ and $S = 4Ns$, and $\Gamma(\cdot)$ and $_1F_1(\cdot,\cdot,\cdot)$ stand for the gamma function and the hypergeometric function, respectively (Yokoyama and Nei 1979; see also Ewens 1964). On the other hand, when S is small, say 40 or less, H can be computed by using the method developed by Watterson (1977) and Li (1978). However, when the value of S is inter-mediate, there is no analytical method available for computing H. Therefore, we used a numerical method recently introduced by Maruyama, Takahata, and Kimura (unpublished). The results obtained are given in Figure 4. These results were obtained in collaboration with Takeo Maruyama. It is clear from this figure that even a small amount of overdominant selection increases the average heterozygosity drastically compared with that for neutral genes. Therefore, it is very difficult to explain protein polymorphism in terms of overdominant selection.

In this connection, however, it should be pointed out that under symmetric overdominant selection the probability of fixation of a mutant gene is somewhat higher than that for neutral genes and thus a smaller mutation rate than that for neutral genes is sufficient to explain a given rate of gene substitution (Nei and Roychoudhury 1973). A smaller rate of mutation reduces the excess amount of heterozygosity generated by overdominant selection. Therefore, we studied the rate of gene sub-stitution and average heterozygosity simultaneously. Our preliminary

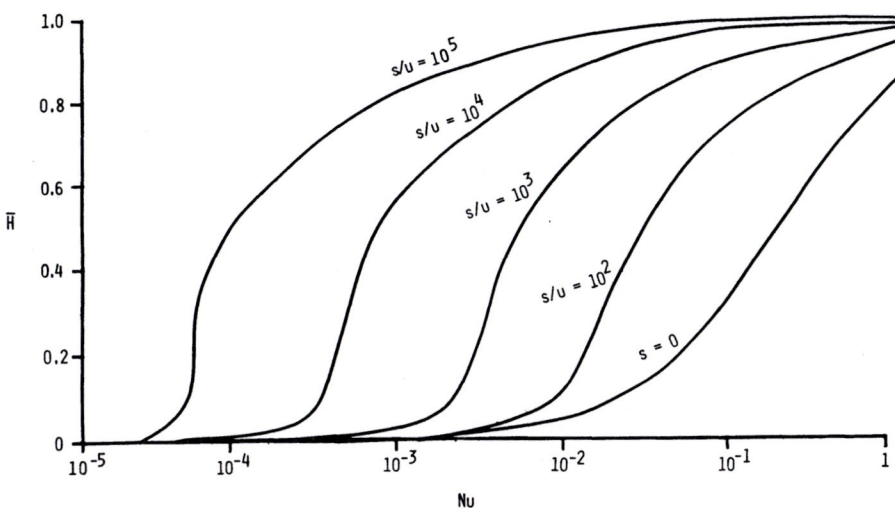

Figure 4. Relationship between population size (*N*) and average hetero-zygosity (*H*) for overdominant genes. *u* = mutation rate. *s* = selection coefficient for homozygotes.

results are presented in Table 1. This table shows that for a fixed value of $4Nv$ overdominant selection increases both the rate of gene sub-stitution and average heterozygosity compared with the case of neutral mutations. However, the effect of overdominant selection on average heterozygosity is greater than that on the rate of gene substitution. This can be seen by computing the expected heterozygosity from the observed rate of gene substitution under the assumption of neutral mu-tations. The expected heterozygosity is given in the last column in Table 1. It is clear that this value is much higher than the observed heterozygosity in the presence of overdominant selection. In other words, for a given rate of gene substitution, overdominant mutations produce a higher level of heterozygosity than neutral mutations. This indicates that overdominant selection is less satisfactory than the neutral theory for explaining protein polymorphism.

Sequentially advantageous mutations: The second model we have studied is that of advantageous mutations. In neo-Darwinism gene sub-stitution is assumed to occur when a new advantageous mutation is intro-duced or when an environmental change causes a previously disadvanta-geous mutation to become advantageous. In collaboration with Ranajit Chakraborty and Paul Fuerst, I studied the relationship between the rate

Table 1. Rate of gene substitution (α) and average heterozygosity (H) for overdominant mutations. N: Effective population size . v: Mutation rate. $\bar{s}$: Mean selection coefficient. These results were obtained by computer simulations.

$4Nv$	$2N\bar{s}$	$2N\alpha$	Observed heterozygosity (H)	H_n*
1. Neutral genes				
0.024	0	0.013	0.023	0.025
0.120	0	0.060	0.118	0.105
2. Constant selection				
0.002	10	0.007	0.084	0.014
0.120	60	0.124	0.753	0.199
3. Varying selection				
0.002	10	0.008	0.040	0.016
0.120	60	0.146	0.696	0.226

*H_n = Average heterozygosity computed from the rate of gene substitution under the assumption of neutrality of genes, i.e. $H_n = 4N\alpha/(1 + 4N\alpha)$.

of gene substitution and average heterozygosity under this type of se-lection. The model we used is as follows: In every generation $2Nv$ advantageous mutations were introduced but only a fraction of them were incorporated into the population because of initial random genetic drift. This fraction is the probability of fixation and equal to $2s$, where s is the selective advantage of the mutant gene (Haldane 1927). In other words, $4Nvs$ mutations were incorporated into the population. In prac-tice, the $4Nvs$ values we used were 5×10^{-5} and 10^{-4}. We assumed that when a new mutation is incorporated, the gene frequency has reached 0.001. After this point, the gene frequency was assumed to change determinis-tically. We also assumed that the new mutant allele is always different from the preexisting alleles and advantageous by s compared with the most fit allele in the population. When the frequency of the mutant allele reached 0.999, the allele was assumed to have been fixed. This process was continued for 300,000 generations, and in every 600th gen-eration the allele frequencies were recorded and fixation of genes (actually codons) was examined. Using the allele frequencies thus obtained, the average heterozygosity was computed to be compared with the value expected for neutral mutations. The average heterozygosity for neutral mutations was computed by equating the rate of gene substi-tution to mutation rate and assuming $N = 500$.

Table 2. Average heterozygosity and proportion of polymorphic loci
for neutral and advantageous mutations when the rate of gene
substitution is fixed. A locus is defined as polymorphic
when the frequency of the most common allele is equal to
or larger than 0.9.

	Neutral mutations	Advantageous mutations
Substitution rate = 5×10^{-5}		
Average heterozygosity	0.0909	0.0013
Polymorphic loci	0.3690	0.0040
Substitution rate = 1×10^{-4}		
Average heterozygosity	0.1667	0.0024
Polymorphic loci	0.6019	0.0140

The average heterozygosities obtained from the simulation are given
in Table 2. It is clear that for a given rate of gene substitution the
heterozygosity for advantageous mutations is extremely low compared with
that for neutral mutations. It should be noted that if we increase the
population size (N), the difference becomes even larger. It is also
clear that the average heterozygosity relative to the rate of gene substitution under this hypothesis is very low compared with the observed
level. We may thus conclude that the hypothesis of sequentially advantageous mutations is not adequate to explain the protein polymorphism in
natural populations. This is in agreement with the conclusion reached
by Maruyama (1972) and Nei (1975, p. 174).

Slightly deleterious mutations: As mentioned earlier, the estimates of average heterozygosity so far obtained are all about 0.3 or
lower, though some organisms apparently have a large effective population size. From this observation, Ohta (1973) proposed that a majority
of polymorphic alleles are slightly deleterious compared with a type
allele and in a large population a mutation-selection balance is established. She believes that the existence of an apparent upper bound of
average heterozygosity is due to this mutation-selection balance. Mathematical models incorporating these features were recently studied by
Ohta (1977), Li (1977, 1978, 1979a), and Kimura (1979b). The results obtained from these studies indicate that the upper limit of average heterozygosity in natural populations can indeed be explained by the mutation-

selection balance, but under this type of selection the rate of gene substitution will no longer be constant for a wide range of organisms. Furthermore, the allele frequency distribution will not be U-shaped in large populations, unlike the observed distributions. Because of these properties we believe that Ohta's hypothesis of slightly deleterious mutations is less satisfactory than the bottleneck hypothesis (Chakraborty et al. 1980). Of course, when selection coefficient is extremely small for the majority of mutations, the allele frequency distribution will be U-shaped with an appropriate value of $4Nv$ (Li 1978). However, even this small magnitude of selection seems to affect the rate of gene substitution substantially (Kimura 1979). Theoretically, the selection coefficient for slightly deleterious mutations should be distributed continuously from 0 to a certain positive value, as claimed by Ohta and Kimura. In practice, however, if selection coefficient is extremely small, the effeet of fluctuation of selection intensity which will be discussed in the following, will be more important than the mean effect, and the behavior of mutant genes will be similar to that of neutral genes (Nei and Yokoyama 1976). If this is the case, very slightly deleterious mutations can be regarded as neutral genes even if $Ns > 1$.

Varying selection intensity: Strictly speaking, the selection coefficient for a genotype should not be the same for all local populations and for all generations, since the environment almost never stays constant. There are a large number of ways to formulate the effect of varying selection intensity (cf. Karlin and Lieberman 1974; Hedrick et al. 1976; Felsenstein 1976; Nei and Yokoyama 1976; Gillespie 1978). Under certain mathematical models a stable equilibrium of gene frequency may be obtained in an infinite population (Levene 1953; Dempster 1955; Haldane and Jayakar 1963). Gillespie and Langley (1974) extended these models and proposed the hypothesis that random fluctuation of selection intensity is the major factor for the maintenance of protein polymorphism. Furthermore, Gillespie (1977) has shown that under certain assumptions the allele frequency distribution *in an infinite population* can have a form similar to that for neutral mutations *in a finite population*.

In practice, of course, this similarity does not mean that the hypotheses of neutral mutations and fluctuating selection intensities result in the same population consequences. Actually, Gillespie's (1977) model is quite unrealistic, since no mutation and no random genetic drift due to finite population size are considered. If these factors are considered, the allele frequency distribution becomes entirely different. Indeed, Nei and Yokoyama (1976) and Takahata and Kimura (1979)

have recently shown that when these factors are considered, random fluctuation of selection intensity reduces genetic variability considerably
compared with the case of neutral mutations (see also Hedrick 1974).
In other words, in a population of realistic size random fluctuation
of selection intensity seems to be a diversity-reducing selection rather
than a diversity-enhancing selection. This view, clearly stated in Nei
and Yokoyama's (1976) paper, is essentially the same as those of Fisher
and Ford (1947) and Wright (1948) but different from those of many
recent authors.

It should be noted, however, that the effect of random fluctuation
of selection intensity is a secondary factor compared with the mean
effect. Only when the mean selection intensity is small relative to the
standard deviation, will this factor be important. Of course, the mean
selection intensity for allozymes is likely to be very small in many
cases, and thus it is possible that the observed heterozygosity smaller
than the neutral expectation is partly due to this factor, as noted by
Nei (1975, p. 167). Unfortunately, however, we have few data on the
actual magnitude of fluctuation of selection intensity.

Powell's (1971) and McDonald and Ayala's (1974) data on average
heterozygosities in constant and heterogeneous environments in Drosophila
are often cited as evidence for supporting the view that varying selection intensity results in a balancing or diversity-enhancing selection.
Indeed, according to their data the populations maintained in a heterogeneous environment show a higher average heterozygosity than those maintained in a homogeneous environment. However, a close examination of
their data indicates that in both environments the average heterozygosity
declined faster than the rate expected under pure genetic drift.
McDonald and Ayala state that in the natural population of *D. pseudo-
obscura* from which the original sample was obtained the average heterozygosity for the 20 polymorphic loci they examined was 0.212 and that
the size of their experimental population was never smaller than
500. Therefore, the maximum reduction in average heterozygosity due to
drift during the experiment (12 ~ 15 generations) is expected to be
$0.212 \times (1 - 1/1000)^{15} = 0.209$. However, the average heterozygosity
for the 14 populations grown in heterogeneous environments was 0.195 at
the end of the experiment, whereas the average heterozygosity for the
four populations grown in homogeneous environments was 0.146. Therefore, the heterogeneous environments did not retard but actually acce-
lerated the reduction of heterozygosity. In Powell's experiment the
amount of the reduction in heterogeneous environments is more pronounced.
In both experiments, however, homogeneous environments produced a more

drastic reduction in heterozygosity. The reason for this is not clear. At any rate, Powell, McDonald, and Ayala's results cannot be regarded as evidence for diversity-enhancing selection.

Recently, Powell and Taylor (1979) emphasized the importance of habitat choice in maintaining genetic variability. In this model each genotype is supposed to choose the habitat which is most suited to the genotype. They provided some indirect evidence for this type of selection in Drosophila. It should be noted, however, that natural populations are polymorphic at many loci (10 - 60 percent of the structural genes) and thus the number of possible genotypes is enormously large. In this case it is not easy to see how habitat selection occurs and how effective it is as a diversity-enhancing selection.

In the past many population geneticists have been interested in modeling diversity-enhancing selection that arises from varying environments (see the papers cited in Hedrick et al. 1976). Some of the models are concerned with the temporal variation of selection intensity, whereas the others deal with the spacial variation (multi-niche or habitat selection). Apparently these models have been developed by the influence of the old view that most of the polymorphisms in nature must be stable since all populations have existed for a long time. Actually this view is illogical, because polymorphic alleles may not be old even if the population is old. Furthermore, it is important to realize that the average heterozygosity for protein loci is generally lower than the value expected under the neutral theory. Therefore, what we really need is not a model of diversity-enhancing selection but a model of diversity-reducing selection if any selection is to be considered (Nei 1975).

General Conclusion

At the outset I mentioned that the neutral theory should be tested statistically since the theory refers to the majority of polymorphic alleles. With this view in mind, we have conducted an extensive statistical test but have not been able to reject the neutral theory, particularly when the bottleneck effect is taken into account. However, this does not mean that all polymorphic alleles are neutral or nearly neutral. The power of the tests used is not very high, and our conclusion is partially derived from additional qualitative arguments. Therefore, it is still possible that a substantial proportion of polymorphic alleles are subject to some form of selection. In this connection we note that there are a number of data on protein polymorphism which are hard to interpret without considering the effect of selection (e.g. Koehn

1969; Frelinger 1972). Nevertheless, our study, which I believe is the most extensive statistical study so far conducted, has shown that the pattern of protein polymorphism and molecular evolution is not much deviated from that expected under the neutral theory. This indicates that stochastic factors are very important in molecular evolution whether selection is operating or not, and that the neutral theory is useful for predicting the process of molecular evolution.

Two decades ago Mayr (1959) questioned the contribution of mathematical genetics (which he called beanbag genetics) to evolutionary theory. He claimed that in the development of the synthetic theory of evolution or neo-Darwinism the contribution of naturalists such as Simpson and Dobzhansky was much greater than that of mathematical geneticists such as Fisher, Wright, and Haldane. In his paper entitled "A defense of beanbag genetics" Haldane (1964) corrected Mayr's misunderstandings and clarified the roles mathematical population genetics played in the conceptual development of neo-Darwinism. In showing the utility of mathematical theory in data analysis, however, he could not find many good examples. In the last ten years the situation has changed drastically. We now have a large amount of data on molecular evolution, which have to be analyzed by using the theory of beanbag genetics, particularly the stochastic theory. It is expected that in the near future this theory will be essential in understanding all fundamental aspects of evolution.

SHIFTING-BALANCE THEORY

Let us now examine the applicability of Wright's shifting-balance theory of evolution to molecular data. This theory requires three conditions. (1) Populations are subdivided into a large number of demes among which gene migration occurs with a certain probability. (2) Most of the loci are polymorphic in all generations and evolution occurs by gene frequency shift rather than by complete gene substitution. The genetic polymorphism is maintained by some sort of balancing selection. (3) Gene interaction among different loci is prevalent.

The first condition is clearly satisfied in most organisms, since they are composed of many local populations among which gene exchange occurs. The second requirement is based on Wright's (1932) conviction that most loci are polymorphic in natural populations. His conviction was derived from the observation that whenever artificial selection was applied to a quantitative character, there was almost always a response

to it.   At the protein level examined by electrophoresis, however, a
high proportion of loci are monomorphic rather than polymorphic.   In
most mammals the proportion of polymorphic loci is less than 50 percent
(Fuerst et al. 1977).   In tropical Drosophila species this proportion
is somewhat higher but not close to 100 percent.   However, electrophoresis does not detect all amino acid substitutions in protein, so that
this itself does not create any serious problem to his theory, as Wright
(1978) noted.   Indeed, mainly because of this plausible genetic variability at the amino acid sequence level Wright thought that protein
polymorphic data support his theory.

However, his theory is not supported by data on long-term molecular
evolution.   Comparison of amino acid sequences of proteins among different species indicates that the genetic change of populations occurs not
through gene frequency shift as Wright assumed but through complete gene
substitution.   Furthermore, the process of gene substitution can be
roughly described by the Poisson process in probability theory, as mentioned earlier.   Therefore, amino acid substitution in evolution seems
to occur independently of the environmental condition.   The gene interaction among structural loci has not been studied very well, but in
general the interaction seems to be very weak if not absent.   Thus, the
amino acid substitution in one polypeptide apparently occurs almost independently of that in another polypeptide (Dayhoff 1972).   This seems
to be so even with the polypeptides that constitute the same protein
such as hemoglobin α and β chains (Langley and Fitch 1974).   Furthermore, if gene interaction is prevalent among protein loci, we would expect a substantial amount of linkage disequilibria among these loci.
Studies on this problem by Kojima et al. (1970), Mukai et al. (1971),
Langley et al. (1974), and others do not support this prediction.   We
also note that gene substitution occurs roughly at a constant rate irrespectively of the organism, whether the organism is rapidly evolving or
a living fossil at the morphological level (Kimura and Ohta 1974; Wilson
et al. 1977).   Therefore, we can conclude that the shifting-balance
theory does not apply to molecular evolution.

Of course, Wright's shifting-balance theory is intended to be
applied to morphological evolution, and thus molecular data do not really
refute his theory.   Unfortunately, we know very little about the relationship between morphological change and gene frequency change in evolution.   It is true that there is a large component of genetic variation
in most quantitative characters in natural populations, and thus the loci
controlling quantitative characters must be highly polymorphic.   It is
also possible that many of these gene loci have some epistatic interac-

tion. For example, many quantitative characters are apparently subject
to optimum model selection (Fisher 1930; Wright 1935). However, these
observations are not proof of the shifting-balance theory. Optimum
model selection is known generally to lead to fixation of genes in the
absence of mutation (Wright 1935; Lewontin 1964). Therefore, if optimum
model selection is operating, the genetic variability must be maintained
by the balance between mutation and selection (Kimura 1965). It is also
possible that some quantitative characters such as stature and dermal
ridge count in man may not be directly related to fitness except when
the values of the characters are extremely different from the mean in
either positive or negative direction. In this case a considerable
amount of genetic variability may be maintained by mutation-drift balance
in large populations (Chakraborty and Nei, unpublished). As long as a
sufficient amount of genetic variability exists in a population, the
mean of the quantitative character would change relatively rapidly when
the optimum value shifts because of environmental change. In this case,
however, the mean change would occur mainly because of directional selection, and no shifting-balance would be required. In other words, this
type of mean change would occur whether populations are subdivided or
not. Furthermore, the mean change may be brought about either by gene
frequency shift or by complete gene substitution at individual loci.

In some morphological or physiological characters the importance
of gene interaction among different loci has been demonstrated. A good
example is that of heterostyly in Primula. Long style and short style
in this plant are controlled by a pair of alleles at a locus, but there
are two more loci, which control the pollen incompatibility and anther
length (cf. Bodmer and Edwards 1962). However, it is not clear whether
the evolution of this type of interacting gene system is really facilitated by subdivision of populations or not.

STOCHASTIC FACTORS IN MORPHOLOGICAL EVOLUTION

In neo-Darwinism the most important evolutionary force is natural
selection, and mutation and genetic drift play only a minor role. In
this theory natural populations are believed to contain genetic variability enough to cope with sudden environmental change, so that the rate
of evolution is primarily determined by the change in environment and
the intensity of natural selection. Molecular data, however, do not
appear to support this view. At the molecular level mutation seems to
be the primary force of evolution, and a large role of genetic drift

cannot be denied, whether selection is important or not.   Various statistical properties of molecular evolution and protein polymorphism are
roughly in agreement with the predictions from Kimura's neutral mutation-
random drift theory.   Of course, there must be a certain proportion of
advantageous mutations.   Otherwise, no adaption can occur.

One can then ask the question: is neo-Darwinism still true with
morphological evolution? My answer to this question is "Probably so to
a large extent but some modifications are necessary." Neo-Darwinism was
constructed largely on the knowledge of morphological evolution, and
there is no question about the importance of natural selection in the
formation of intricate morphological characters such as human eyes and
brains.   However, are all individual differences in morphology and physiology adaptive as claimed by neo-Darwinians? On this earth more than
4 billion people are living, and all of them except identical twins are
different with respect to various morphological and physiological characters. Are all these differences adaptive? Is random genetic drift
unimportant for generating morphological and physiological diversities
among organisms except when the population goes through a bottleneck,
as Mayr (1963) claims? I doubt it. It seems to me that in some morphological characters a substantial part of the variation in a population
is non-adaptive. For example, the sternopleural or abdominal bristle
number of *Drosophila melanogaster* does not seem to be directly related
to fitness except the extreme values in both directions (Clayton and
Robertson 1957). Robertson (1967) conducted upward artificial selection
for six generations with respect to sternopleural bristle number and
obtained a rapid response to the selection. He then relaxed the selection and examined the change in mean bristle number in the following
generations for nearly two and a half years (about 40 generations). In
the first few months about one-fifth of the selection gain was lost, but
thereafter no visible change was observed. However, when downward selection was applied to this line, there was a rapid response. This indicates that this line had enough genetic variability when upward selection was relaxed, but natural selection ceased to operate a few months
after relaxation of the selection. A similar result was obtained in a
different experiment in which downward artificial selection was conducted.
From these experiments he concluded that the genes at a high proportion
of the loci responsible for the bristle number must be neutral in their
effects on fitness.

Variation in the dermal ridge count in man seems to be as trivial
as that of Drosophila bristle number. This character is highly herita-
ble (nearly 100 percent heritability; Holt 1961), and there is a large

amount of genetic variation among human races. The dermal ridge count is known to be highly correlated with the total number of tri-radii on fingers (PII, 2 × frequency of whorls + frequency of loops). This number is 20 in non-ape primates, whereas it is about 13 in man, 14 in chimpanzee, 18 in gorilla, and 7 in orangutan. It seems that in apes and man natural selection for this character has been relaxed, and the number is drifting largely by mutation and genetic drift (Chakraborty and Nei, unpublished).

There are many other such characters which do not appear to be under strong selection pressure. For example, human stature does not seem to be directly related to fitness except extremely short or tall statures. It is possible that the individuals whose stature is not far from the mean are virtually identical in fitness and the genetic variation within this range is maintained largely by the balance among mutation, genetic drift, and weak selection, if any. In other words, the relation between phenotypic value and fitness may not be so rigid and a large proportion of individuals may survive or reproduce with an equal or nearly equal probability. In this view the genetic variability existing in a population is simply the product of past evolution and is not designed to be used as the material for future evolution, as often assumed in neo-Darwinism. Some neo-Darwinians maintain the extreme view that the maintenance of a large amount of genetic variability is advantageous and thus natural selection operates to increase the amount of genetic variability. I doubt that any organism, even man, is so teleolistic or altruistic as to be able to judge the amount of genetic variability in his population and consciously increase it. Some authors believe that overdominant selection or some other balancing selection fulfills the purpose. I disagree. Natural selection is nothing but a consequence of the reaction of different genotypes to the environment, and there is no teleological orientation to increase or decrease genetic variability. If it happens to increase the genetic variability, it is simply a byproduct of genotypic reaction to the environment.

Even the genetic variability between populations may not always be adaptive. The Ainu living in northern Japan are morphologically different from the Japanese, their male body being quite hairy. However, it is not clear what kind of selective advantage their hairiness confers to the Ainu. It is possible that this character was brought about by mutation in their ancestral population and the individuals with this mutant gene or genes later formed a new group, which further later has become the Ainu population. In the past several decades anthropologists, evolutionists, and recently sociobiologists have tried to explain every

detail of morphological, physiological, and behavioral differences between races in terms of natural selection. However, some of the morphological differences may well be due to non-adaptive genetic change.

It should be noted that the possibility of non-adaptive change of
morphological characters was recognized even by Charles Darwin (1872).
He stated: "Variation neither useful nor injurious would not be
affected by natural selection, and would be left either a fluctuating
element, as perhaps we see in certain polymorphic species, or would
ultimately become fixed, owing to the nature of the organism and the
nature of the conditions." Later a number of authors discussed the
possibility of neutral evolution or variation (e.g., Gulick 1905; Wright
1932). (In his later writings (e.g., Wright 1971), Wright disregarded
the importance of genetic drift except as an aid for attaining a better
gene combination in his shifting-balance theory.) However, with the
rise of neo-Darwinism this view was completely obliterated. Thus, Mayr
(1963, p. 207) stated: "Entirely neutral genes are improbable for
physiological reasons. Every gene elaborates a 'gene product', a chemical
that enters the developmental stream. It seems unrealistic to me to
assume that the nature of the particular chemical (enzyme or other
product) should be without any effect whatsoever on the fitness of the
ultimate phenotype." "Selective neutrality can be excluded almost automatically wherever polymorphism or character clines are found in natural
populations." This view has been shared by a large number of authors.
As I mentioned earlier, however, I do not think that the activity difference between two forms of enzymes always results in fitness difference
in finite populations. Many higher organisms have a high degree of phenotypic plasticity and are tolerant to a certain degree of environmental
variation. In Waddington's (1957) terminology many characters are well
canalized despite the fact that natural populations contain a large
amount of genetic variability.

At this point I note that Mayr's (1963) definition of neutral genes
is quite vague. From the sentences quoted above it is clear that he
defines neutral genes as those which do not have any effect on fitness.
In other words, Mayr's neutral genes seem to be functionless genes.
Actually this is not the definition of neutral genes in population
genetics. As mentioned earlier, neutral alleles may be vitally important for the survival of the individual, but if they are equally important, they are called neutral alleles. On page 212 he states: "Perhaps
the greatest single source of randomness and indeterminacy in evolution
is the selective equivalence of genotypes." Mayr apparently does not
call our neutral alleles or genotypes neutral, but seems to recognize

the importance of random genetic drift for determining the frequencies of these alleles or genotypes. This suggests that his denial of the important role of genetic drift in evolution is largely due to his erroneous conception of neutral genes.

Many quantitative characters seem to have a large component of genetic variance, and when environmental changes occur this variance could be used for the future evolution whether it is selectively or neutrally maintained in the original environment. In this case natural selection would certainly be an important factor for determining the rate of evolution. However, the genetic variation existing in a population would not always be sufficient for completing adaptation to a new environment. In this case the speed of adaptation or the rate of evolution will depend on all factors of natural selection, mutation, and genetic drift. For example, American Indians apparently migrated to the New World from Asia about 30,000 years ago and probably reached the tropical region by at the latest about 13,000 years ago. They are genetically more different from the present Asian races than Oceanian Negritoes are (Nei and Roychoudhury 1980). Yet their skin color is not as dark as Negritoes' or African Negroids'. It is possible that 13,000 ~ 30,000 years were not enough for new mutations for dark pigmentation to be accumulated. Similarly, in the evolution of such characters as giraffe's neck and elephant's snout not only selection intensity but also mutation rate might have determined the rate of evolution. In bacteria it is well known that adaptation to new environments such as the presence of drugs or new substrates occurs by both mutations and selection (Lederberg and Lederberg 1952; Rigby et al. 1974). It seems to me that morphological evolution is controlled by all three evolutionary forces, i.e., natural selection, mutation, and genetic drift, and the relative contributions of these factors vary with organism and evolutionary circumstance. Under certain circumstances the latter two factors may be more important than the first. In his book *Chance and Necessity*, Monod (1971) discussed the significance of mutation in evolution. Recognizing that occurrence of mutation has nothing to do with the teleonomy of an organism, he concluded "chance *alone* is at the source of every innovation, of all creation in the biosphere. Pure chance, absolutely free, but blind, at the very root of the stupendous edifice of evolution." Chance seems to be important even after occurrence of mutation.

Summary

(1) Statistical tests of the neutral mutation hypothesis have been conducted by using data on protein polymorphism from more than 130 species. In these tests agreement between theory and data is examined about the relationships between the means and variances of heterozygosity and genetic distance, the relationship between genetic identity and correlation of heterozygosity between populations, the distribution of allele frequencies, etc. These tests have shown that most data on protein polymorphism can be accounted for by the neutral theory but in a significant proportion of species there is an excess of rare alleles. This excess of rare alleles seems to be best explained by the bottleneck effect.

(2) It is indicated that any reasonable hypothesis to explain protein polymorphism should also be able to explain the rate of gene substitution in long-term evolution. From this point of view various alternative hypotheses are examined, and it is concluded that diversity-enhancing selection such as overdominant selection or certain types of selection in heterogeneous environments is not adequate for explaining the level of heterozygosity and the rate of gene substitution simultaneously, since it gives a much higher level of heterozygosity than the observed one for a given rate of gene substitution. On the other hand, sequentially advantageous selection gives a too low level of heterozygosity. The current data on average heterozygosity and rate of gene substitution can be explained either by the neutral mutation theory with bottleneck effects or by the type of fluctuating selection modeled by Nei and Yokoyama.

(3) Applicability of Wright's shifting-balance theory of evolution to molecular data is examined. Molecular data do not appear to support his theory.

(4) The role and evidence of stochastic factors in the evolution of morphological characters are reviewed. It seems that under certain circumstances mutation and random genetic drift play an important role in the differentiation of morphological characters among populations.

ACKNOWLEDGEMENTS

This work was supported by research grants from the U.S. National Institute of Health and the U.S. National Science Foundation. An original version of this paper was presented in a symposium on Stochastic Processes in Evolution, Society for the Study of Evolution, Loyola University, New Orleans, Louisiana, June 1, 1976.

REFERENCES

Ayala, F. J. 1972. Darwinian versus non-Darwinian evolution in natural populations of *Drosophila*.
Proc. 6th Berkeley Symp. Math. Stat. Prob. V:211-236.

Bodmer, W. F. and A. W. F. Edwards. 1962. Linkage and recombination in evolution.
Adv. Genet. 11:1-100.

Chakraborty, R. and M. Nei. 1976. Hidden genetic variability within electromorphs in finite populations.
Genetics 84:385-393.

Chakraborty, R. and M. Nei. 1977. Bottleneck effects on average heterozygosity and genetic distance with the stepwise mutation model.
Evolution 31:347-356.

Chakraborty, R., P. A. Fuerst, and M. Nei. 1978. Statistical studies on protein polymorphism in natural populations. II. Gene differentiation between populations.
Genetics 88:367-390.

Chakraborty, R., P. A. Fuerst, and M. Nei. 1980. Statistical studies on protein polymorphism in natural populations. III. Distribution of allele frequencies and the number of alleles per locus.
Genetics (in press)

Clayton, G. A. and A. Robertson. 1957. Mutation and cumulative variation.
Amer. Nat. 89:151-155.

Dayhoff, M. O., ed. 1972. *Atlas of Protein Sequence and Structure.* Vol. 5.
Natl. Biomed. Res. Found., Washington, D.C.

Darwin, C. 1872. *The Origin of Species.* 6th ed. D. Appleton, London.

Dempster, E. R. 1955. Maintenance of genetic heterogeneity.
Cold Spring Harbor Symp. Quant. Biol. 20:25-32.

Ewens, W. J. 1964. The maintenance of alleles by mutation.
Genetics 50:891-898.

Felsenstein, J. 1976. The theoretical population genetics of variable selection and migration.
Ann. Rev. Genet. 10:253-280.

Fisher, R. A. 1922. On the dominance ratio.
Proc. Roy. Soc. Edinburgh 42:321-341.

Fisher, R. A. 1930. *The Genetical Theory of Natural Selection.*
Clarendon Press, Oxford.

Fisher, R. A. and E. B. Ford. 1947. The spread of a gene in natural conditions in a colony of the moth *Panaxia dominula* L.
Heredity 1:143-174.

Fitch, W. M. and E. Margoliash. 1967. A method for estimating the number of invariant amino acid coding positions in a gene using cytochrome c as a model case.
Biochem. Genet. 1:65-71.

Ford, E. B. 1975. *Ecological Genetics.* 4th ed. Chapman and Hall Ltd., London.

Frelinger, J. A. 1972. The maintenance of transferrin polymorphism in pigeons.
    Proc. Natl. Acad. Sci. US 69:326-329

Fuerst, P. A. and R. E. Ferrell. 1980. The stepwise mutation model: an experimental evaluation utilizing hemoglobin variants.
    Genetics (in press)

Fuerst, P. A., R. Chakraborty, and M. Nei. 1977. Statistical studies on protein polymorphism in natural populations. I. Distribution of single-locus heterozygosity.
    Genetics 86:455-483.

Gillespie, J. H. 1977. Sampling theory for alleles in a random environment.
    Nature 266:443-445.

Gillespie, J. H. 1978. A general model to account for enzyme variation in natural populations. V. The SAS-CFF model.
    Theoret. Popul. Biol. 14:1-45.

Gillespie, J. H. and C. H. Langley. 1974. A general model to account for enzyme variation in natural populations.
    Genetics 76:837-848.

Gulick, J. T. 1905. *Evolution, Racial and Habitudinal.* Publ. 25.
    Carnegie Institution of Washington.

Haldane, J. B. S. 1927. The mathematical theory of natural and artificial selection. Part V.
    Proc. Camb. Philos. Soc. 23:838-844.

Haldane, J. B. S. 1964. A defense of beanbag genetics.
    Perspectives in Biology and Medicine 7:343-359.

Haldane, J. B. S. and S. D. Jayakar. 1963. Polymorphism due to selection of varying direction.
    J. Genet. 58:237-242.

Hedrick, P. W. 1974. Genetic variation in a heterogeneous environment. I. Temporal heterogeneity and the absolute dominance model.
    Genetics 78:757-770.

Hedrick, P. W., M. E. Ginevan, and E. P. Ewing. 1976. Genetic polymorphism in heterogeneous environments.
    Ann. Rev. Ecol. Syst. 7:1-32.

Holt, S. B. 1961. Quantitative genetics of finger-print patterns.
    Brit. Med. Bull. 17:247-250.

Karlin, S. and U. Lieberman. 1974. Random temporal variation in selection intensities: Case of a large population size.
    Theoret. Popul. Biol. 6:355-382.

Kimura, M. 1965. A stochastic model concerning the maintenance of genetic variability in quantitative characters.
    Proc. Natl. Acad. Sci. US 54:731-736.

Kimura, M. 1968. Evolutionary rate at the molecular level.
    Nature 217:624-626.

Kimura, M. 1979 . The neutral theory of molecular evolution.
    Scientific American 241:98-126.

Kimura, M. 1979 . Model of effectively neutral mutations in which selective constraint is incorporated.
Proc. Natl. Acad. Sci. US 76:3440-3444.

Kimura, M. and J. F. Crow. 1964. The number of alleles that can be maintained in a
finite population.
Genetics 49:725-738.

Kimura, M. and T. Maruyama. 1971. Pattern of neutral polymorphism in a geographically structured population.
Genet. Res. 18:125-131.

Kimura, M. and T. Ohta. 1971. Protein polymorphism as a phase of molecular evolution.
Nature 229:467-469.

Kimura, M. and T. Ohta. 1973. Mutation and evolution at the molecular level.
Genetics 73 (Suppl.):19-35.

Kimura, M. and T. Ohta. 1974. On some principles governing molecular evolution.
Proc. Natl. Acad. Sci. US 71:2848-2852.

Koehn, R. K. 1969. Esterase heterogeneity: Dynamics of a polymorphism.
Science 163:943-944.

Kojima, K., J. Gillespie, and Y. N. Tobari. 1970. A profile of Drosophila species'
enzymes assayed by electrophoresis. I. Number of alleles, heterozygosities, and
linkage disequilibrium in glucose-metabolizing systems and some other enzymes.
Biochem. Genet. 4:627-637.

Langley, C. H. and W. M. Fitch. 1974. An examination of the constancy of the rate
of molecular evolution.
J. Mol. Evol. 3:161-177.

Langley, C. H., Y. N. Tobari, and K. Kojima. 1974. Linkage disequilibrium in
natural populations of *Drosophila melanogaster*.
Genetics 78:921-936.

Latter, B. D. H. 1975. Influence of selection pressures on enzyme polymorphisms
in Drosophila.
Nature 257:590-592.

Lederberg, J. and E. M. Lederberg. 1952. Replica plating and indirect selection
of bacterial mutants.
J. Bacteriology 63:399-406.

Levene, H. 1953. Genetic equilibrium when more than one ecological niche is
available.
Amer. Nat. 87:331-333.

Lewontin, R. C. 1964. The interaction of selection and linkage. II. Optimum models.
Genetics 50:757-782.

Lewontin, R. C., L. R. Ginzburg, and S. D. Tuljapurkar. 1978. Heterosis as an
explanation for large amounts of genic polymorphism.
Genetics 88:149-170.

Li, W.-H. 1976. A mixed model of mutation for electrophoretic identity of proteins within and between populations.
Genetics 83:423-432.

Li, W.-H. 1977. Maintenance of genetic variability under mutation and selection pressures in a finite population.
Proc. Natl. Acad. Sci. US 74:2509-2513.

Li, W.-H. 1978. Maintenance of genetic variability under the joint effect of mutation, selection and random drift.
Genetics 90:349-382.

Li, W.-H. 1979 . Maintenance of genetic variability under the pressure of neutral and deleterious mutations in a finite population.
Genetics 92:647-667.

Li, W.-H. 1979 . Variance of genetic distance and correlation of heterozygosity between populations under the pressure of stepwise mutation.
Theoret. Popul. Biol. 15:171-190.

Li, W.-H. and M. Nei. 1975. Drift variances of heterozygosity and genetic distance in transient states.
Genet. Res. 25:229-248.

Li, W.-H. and M. Nei. 1977. Persistence of common alleles in two related populations or species.
Genetics 86:901-914.

Maruyama, T. 1972. A note on the hypothesis: protein polymorphism as a phase of molecular evolution.
J. Mol. Evol. 1:201-219.

Mayr, E. 1959. Where are we?
Cold Spring Harbor Symp. Quant. Biol. 24:409-440.

Mayr, E. 1963. *Animal Species or Evolution*.
Harvard Univ. Press, Cambridge, Mass.

McDonald, J. F. and F. J. Ayala. 1974. Genetic response to environmental heterogeneity.
Nature 250:572-574.

Monod, J. 1971. *Chance and Necessity*. Translated by A. Wainhouse. Originally published in France as *Le Hasard et la Nécessité* by editions du Seuil, Paris, 1970. Alfred A. Knopf, Inc., New York.

Mukai, T., L. E. Mettler, and S. I. Chigusa. 1971. Linkage disequilibrium in a local population of *Drosophila melanogaster*.
Proc. Natl. Acad. Sci. US 68:1065-1069.

Nei, M. 1975. *Molecular Population Genetics and Evolution*.
North Holland, Amsterdam.

Nei, M. 1976. Mathematical models of speciation and genetic distance.
In: *Population Genetics and Ecology*. S. Karlin and E. Nevo, eds.
Academic Press, New York. 723-765.

Nei, M. 1978. The theory of genetic distance and evolution of human races.
Japan. J. Hum. Genet. 23:341-369.

Nei, M. and W.-H. Li. 1975. Probability of identical monomorphism in related species.
Genet. Res. 26:31-43.

Nei, M. and W.-H. Li. 1976. The transient distribution of allele frequencies under mutation pressure.
Genet. Res. 28:205-214.

Nei, M. and W.-H. Li. 1980. Non-random association between electromorphs and inversion chromosomes in finite populations.
Genet. Res. (in press)

Nei, M. and A. K. Roychoudhury. 1973. Probability of fixation and mean fixation time of an overdominant mutation.
Genetics 74:371-380.

Nei, M. and A. K. Roychoudhury. 1974. Genic variation within and between the three major races of man, Caucasoids, Negroids, and Mongoloids.
Amer. J. Hum. Genet. 26:421-443.

Nei, M. and A. K. Roychoudhury. 1980. Genetic relationship and evolution of human races.
(submitted)

Nei, M. and Y. Tateno. 1975. Interlocus variation of genetic distance and the neutral mutation theory.
Proc. Natl. Acad. Sci. US 72:2758-2760.

Nei, M. and S. Yokoyama. 1976. Effects of random fluctuation of selection intensity on genetic variability in a finite population.
Japan. J. Genet. 51:355-369.

Nei, M., T. Maruyama, and R. Chakraborty. 1975. The bottleneck effect and genetic variability in populations.
Evolution 29:1-10.

Nei, M., R. Chakraborty, and P. A. Fuerst. 1976 . Infinite allele model with varying mutation rate.
Proc. Natl. Acad. Sci. US 73:4164-4168.

Nei, M., P. A. Fuerst, and R. Chakraborty. 1976 . Testing the neutral mutation hypothesis by distribution of single-locus heterozygosity.
Nature 262:491-493.

Nei, M., P. A. Fuerst, and R. Chakraborty. 1978. Subunit molecular weight and genetic variability of proteins in natural populations.
Proc. Natl. Acad. Sci. US 75:3359-3362.

Ohta, T. 1973. Slightly deleterious mutant substitutions in evolution.
Nature 246:96-98.

Ohta, T. 1975. Statistical analyses of Drosophila and human protein polymorphisms.
Proc. Natl. Acad. Sci. US 72:3194-3196.

Ohta, T. 1977. Extension to the neutral mutation random drift hypothesis.
Proc. 2nd Taniguchi Intl. Symp. Biophysics.

Powell, J. R. 1971. Genetic polymorphisms in varied environments.
Science 174:1035-1036.

Powell, J. R. and C. E. Taylor. 1979. Genetic variation in ecologically diverse environments.
Amer. Scientist 67:590-596.

Ramshaw, J. A. M., J. A. Coyne, and R. C. Lewontin. 1980. The sensitivity of gel electrophoresis as a detector of genetic variation.
Genetics (in press)

Rigby, P. W. J., B. D. Burleigh, Jr., and B. S. Hartley. 1974. Gene duplication in experimental enzyme evolution. *Nature* 251:200-204.

Robertson, A. 1967. The nature of quantitative genetic variation. In: *Heritage from Mendel*. R. A. Brink, ed. Univ. of Wisconsin Press, Madison, Wisconsin. 265-280.

Soulé, M. 1976. Allozyme variation: its determinants in space and time. In: *Molecular Evolution*. F. J. Ayala, ed. Sinauer Associates, Sunderland, Mass. 60-77.

Takahata, N. and M. Kimura. 1979. Genetic variability maintained in a finite population under mutation and autocorrelated random fluctuation of selection intensity. *Proc. Natl. Acad. Sci. US* 76:5813-5817.

Waddington, C. H. 1957. *The Strategy of the Genes*. Allen and Unwin, London.

Watterson, G. A. 1977. Heterosis or neutrality? *Genetics* 85:789-814.

Wilson, A. C., S. S. Carlson, and T. J. White. 1977. Biochemical evolution. *Ann. Rev. Biochem.* 46:573-639.

Wright, S. 1931. Evolution in Mendelian populations. *Genetics* 16:97-159.

Wright, S. 1932. The roles of mutation, inbreeding, crossbreeding, and selection in evolution. *Proc. 6th Intl. Cong. Genet.* 1:356-366.

Wright, S. 1935. The analysis of variance and the correlation between relatives with respect to deviations from an optimum. *J. Genet.* 30:243-256.

Wright, S. 1938. Size of population and breeding structure in relation to evolution. *Science* 87:430-431.

Wright, S. 1948. On the roles of directed and random changes in gene frequency in the genetics of populations. *Evolution* 2:279-294.

Wright, S. 1949. Adaptation and selection. In: *Genetics, Paleontology, and Evolution*. G. L. Jepson, G. G. Simpson, and E. Mayr, eds. Princeton Univ. Press, Princeton, N.J. 365-389.

Wright, S. 1971. Random drift and the shifting balance theory of evolution. In: *Mathematical Topics in Population Genetics*. K. Kojima, ed. Springer-Verlag, Berlin. 1-31.

Wright, S. 1978. *Variability Within and Among Natural Populations*. Vol. 4 of: *Evolution and the Genetics of Populations*. Univ. of Chicago Press, Chicago.

Yokoyama, S. and M. Nei. 1979. Population dynamics of sex-determining alleles in honey bees and self-incompatibility alleles in plants. *Genetics* 91:609-626.

Zuckerkandl, E. and L. Pauling. 1965. Evolutionary divergence and convergence in proteins. In: *Evolving Genes and Proteins*. V. Bryson and H. J. Vogel, eds. Academic Press, New York. 97-166.

NATURAL SELECTION AND CONTINUOUS VARIATION

Alan Robertson
Genetics, University of Edinburgh, Scotland

Introduction

In his paper to this meeting, Dr. Lewontin stresses the difficulty in using some of the classical formulae of population genetics, even when we deal only with a single locus at which the genotypes can be accurately identified. One of the problems is the difficulty of transferring the concept of fitness from the context of changes of gene frequency within the population, to changes of the ability of the population as a whole to survive - a problem made more complicated by the possibility of frequency dependent selection. He indicated, very briefly, the way in which there are difficulties in discussing natural selection for continuous characters, and I would like to devote the greater part of my talk to this particular problem.

The basic genome of an individual controls in some measure its phenotypic development. In so far as this affects the ability of the individual to pass genes into the next generation, the phenotypic variation is then reflected in a genetic change in the population and perhaps also in a modification of the apparent rules for transforming a genotype into a phenotype - as exemplified by the evolution of dominance and of canalization.

First let me summarise our present knowledge about the genetic control of continuous characters. Ideally, we wish to describe the genetic variation in terms of the effects of substitution of the segregating alleles at different loci, of the frequency of such alleles in the population, of the interaction between alleles at different loci and, finally, the existence of linkage disequilibrium between them. In a sense, our knowledge is surprisingly scanty. Our understanding of gene action is perhaps coloured by the fact that we generally choose for our analyses characters which are not particularly relevant to fitness, for example, bristle characters in Drosophila, and we analyse selected lines. We usually find that a high proportion of the differences between such lines can be accounted for by the additive action of genes, which is hardly surprising because precisely such genes will be altered in gene frequency by artificial selection. But there is also now much evidence from random breeding populations that a high proportion of the genetic variation in such characters is of the additive kind. One might expect that in moving to characters with a closer connection with fitness, such as viability or fertility, interaction both within and between loci would play a large role. However, although evidence of dominance and recessivity is clear in such characters from the effect of inbreeding, when we consider, for instance, analyses such as have been made on yield in maize (which must be closely connected with natural fitness), we find that in the majority (whether of crosses between inbred lines, or analyses of random breeding populations) a considerable proportion of the genetic variance is of this simple kind.

As yet we know comparatively little about the nature of this genetic variation

in terms of gene effects and frequencies. Thoday (1979) has analysed differences
between highly selected lines using modifications of the standard linkage techniques with single genes. He found clear evidence for major genes affecting
bristle characters, and has been able to map them on the chromosome. We, in
Edinburgh, have done some experimentation in this direction and have also considered the fundamental properties of this technique by simulation methods,
assuming that the distribution of gene effects is such that there will be more loci
with small effects than with large. It seems that the method will tend to give a
too simple answer - to suggest that a few loci may be involved when there really may
be many. Perhaps it is wrong to ask how many loci are involved in a particular
quantitative character, the only sensible description being in terms of the proportion of the response which can be accounted for by the major loci. But from my
own work I feel fairly sure that a small number of loci, say less than 10, usually
account for the greater part of response in my selection lines. For example, in
lines selected for sternopleural bristles, about a half of the differences between
high and low lines is due to the third chromosome. Further, when this chromosome
is analysed, more than half the effect is found to be concentrated into about one
sixth of its total map length.

I would note one peculiarity of models in which "the smaller the effect, the
greater the number of loci." The statistical concept of the effective number of
genes is not very useful. Suppose we have a distribution such that the number of
loci with a certain range of effect is inversely proportional to the effect itself.
If we ranked the loci according to their effect, the distribution would be a geometric one e.g. 16, 8, 4, 2, 1, 0.5 etc. The peculiarity of such a distribution is
that the effective number of units, expressed from the well-known Wright-Castle
formula as $(\Sigma a)^2 / \Sigma a^2$, is not affected by selection. In the example, the effective
number of loci is 3. But, if we take out that with the largest effect, as we might
by fixing it by selection, the number of effective loci contributing to the variation remains the same.

We have little direct evidence about the frequency of alleles at such loci in
wild random breeding populations. There is some indirect evidence that the genes
which we eventually fix in our selection lines are probably not rare variants in
populations. If they were, the effect of an initial bottleneck in population size
on the final limit to selection would be great, since a sub-population derived from,
perhaps, a single pair mating would be lacking the majority of such rare favourable
alleles, and we do not find this. Thus a situation in which we might be fixing rare
variants at one set of loci in selecting upwards, and at a completely different set
of loci in selecting downwards, seems to be ruled out. The general picture of
variation between populations that we have from loci affecting biochemical polymorphisms is of degree, but not in kind - of differences in gene frequency between
populations, but only rarely the fixation of one alternative in one and another in

another. It seems probable that the same is true for quantitative variation. Thus
the limit to selection for lines derived from mixtures of wild populations seems to
be not markedly greater than for lines from a single source, suggesting that the
loci contributing to the response are the same in different populations (Lopez-
Fanjul and Hill, 1973).

The Statistical Approach

We are therefore reduced to treating the quantitative variation statistically,
for which there is a well understood framework in terms of the concepts of the additive genetic variance and of the heritability of the character. This leads to the
well known formula for the expected change in the population produced by a given
amount of selection

$$\Delta G = h^2 \Delta P$$

where ΔG is the expected genetic change produced by a selection differential, ΔP, in
a character with heritability h^2. In deriving this equation in terms of the effects
of individual loci, the argument splits clearly into two steps. In the first, we
predict the expected difference of gene frequency in selected parents from that in
unselected individuals from the selection differential applied. In the second, we
predict the change in the population mean as a consequence of this change in gene
frequency. The well known concept of the "average effect of a substitution"
appears in both steps if the selection is carried out in a random breeding population. But it is not sufficiently appreciated that this classical equation is very
limited in relevance - it holds only when the selection has been applied directly
to the character observed and not through any other character. Thus if we merely
observe selection differentials in several measurements and do not know how they
came about, we are able to predict the consequent change only if we know that
selection was applied solely to these characters. This presents difficulties in
the analysis of the effects of natural selection.

In theory, we may be able to overcome this problem. The well known fundamental theorem of natural selection states that the expected change in relative fitness is equal to the variance in fitness itself. This can be considered as a
special case of what I have called the secondary theorem of natural selection - that
the expected change in a metric character produced by any selection process is equal
to the genetic covariance between the character concerned and relative fitness.
This is true only if that selection is applied to individuals on the basis of their
own phenotype and is not in any way related to that of their parents. This equation
has been of some value in predicting the consequences of selection carried out by
animal breeders, in a somewhat subjective manner, but is difficult to apply in wild
populations in which the genetic relationship between individuals is not known.

We may presume that the majority of species are in a kind of equilibrium with
their environment, though this may not be true for those whose environment has been
radically altered by domestication. Leaving this point on one side, we might expect

that fitness itself, in a population at equilibrium, could not be improved by artificial selection. Further it would follow that selection for any character other
than fitness must lead to a decrease in fitness, irrespective of the direction of
selection. If the gene frequencies in the population are at their optimum value,
then any changes must be for the worse. The current theory of quantitative inheritance is essentially a linear one - it is based on the assumption of a linear regression of gene frequency on phenotypic value, and on a linear effect of change of
gene frequency on population mean in the next generation. However, for a population
assumed at equilibrium, all changes in gene frequency must reduce fitness and we are
therefore dealing with a quadratic rather than a linear model. As far as I know,
there is no existing theory which could lead to a prediction of the expected changes
in fitness consequent upon artificial selection.

If the population is at equilibrium, any change in gene frequencies will cause
a decline in fitness. Correspondingly we may expect that for the majority of metric
characters, individuals which are intermediate will have the highest fitness. We
are not short of models to account for this - we merely lack critical evidence to
distinguish one from another. We may consider the problem in terms of two extreme
models:

1) The homeostatic model - in which loci have an additive effect on the metric
   character, with the heterozygote superior in fitness for reasons which have
   nothing to do with this particular character. Here it is easy to show that the
   fitness of individuals will be at a maximum at the population mean for the
   character, and that selection will reduce fitness.

2) In the other extreme "optimum" model we assume that the genes which control the
   character affect fitness solely through the character - that individuals which
   deviate from the population mean lack fitness because of that deviation. I
   would comment here on a somewhat philosophical problem. In the verbal discussion of such evolutionary problems we talk in terms of characteristics such
   as, for instance, body size. As quantitative geneticists, however, we manipu-
   late measurements and so we have to be very precise about exactly how our
   measurements are taken.

I would suggest that this model is extreme to the point of absurdity - that it
denies the possibility of pleiotropy between measurements (which is in fact every-
where in development). In effect, it divides the individual into compartments within which a particular set of genes operate and outside which they have no effect.
It also divides phenomena, which are really at the same level, arbitrarily into
cause and effect. We consider the genes affecting the character operating under the
constraint of the given relationship between the character and fitness. But we must
then ask how this relationship came about. If it is a consequence of the other
characters of the organism these too may be under genetic control, so that the relationship of the character with fitness might respond to selection as well.

In both models, then, fitness will decline as the individual measurements deviate from the population mean, and the population mean fitness will decline with selection. In consequence, the population mean will return to its original value when the artificial selection is relaxed. Is it then possible to distinguish between the two or to obtain information that will enable us to sophisticate the model? The "optimum" model contains implications of interactions between loci with respect to fitness. An allele with a positive affect on the character will be at a disadvantage if the remainder of the genotype is above average for the character, and vice versa. This might be detectable experimentally. As a further consequence of this epistasis, negative linkage disequilibrium, between alleles at linked loci affecting the character in the same direction, would be expected. This has the effect of producing an excess of chromosomes close to the mean for the character concerned, given the name of "relational balance" by Mather many years ago.

The model has been modified in two ways. Wright (1935) was, I think, the first to show that the optimal model for a single character is genetically unstable in that it leads to the fixation of every locus but one. Bulmer (1971) confirmed this but was able to show that, if the fitness function had not one but two optima, stability of the whole genotype might ensue. Latter (1970) and, more recently, Lande (1976) have considered the balance between new mutation at the loci affecting the character and the pressure towards fixation with a model with a single optimum, and Lande has suggested that this model is in fact in accordance with experimental data. More recently he has extended the model to cover simultaneous selection for many characters, so that the fitness function is a multivariate function of many measurements. Each new mutation may be expected to affect the different measurements in a specific way. He is therefore overcoming the problem I mentioned earlier of the genetic control of the fitness function for a single character, but at the expense of so complicating the model that I cannot see that it can be confronted with evidence.

Experimental Evidence

(i) The effect of artificial selection on fitness

Considering the number of experiments devoted to artificial selection in laboratory animals, surprisingly few have involved a precise measurement of the correlated effect on fitness. In such experiments, fitness might be expected to decline, not only as a consequence of the change in gene frequencies brought about by artificial selection, but also because of the direct effect of inbreeding due to the small number of selected parents used. It is therefore necessary to compare selected lines with controls of the same effective population size. Latter and Robertson (1962) considered the effect of artificial selection for two bristle characters (sternopleural and abdominal) and wing length, using as a measure of fitness a composite of viability, mating success and fertility. Although fitness always declined relative to the base population, there was not always a significant decline relative to the control. For instance, at generation 5, when the wing length lines had moved by about three genetic standard deviations, three of the lines did not differ significantly from the controls in fitness although all four did at generation 10. For the abdominal lines the average decline in fitness below the controls at generation 5 was only 30% with one of the lines not differing significantly from the controls and remaining at the control level up to the 20th generation. If we invoke the homeostatic model to explain these results, they are consistent with an average selective disadvantage, of homozygotes relative to heterozygotes, of 0.5%.

Verghese and Nordskog (1968) examined lines of chickens selected in both directions for egg weight and body weight, and compared their fitness with that of controls with the same level of inbreeding. At the sixth generation of selection, the average fitness had declined by some 20% below the controls - the response to selection in both characters was then over two genetic standard deviations.

Chance linkage between loci affecting the metric character and recessive genes affecting fitness may also produce a decline in fitness in selected lines. However simulation work by Sved (1977) would suggest that, in general, linkage effects are not likely to be large though they may be in particular instances.

(ii) Relaxation of selection

It is easy to observe the effect of relaxation of selection on the response achieved. Where this has been done in a critical manner, there is often a fairly rapid initial loss of response followed by a very slow return to the initial values, and there are many cases of selected lines reaching a position of stability removed from the original. There are two important elements in the design of such experiments. First the relaxation must be imposed before the selection has gone too far. If some loci have been fixed by the selection, they cannot return to their initial gene frequency. Secondly, such experiments are very susceptible to contamination - individuals in selected populations would be somewhat less fit than ordinary wild types and any invader at an advantage. It is therefore necessary to have some genetic marker in such lines so as to avoid contamination. In the experiment of Latter and Robertson, when lines selected for abdominal bristles for 5 generations were relaxed, on average 20% of the response was lost in 10 generations of relaxation. For sternopleural bristles, the high lines, when relaxed at generation 5 for a period of 25 generations, lost only 14% of the selection gain whereas the low lines lost 40%. This was in agreement with the greater loss of fitness in the low lines.

The general picture of the effect of relaxation (of a fairly immediate loss followed by a long period with little or no change) certainly suggests that the process is not homogeneous. This is an argument against the simple-minded optimal model of selection operating on a single character. It would however be consistent with either the homeostatic model or with Lande's model of a multivariate fitness function.

(iii) <u>The relationship of fitness to deviation from the population mean</u>

Although it is generally accepted that individuals with intermediate values will be higher in fitness there are not many critical measurements of this relationship, certainly not in relation to all aspects of fitness.   Lerner and Gunns (1952) confirmed the previous observations in poultry that eggs of intermediate size have the highest hatchability. But the interpretation was complicated by the fact that in older hens laying larger eggs, the position of the optimum value increased so that the hatchability was not directly related to the measurement. In an interesting experiment, Kearsey and Barnes (1970) showed that genotypes intermediate for sternopleural bristles in Drosophila had the highest larval viability.   Here again we have a situation which cannot be interpreted simply under the model, because the selection has taken place before the character exists.

(iv) <u>Interaction between loci for fitness</u>

I commented earlier that the optimal model involved an interaction for fitness between loci affecting the character in such a way that the fitness differentials between different alleles having an affect on the character would depend on the background genotype for the character. An allele having a positive effect on the character would increase fitness in a low character background and decrease it in a high. There are two methods of examining this. The first uses the chromosomes selected for the metric character but not otherwise marked, and examines the effect of natural selection in different backgrounds. My colleagues and I have carried out such experiments in Edinburgh, in which we have kept populations segregating for a high and a low third chromosome (for instance) in a high or low background for the rest of the genotype. The results are somewhat mixed. We have however several cases in which populations which are genetically variable for the character concerned (in the sense that they will respond to artificial selection) appear to be stable under natural selection although they deviate by many genetic standard deviations from the base population. This then constitutes strong evidence against the simple optimal model. In another kind of experiment, which I am not aware of having been done, one could examine the relative fitnesses of chromosomes with different values for a metric character against a standard marker chromosome, in which crossing over has been suppressed, and to ask whether the observed fitnesses of chromosomes are dependent on their own genotype for the measured character and whether this depends on the genetic background.

(v) <u>Linkage disequilibrium for quantitative characters</u>

A consequence of the optimal model is a negative disequilibrium between alleles affecting the character in the same direction. Bearing in mind our general ignorance about the individual loci affecting specific characters, there have, I think, been no efforts to look for such disequilibrium at the level of the character itself. It is very difficult to distinguish a situation in which there is linkage disequilibrium from one in which linkage is at random with respect to the character. In the latter case one might expect fixation to occur rapidly at those pairs of loci which were in positive linkage disequilibrium in the population (and which would therefore be fixed as single units) whereas pairs of loci in negative disequilibrium would be dependent on the occurrence of the "right" cross-over to respond to selection.   As far as biochemical loci are concerned, there have in the recent past been many examinations of wild populations of Drosophila and the general consensus of the evidence must be that, apart from that associated with specific inversions, evidence of disequilibrium is conspicuously lacking (Langley, Ito and Voelker, 1977).

References

Bulmer, M.G. (1971). Stable equilibria under the two-island model. Heredity 27, 321-330.

Kearsey, M.G. & Barnes, B.W. (1970). Variation for metrical characters in Drosophila populations. II. Natural Selection. Heredity 25, 11-21.

Lande, R. (1976). The maintenance of genetic variability by mutation in a polygenic character with linked loci. Genet.Res. 26, 221-235.

Langley, C.H., Ito, K. & Voelker, R.A. (1977). Linkage disequilibrium in natural populations of Drosophila melanogaster. Genetics 86, 447-54.

Latter, B.D.H. (1970). Selection in finite populations with multiple alleles. II. Centripetal selection, mutation and isoallelic variation. Genetics 66, 165-86.

Latter, B.D.H. & Robertson, A. (1962). The effects of inbreeding and artificial selection on reproductive fitness. Genet.Res. 3, 110-38.

Lerner, I.M. & Gunns, C.A. (1952). Egg Size and Reproductive Fitness. Poultry Sci. 31, 537-44.

Lopez-Fanjul, C. & Hill, W.G. (1973). Genetic differences between populations of Drosophila melanogaster. II. Laboratory and wild populations. Genet.Res. 22, 69-78.

Sved, J.A. (1977). Opposition to artificial selection caused by natural selection at linked loci. In Proc.Int.Conf. on Quantitative Genetics, Ames, Ia.

Thoday, J.M. (1979). Polygene Mapping: Uses and Limitations. pp.219-237 in Quantitative Genetic Variation. ed. Thompson & Thoday, Academic Press, New York.

Verghese, N.W. & Nordskog, A.W. (1968). Correlated responses in reproductive fitness to selection in chickens. Genet.Res. 11, 221-239.

Wright, S. (1935). Evolution in populations in approximate equilibrium. Genetics 20, 257-66.

SOME MODELS FOR THE EVOLUTION OF ADAPTIVE TRAITS

Simon A. Levin

Section of Ecology and Systematics
Cornell University
Ithaca, New York 14853

Introduction

The elegance and persuasiveness of Darwinian thought strikes a sympathetic chord
with ecologists and natural historians, who see in the beauty of nature remarkable
examples of organisms "adapted" to their environments. The subtlety of the *process*
of adaptation is however too often ignored , and the notion of *optimization* mis-
takenly equated with adaptation. Lewontin (1977) reminds us that "adaptation, for
Darwin, was a process of becoming rather than a state of final optimality." As
pointed out elsewhere (Levin 1978), "environments change, not only due to extrinsic
causes, but also as a result of adaptation already effected. The evolutionary response is to the present, and carries with it no guarantee that any sort of optimum
will be attained. Evolution is something which simply happens, rather than a calculated, far-seeing program for optimization."

In the presence of changing environments, ambiguity arises even in the definition of what an "optimal" strategy means, because the question of an appropriate
time horizon enters. Further, when those environments change in response to variations in gene frequency, fitnesses are frequency-dependent and it generally is
impossible to locate reasonable candidates for optimization.

Sensibly used, optimization theory is not without value. For example, when
concerned with an organism immersed in an environment reasonably independent of the
individual's physiological "strategy," one may make effective use of optimization
solutions to what are in effect engineering problems. Further, even without the
assumption that evolution has optimized anything, *strategic* models (see, for example,
Oster and Rocklin 1979) may in some situations be used to set a standard against
which observed solutions may be evaluated. For the population or community ecologist,
however, almost all evolutionary problems of interest involve interactions between

individuals; fitnesses are usually frequency dependent, and hence the conventional optimization arguments are inappropriate.

The contrast between these two situations may perhaps best be illustrated with an example. Cohen (1971, 1976; see also Amir 1979) considers the problem of the optimal timing of reproduction, using a model in which all resources are directed to vegetative growth until some threshold when a switch occurs to purely reproductive growth. Maximization of the reproductive value at age zero leads, under the hypotheses of his model, to determination of a critical value of the threshold, and it is then reasonable to conjecture that this is the value which would evolve under natural selection. In this formulation, interactions between individuals may be ignored and the problem is thus essentially an autecological one.

A problem of ostensibly similar structure relates to the optimal fraction of resources a plant commits to long-range dispersal. Many annual plants (e.g., *Postelsia palmaeformis* (Paine 1979), *Ambrosia artemisiifolia*) divide their reproductive output between meiospores or seeds that drop close to the parent plant and those that are involved in long-range dispersal. The mechanisms vary considerably, but that is not at issue here. For example, in the case of the marine intertidal alga *P. Palmaeformis*, long-range dispersal occurs at the end of a reproductive season, when the adult sporophyte, still carrying a load of reproductive units, is ripped from the shore and destroyed or else floated on the waves. In the latter case, likely with low probability, the plant may be transported over long distances to establish new populations (Paine 1979). This is perhaps not a strategy in the behavioral sense; indeed, it might appear to be the result simply of defective architecture in the sporophyte, its inability to stay attached. Not only is such thinking anthropomorphic, but also it is irrelevant. The fraction of spores so dispersed is to some extent under genetic control, as is the rate at which spores are released prior to the end of the season. Moreover *Postelsia*, as a colonizer of temporary habitats, must invariably become extinct at almost every one of its sites and can survive as a species only by its ability to exploit new opportunities by long-range dispersal. Thus it is reasonable to assume that the fraction of spores (or of some other measure of reproductive effort) put into long distance dispersal has evolved, and further that the fraction so selected is in some sense better than other possible fractions (assuming a relatively stable global environment for the plant). But in what sense is it best?

Mimicking Cohen's approach to the problem of the timing of reproduction, one possible approach (the *optimization* approach) might be to define a yield function f associated with the non-dispersing spores and a similar expected yield g associated with dispersing spores. If S represents the total number of spores in the system and

x is the fraction dispersed, we then obtain a total expected yield associated with
the strategy x:

$$Y(x) = (1-x)\ Sf\ (x,S) + xSg\ (x,S).\tag{1}$$

Note that it is assumed that the yields are functionally dependent upon both the total
number of spores S and upon the fraction dispersed x. Proceeding naively, one may
now find the value x(S) which maximizes Y(x) (assuming, as is reasonable, that the
functions f and g permit such a choice for S fixed), and declare that to be the
optimal strategy. It remains to determine the appropriate value of S to be used in
this analysis; but there are ways to do this, most logically by requiring that
Y(x(S)) = 1.

There are several problems with this approach, some minor (such as that
only expected values are considered) but at least two of major importance:

(1) The one-year yield is not really what is relevant. Dispersing spores run a
    high risk and low probability of success. If they do find a suitable site,
    however, a major part of the payoff involves the chance that the site
    discovered is one which the plant can expect to remain favorable for more
    generations than the source site. Thus the yield must be measured as a
    long-term yield, most ideally as an asymptotic fraction of total population.
    In theory, this works perfectly; but, as usual, in practice things are
    harder. The long-term asymptotic fraction is somewhere between difficult
    and impossible to compute, in part because of density dependence.

(2) Even if a long term yield could be computed, there is no reason to expect
    evolution to maximize it; the reasons are separate from the fact that
    genetic constraints may intrude. The maximum yield will in general occur
    for a value of x at which $f \neq g$; that is, the return on investment would
    not be the same for energy put into dispersal as for that which is not.
    In general, such a strategy would not be *evolutionary stable* (Maynard Smith
    1976); that is, it could be evolutionarily displaced by a strategy that put
    a larger fraction of its energy into the more profitable alternative. This
    is a hand-waving argument, and it would involve much effort and a carefully
    specified model to make it precise. Instead, let us consider an example in
    which the notion of a one-year yield suffices.

There are two extreme situations regarding redistribution by dispersal;
essentially these correspond to the *propagule* and *migrant* pool models discussed by
Slatkin and Wade (1978) and Wade (1978). In the first, the relative rates of
colonization and subsequent growth or spread are such that a single colonization
incident will result in the pre-emption of the site. Whether this involves a single
individual, a single propagule of related individuals, or the offspring from a first

colonist is not germane;the net effect is that the population at an individual site will be monomorphic, but individual sites may differ regarding the prevailing type. One such example is the situation treated by Hamilton and May (1977), to which we shall return later.

At the second extreme, a large number of colonization events are involved at each site; the proportion of colonists of a particular type at a particular site will reflect the proportion of that type in the dispersing pool at large. Individual sites may be highly polymorphic, but all sites colonized will be identical in per cent composition. It is the latter extreme that we consider here. We assume further that colonization rates are sufficiently high that all available sites are saturated during their first year; thus all sites of age 2 or greater will have the same expected yields.

Consider two morphs characterized by densities S and T and "strategies" x and y (the fractions put into dispersal). Then a reasonable model for the densities S', T' in the successor generation would put

$$S' = (1-x) \; SF \; (xS+yT, \; S+T) + xSG \; (xS+yT, \; S+T)$$
$$T' = (1-y) \; TF \; (xS+yT, \; S+T) + yTG \; (xS+yT, \; S+T) \tag{2}$$

where F and G are positive differentiable functions, decreasing in both S and T. I assume $F(0,0) > 1$ and $G(0,0) > 1$, but that both fall below 1 for S or T sufficiently large. It is further assumed that SF and SG both increase in S for T fixed, and similarly, that TF and TG increase in T for S fixed. Finally, F is assumed to be an increasing function, and G a decreasing function of $xS+yT$ for $S+T$ fixed. Thus, for a given total number of spores, as a higher fraction of spores are dispersed, the per capita yield of the non-dispersers will improve and that of the dispersers will decline due to changing competitive effects.

The possible outcomes of the competition between "x" and "y" depend of course on the values x and y; indeed for some pairs of values coexistence is possible. However, what is more instructive is the condition for invasibility of the unique non-trivial equilibrium that each type would reach in the absence of the other. If, for example, $x = \bar{x}$, then the reduced system

$$S' = (1-x) \; SF \; (xS,S) + xSG \; (xS,S) \tag{3}$$

will have a unique, non-trivial equilibrium at a value $S = \bar{S} > 0$. The pair $S = \bar{S}$, $T=0$ then represents an equilibrium for (2), and invasibility is studied in terms of the stability of $(S,T) = (\bar{S},0)$ to small perturbations (with positive T). If $0 < \bar{x} < 1$, there will be another, "better" strategy that can invade $(\bar{S},0)$ unless $F(\bar{x}\bar{S},\bar{S}) = G(\bar{x}\bar{S},\bar{S}) = 1$; on the other hand, a strategy for which $F=G=1$ at equilibrium is indeed protected against invasion.

Whether such an intermediate strategy which equilibrates yields exists, depends in a bit more detail on the functional forms of F and G. For example, if $\bar{S}_0$ denotes the equilibrium associated with $\bar{x}=0$, then this pure non-dispersing strategy will be stable against invasion unless

$$1 = F(0,\bar{S}_0) < G(0,\bar{S}_0). \tag{4}$$

Were (4) not satisfied, then dispersal would never pay and the strategy $\bar{x}=0$ would be optimal. Similarly, let $\bar{S}_1$ be the equilibrium associated with $\bar{x}=1$. Then that strategy will be stable unless

$$F(\bar{S}_1,\bar{S}_1) > G(\bar{S}_1,\bar{S}_1) = 1. \tag{5}$$

If, however, (4) and (5) are satisfied, then there will be a unique intermediate strategy that can outcompete all other types. It is not the choice that maximizes yield, but rather is that which equilibrates the yields F and G at equilibrium, the unique non-trivial solution of the system

$$\begin{aligned} F(\bar{x}\bar{S},\bar{S}) &= 1 \\ G(\bar{x}\bar{S},\bar{S}) &= 1. \end{aligned} \tag{6}$$

The strategy so defined is "evolutionarily stable" in the sense of Maynard-Smith (1976). It indeed may be thought of as "optimal" in that evolutionarily it is better than any other, but this is more a definition than anything else. It is quite a different thing than attempting to define in advance a function for maximization. Indeed, even for $S = \bar{S}$ it is not the case in general that setting $x = \bar{x}$ results in the maximization of

$$\frac{S'}{S} = (1-x) \, F \, (x\bar{S},\bar{S}) + xG \, (x\bar{S},\bar{S}) \, . \tag{7}$$

What is true, however, is that $x = \bar{x}$ maximizes

$$(1-x) \, F \, (\bar{x}\bar{S},\bar{S}) + xG \, (\bar{x}\bar{S},\bar{S}); \tag{8}$$

but this is trivial and basically the definition of the evolutionarily stable strategy (ESS).

As a specific application, suppose that there are a fixed number of identical possible sites, and that each has probability w of being recycled each year: recycling obliterates the resident population but makes the site available for high-yield colonization by dispersers. Then, if α is the probability of a dispersing seed landing safely on one of the sites, the evolutionarily stable strategy -- that is, the one which equilibrates yields -- is to disperse a fraction $\bar{x} = w/(1-(1-w)\alpha)$.

The notion of equilibration of yields is similar in spirit, but different than the idea that evolution will equilibrate *fitnesses* of competing types (Slatkin 1979a); the distinction is that here we are dealing with a single genetic type that partitions its own efforts between two activities. Hamilton and May (1977) and

Motro (1979a,b) consider a closely related problem to the one we have just discussed, in which the "optimal" solution does not equilibrate yields, but is still an ESS. In their definition of the dispersal problem, there are a fixed number of discrete and independent sites that are renewed every year in the sense that the resident adult is an annual. Competition is by contest, rather than by scramble. This contrasts with the situation previously described, in which the total plant megapopulation is comprised of a mosaic of demes; and it therefore negates the reasoning that requires equalization of yields at equilibrium. Model (2) does not apply, because a single function F cannot accurately capture the competitive effects. S. Ellner (pers.comm.) has developed some-what more fully the differences between the situation considered by Hamilton and May (1977) and that described in this paper, and these will be published elsewhere. Comins et al. (1980) extend the original ideas of Hamilton and May to allow more than one individual per site; between site variance is maintained by allowing stochastic effects. Disturbance is introduced explicitly. As the number of individuals per site becomes large, the model becomes essentially the same as the model just described, and the optimal dispersal fraction $\bar{x} = w/(1-(1-w)\alpha)$ is obtained in the limit.

Having observed that the ESS strategy need not equilibrate yields, I must also point out that the ESS itself is not always an appropriate concept, especially when in-dividuals are diploid. This issue is more fully reviewed in the next section.

The population genetic basis of optimization and other approaches.

Optimization arguments persist in evolutionary theory not only because they suit people's tastes, but also because they have some formal basis in Fisher's funda-mental theorem of natural selection and Wright's related concept of the adaptive sur-face. However, although Fisher and Wright derived their notions by rigorous deductive reasoning, the ideas are usually applied without attention to the underlying hypotheses; these are discussed in detail in Levin (1978), and what follows here is a brief précis. A superb recent treatment may be found in Ewens (1979).

The standard mathematical approach to population genetics begins with a set of equations

$$(p_i^k)' = p_i^k \, w_{i.}^k / \bar{w}^k \qquad\qquad , k=1,\dots m; \quad i=1,\dots,n_k \qquad (9)$$

for the gene frequencies p_i^k of the various alleles p_i^k in the kth population. In this representation, unprimed variables represent values in the present generation, and primes in the successor. $w_{i.}^k$, the mean fitness associated with allele i, is given by

$$w_{i.}^k = \sum p_j^k \, w_{ij}^k , \qquad\qquad (10)$$

in which w_{ij}^k is the fitness of the genotype i,j. Further, the mean fitness $\bar{w}^k$ of the kth population is

$$\bar{w}^k = \Sigma p_i^k w_i^k. \qquad . \tag{11}$$

Because densities may vary, to (9) must be appended the equations

$$(N^k)' = N^k \; \bar{w}^k \qquad , \; k=1,\ldots,m. \tag{12}$$

in which N^k is the size of the kth population. In the most general case, the fitnesses w_{ij}^k may depend on densities or frequencies, or may vary with time in other ways.

Proceeding from these equations when the w_{ij}^k are constant, Wright (1949) showed that the change Δp_i^k in p_i^k may be written

$$\Delta p_i^k = p_i^k \; (1-p_i^k) \; (\partial \bar{w}^k / \partial p_i^k)/2\bar{w}^k, \tag{13}$$

where partial derivatives are taken subject to the constraint that

$$p_1^k + \ldots + p_{n_k}^k = 1; \tag{14}$$

i.e., the relative frequencies of the other alleles are held fixed (see discussion in Levin 1978). Arguing from (13), it follows at once that gene-frequency equilibrium can only be achieved if $\bar{w}^k$ is at a critical point as a function of gene frequencies, subject to constraint (14); and it further follows from (9) that that critical point is a maximum. Indeed, Fisher's theorem states further that the rate of change in fitness is approximately proportional to the genic variance of the population:

$$V_g^k = 2 \sum_i p_i^k \; (w_i^k - \bar{w}^k)^2 = \sum_i p_i^k \; (1-p_i^k) \; (\partial \bar{w}^k / \partial p_i^k)^2; \tag{15}$$

and in any case, it may be shown (Mulholland and Smith 1959, Scheuer and Mandel 1959, Kingman 1961a,b) that $\Delta \bar{w}^k$ is strictly positive unless the genic variance is zero. Thus, not only is the mean fitness maximized at equilibrium, but the process of evolution is an orderly one of continuous improvement in $\bar{w}^k$.

The beauty and simplicity of these results carry with them a high price. They do not hold true in general, and yet they are too appealing to abandon completely. When fitnesses are dependent upon the density of the species in question, fitness is still maximized at equilibrium, but only subject to the constraint that the population density is held at its equilibrium value (Anderson 1971, Charlesworth 1971). The Fisher theorem concerning continual improvement in $\bar{w}^k$ no longer applies in general. When interacting populations are considered, with fitnesses allowed to depend upon the densities of all species, it may be shown that each species maximizes its equilibrial mean fitness subject to the constraints that all other species are genetically fixed and that population sizes in all species are fixed (see Ginzburg 1977, Roughgarden 1976,1977).

Under frequency-dependent selection, the situation becomes appreciably worse, and one can easily construct examples (even involving a single species) where mean fitness is minimized at equilibrium. In general, it is certainly no longer true under frequency dependence that mean fitness is maximized at equilibrium; and these fre-quency-dependent situations almost always apply when ecological interactions are under consideration.

Similar problems arise from consideration of multiple loci even when fit-nesses are constant. Ewens (1969 a,b) shows that mean fitness still increases under selection in the absence of epistasis (see also Nagylaki 1976); but under strong epistasis the result again collapses.

For those situations in which mean fitness is maximized at equilibrium with repsect to gene frequency change within the species, subject to suitable constraints, then game theoretic approaches are often useful; the equilibrium may be viewed as a competitive (Nash) equilibrium in the sense of game theory, although, as pointed out by Slatkin and Maynard Smith (1979), this is only a translation that does not simplify analysis at all. Further discussion may be found in Levin (1978). Recall also that there are circumstances under which fitness is not maximized at equilibrium in any sense; moreover, as pointed out in Levin (1978), any equilibrium-based theory may be inadequate.

The evolutionarily stable strategy (Maynard Smith 1976,1977), already discussed in the preceding section, is an equilibrium theory that trades on such game-theoretic notions. One identifies a number of possible "strategies" and a matrix that assigns to each possible strategy a "payoff" related to every potential strategy for a theoretical opponent. The notion of the payoff is often elusive, like the concept of long-term yield in the preceding section.

Given a payoff matrix, a dynamic may be defined which identifies the payoff function with fitness and basically assumes that reproduction is asexual. Given this dynamic, under certain conditions the population will evolve to a homogeneous situa-tion (possibly dependent on initial conditions) in which all individuals play the same strategy. This "winning" strategy is the ESS. Under other conditions, there is no ESS, and coexistence between strategies is possible; although it might be quite logical to define these as coexisting evolutionary stable strategies, this terminology would not be consistent with Maynard Smith's original (1976) usage.

The discussion to this point has been based on *pure* strategies that "breed true" (Maynard Smith 1977). Mixed strategies lead to some problems of interpretation. Further problems arise under consideration of diploid populations, since strategies do not then breed true (see Levin and Udovic 1977, Maynard Smith 1977, Levin 1978). One way around this is to focus attention on allelic "strategies" rather than genotypic strategies; but this is often more easily said than done, and the notion of the gene having a strategy has less popular appeal than allowing a genotype to possess one (but see Dawkins 1976).

What does one do in general when unsure whether any of these approaches applies? The tempting alternative is to revert to the dynamic equations (9-12) themselves, thereby avoiding teleology. Under some conditions (see, for example, Motro 1979a, b; Orzack et al. 1980), when one can specify a genetic basis for a character, such an approach will be successful. More generally, however, one has little knowledge concerning the genetic basis of an ecological trait, which might well be controlled at many loci with complex epistatic interactions between them. Under such conditions, an alternative approach is necessary.

One such approach, which will be utilized in the next two sections, is to define phenotypic dynamics, based to the greatest extent possible upon the laws of genetics, but without specific reference to genetics. In the asexual case, this is quite easily achieved; indeed, often one does so by ignoring effects of the environment, making the genotypic model identical with the phenotypic. In the sexual case the approach requires the assumption that the distribution of offspring phenotypes may be predicted solely from the knowledge of parental phenotypes (and possibly the phenotypes of others in the population). This is indeed an assumption, but perhaps not a crippling one. Slatkin (1979b) describes several other approaches at the phenetic level.

Dispersal and dormancy as adaptive traits.

Populations which inhabit unpredictable environments generally have evolved mechanisms to reduce the variability. Foremost among these mechanisms are dispersal, which spatially averages (see for example Strathman 1974); dormancy, which temporally averages; and the development of perenniality and iteroparity.

Essentially asexual models to study dispersal have been considered by Gadgil (1970), Roff (1975), Hamilton and May (1977) and Motro (1979a). The latter two I have already discussed; Roff (1975) and Motro(1979b) both also consider simple single-locus diploid genotypic models. The situation considered by Gadgil (1970) and

Roff (1975) is most similar to that discussed in the remainder of this section.
Available habitats are not immediately saturated by a single individual or its progeny,
as contrasted with (2) and the models of Hamilton and May (1977) and Motro (1979 a,b),
and only a fraction of sites are renewed annually. Such dynamics are most appropriate
to the study of adaptive strategies in patchy environments (Levin and Paine 1974,
Paine and Levin 1980) in which most species are opportunists that are doomed locally
and survive only by dispersal or dormancy.

   Gadgil (1970), in studying this situation, employs a model of competition
between non-interbreeding types that differ only in their rates of dispersal per unit
time; the model is essentially equivalent to one of an annual plant, because all individuals of a given type are considered identical in characteristics, independent of
their age. In the model, local population densities of a variety of morphs are recorded at each of a number of sites and allowed to change over time through dispersal
and density-dependent local growth. Interest focuses on the asymptotic behavior of
the system, the assumption being that the model mimics evolution and that if there is
a winner, it would also be evolution's choice *from among those considered*. Several
interesting conclusions are drawn, but purely on the basis of simulation studies.
The simulations suggest that there is a "fittest" type, and some broad generalizations
about the relationship of this type to environmental variability are inferred. However, because of the limitations of simulation studies, it is not possible to transform
these generalizations into precise statements, nor to sort out model dependence.

   Roff (1975), considering basically the same situation, takes a radically
different approach. In his simplest model, he assumes no genetic determination of
dispersal except that a fixed fraction of the population disperses per unit time;
genetically, each individual is identical. Because evolution is not explicit in his
model and he requires some criterion to evaluate the "relative selective values of
different dispersal rates," he chooses that dispersal rate that "will tend to minimize
a population's chance of extinction." On the basis of simulations, he further argues
that minimization of extinction is achieved by maximization of population size. Roff
states "whilst this criterion obviously describes the situation which is best for the
population as a whole, it is by no means clear that individual selection will favour
such a situation." In later sections of the paper, Roff considers genetic models
that demonstrate how a polymorphism might be maintained -- and shows that individual
selection does not lead to maximization of mean population size.

   With Dan Cohen and several collaborators, I have been studying the evolution
of dispersal and dormancy strategies in patchy and heterogeneous environments, basically
using extensions of the approach of Gadgil. The general framework will be presented
in work with Alan Hastings (Levin, Cohen and Hastings 1980). Further elaborations,
motivated by special attention to the characteristics of ragweed (*Ambrosia*

artemisiifolia), represent joint work with David Andow, Karl Beres, Brian Chabot, Stephen Ellner, and Louis Gross. In the *Ambrosia* model, two classes of dormancy are distinguished -- enforced and secondary.

In the work with Cohen and Hastings, a number of preliminary conclusions are emerging concerning the relation of the selected strategy to patterns of environmental variation. Indeed, when both dispersal and dormancy are allowed, under some conditions stable coexistence of alternative types is possible. However, although the equations for the dynamics of these systems may be written explicitly, analysis is (as predicted by Gadgil 1970 for the simpler versions) extremely difficult. For example, in the simplest version of the model, and ignoring dormancy, we have shown that the dynamics of the system for annuals may be approximated by the system of equations

$$\frac{\partial n_i}{\partial t} + \frac{\partial n_i}{\partial a} = [r_i (\underset{\sim}{n}, a, t) - D_i (a)]n_i + \alpha \int_0^\infty D_i(a)\, P\,(a,t)\, n_i\,(a,t)\, da;$$

$$(16)$$

$$n_i (0,t) = 0; \quad i=1, \ldots, m \quad .$$

Here, $\underset{\sim}{n} = (n_1, \ldots, n_m)$ is the vector of species densities in patches of age a, D_i is a dispersal rate for species i, and P defines the age structure of available patches. $r_i(\underset{\sim}{n},a,t)$ is the density dependent local yield function, and $0<\alpha<1$ is the relative probability that a dispersal episode will be successful. Dispersal is assumed to involve random redistributions over available patches. One may simplify even further by assuming that for all i, r_i is the same function and depends on $\underset{\sim}{n}$ alone, and that D_i is independent of the age of the patch. One still obtains a system of nonlinearly coupled partial differential-integral equations, and of a peculiar type in which the integration is over a fixed interval. Very little work of a mathematical nature has ever been done on such systems, and indeed even in the case m=1 existence, uniqueness, and smoothness properties have only recently been established for special cases (Elderkin 1979). Since we are concerned not only with systems, but in theory with infinitely many possible equations, analysis is not proceeding as quickly as one might hope. Some progress, however, has been made.

The models described so far are phenomenological, and make no attempt to consider the morphological and physiological bases of these strategies. The work on ragweed, which is primarily phenomenological, does attempt, however, to relate strategies to seed size. A more explicit consideration along these general lines represents the thesis work of Stephen Ellner at Cornell, who is investigating with such theoretical models under what circumstances heterocarpy is favored over homocarpy or a mixture of monocarpic seeds. His focus is on the liguliflorus annual composites of the *Picris amalecitana* complex.

Dispersal polymorphism also provides the focus of the excellent review by Harrison (1980), who has studied the selective advantages and disadvantages of normal and flightless insect morphs in relation to habitat characteristics. Almost certainly, consideration of problems of this kind cannot ignore the diploid nature of the genetic system. Explicit single-locus genetic models (e.g., Motro 1979b) or multi-locus models which invoke modifier loci (e.g., Gillespie 1979) can sometimes serve admirably at least as metaphors of the dynamics, especially when consideration is restricted to a few alternative morphs (e.g., winged and wingless). When, as in the case of dispersal strategies, interest is upon a variable that may take any of a con-tinuum of values, the trait must be considered as metric, a *quantitative* character controlled at a large number of loci. A promising approach is then to construct models purely at the phenotypic level, as in Kimura (1965), Slatkin (1970), Lande (1976), Slatkin and Lande (1976), and Karlin (1979). This is quite difficult to do in the context of the problems posed in this section, because selection coefficients would necessarily be functionals involving the frequency distribution of phenotypes in the population at large. Instead, in the next section, an application of this basic approach to a somewhat different ecological evolutionary problem is discussed.

Predator pressure and aspect diversity.

Endler (1978) reviews data and theories concerning color and other poly-morphisms in animal populations. Observed genetically-based polymorphisms are in-fluenced both by sexual selection and by visual selection by predators. Predation plays an important role both in influencing selection for crypsis and by apostatic selection based on the predator's tendency to form search images for frequently-en-countered prey. The notion that apostatic selection is important in maintaining *aspect* diversity is discounted by Endler for wild populations of guppies (*Poecilia reticula* Peters), but has been advanced in other settings by Rand (1967) and Ricklefs and O'Rourke (1975).

With Lee Segel (Levin and Segel 1980), I have been investigating mathematical models for the evolution of aspect diversity using a phenotypic model for quantitative inheritance. Assuming for simplicity perfect heritability (one can easily modify the basic equations to weaken this assumption; see Slatkin and Lande 1976), and that the patterns of interest may be quantified by the single *aspect* variable z, and ignoring the problem of background matching (this can also be introduced), our equa-tions (Levin and Segel 1980) take the form

$$\frac{\partial v(z,t)}{\partial t} = -f(v(z,t))e(z,t)+\iint v(\eta,t)v(\xi,t)\alpha(\eta,\xi)\frac{r(\eta,W(\eta,t))}{W(\eta,t)} \phi(\frac{\eta+\xi}{2},z)d\xi d\eta \qquad (17)$$

$$\frac{\partial e(z,t)}{\partial t} = -e(z,t)m(V(z,t))+c(z,t)-s(v(z,t))e(z,t)+\int\psi(\eta,z)e(\eta,t)s(v(\eta,t))d\eta \qquad (18)$$

where

$$W(\eta,t) = \int\alpha(z,\xi)v(\xi,t)d\xi, \qquad (19)$$

$$V(z,t) = \int\theta(z,\xi)v(\xi,t)d\xi, \qquad (20)$$

and

$$\int\alpha(x,y)dy = \int\phi(x,y)dy = \int\psi(x,y)dy = \int\theta(x,y)dy = 1 \text{ for all } x. \qquad (21)$$

In these equations, $v(z,t)$ is the distribution of "prey" with regard to (genetically determined) aspect z at time t, and $e(z,t)$ is the distribution of predators with regard to their search image z. The first term on the right of equation (17) represents the loss due to predation, and incorporates a functional response; the second term, the mating term, includes a mate preference function $\alpha(\eta,\xi)$ and a fecundity $r(\eta,W(\eta,t))$ for females of type η; r is dependent upon the number of W of available mates, weighted by their desirability. The inclusion of the function ϕ, which is the *offspring distribution kernel*, is based on the implicit assumption that the offspring distribution can be predicted if the parental types are known.

The first two terms on the right of (18) represent switching by the predators to alternative prey other than those under explicit consideration; the latter two terms represent direct switching of search image among the various aspect values. Both types of switching are assumed to be controlled by the relative desirability of particular search images as represented by the density of prey having those aspects; however, the presumably more dramatic decision to abandon the class of prey entirely, as reflected in the first term, is allowed to depend on a weighted average $V(z,t)$ of prey likely to be encountered under "short range" switching, rather than on simply the local density $v(z,t)$. V and v become identical if θ is taken to be the δ-function.

Segel and I have been interested in what asymptotic distributions of aspect will result from the system (17)-(18). Under what conditions will spikes develop in which one or a few aspect types are selected for? When the spike solutions may be shown to be unstable, how much diversity in aspect will evolve? When will stationary distributions develop, and when spatio-temporal ones? When will a uniform distribution, in which all possible types are equally represented, emerge?

In Levin and Segel (1980), we begin a study of these questions for certain special cases of (17)-(18) by analyzing the stability of uniform solutions. It is shown that as the controlling parameters are varied, uniform solutions become unstable and non-uniform ones bifurcate from these. These bifurcating solutions may be either time-varying or time-invariant. Because we are interested in questions of limiting similarity, it is not sufficient to study only this linear phenomenon, but we must eventually be concerned with the nonlinear behavior of the system as well.

This example of the usage of phenotypic dynamics represents only a brief introduction to the problem, but I hope it will be apparent that systems of this type are not only rich objects for mathematical study but also provide promising approaches to problems concerning the evolution of ecological parameters.

Summary.

There is considerable motivation to understand how evolution has shaped ecological parameters. A popular tool among ecologists, but one which cannot usually be justified, is optimization theory. Optimization arguments derive their legitimacy from the classical work of Fisher and Wright, in particular their development of the notions of the Fundamental Theorem of Natural Selection and the Adaptive Landscape. However, those results are strictly applicable only under very restrictive conditions, and must be weakened or abandoned entirely as density- and frequency-dependence of fitnesses and multi-locus effects are considered.

Two ecological evolutionary problems are discussed briefly in this paper, and methods emphasized which are non-teleological for studying the evolutionary process. In the first, the consideration of dispersal as an adaptation to unpredictable environments, it is shown that optimization methods (as have been discussed for example by Roff 1975) lead to incorrect answers; and the suggestion is made that, at   least for asexual populations, evolution may be expected in many situations to equalize the long-term returns on investment of energy put into dispersal and that which is not. Equilibration of long-term yields (not to be confused with equilibration of fitnesses, Slatkin 1979a) is a special case of the *evolutionarily stable strategy* of Maynard Smith (1976), an apparently more general concept.

Sexual reproduction, involving diploid genetics, is more difficult to analyze, especially if many loci are involved; in these cases, other methods are usually necessary. A promising approach when dealing with quantitative characters is based on purely phenotypic dynamic equations such as used by Slatkin (1970). An example of this method is given for the analysis of the effect of apostasis by predators upon the maintenance of aspect diversity in prey species.

Acknowledgment.

I am grateful to the National Science Foundation for its support under grant MCS-7701076, and to the John Simon Guggenheim Memorial Foundation and the Department of Mathematics and the Institute of Animal Resource Ecology of the University of British Columbia for their support and hospitality during my sabbatical stay there.

REFERENCES

Amir, S., On the optimal timing of reproduction. Amer.Natur. 114:461-466, 1979.

Anderson, W.W., Genetic equilibrium and population growth under density-regulated selection. Amer.Natur. 105:489-498, 1971.

Charlesworth, B., Selection in density-regulated populations. Ecology 52:469-474, 1971.

Cohen, D., Maximizing final yield when growth is limited by time or by limiting resources. J.Theor.Biol. 33:299-307, 1971.

Cohen, D., The optimal timing of reproduction. Amer.Natur. 110:801-807, 1976.

Comins, H.N.,W.D. Hamilton, and R.M. May, Evolutionary stable dispersal strategies. Theor. Pop.Biol., to appear.

Dawkins, R., The Selfish Gene. New York, Oxford University Press. 1976. 224+xi pp.

Elderkin, R.H., Analysis of an age-dependent, nonlinear model of seed dispersal, ms., 1979.

Endler, J.A., A predator's view of animal color patterns. Evol.Biol. 11:219-364, 1978.

Ewens, W.J., A generalized fundamental theorem of natural selection. Genetics, 63: 531-537, 1969a.

Ewens, W.J., Mean fitness increases when fitnesses are additive. Nature 221:1076, 1969b.

Ewens, W.J., Mathematical Population Genetics. Springer Verlag, Berlin-Heidelberg-New York. 1979. 325+xii pp.

Gadgil, M., Dispersal: population consequences and evolution. Ecology 52:253-260, 1971.

Gillespie, J.H., The role of migration in the genetic structure of temporally and spatially varying environments. III. Migration modification (ms.), 1979.

Ginzburg, L.R., The equilibrium and stability for n alleles under the density-dependent selection. J. Theor. Biol. 68:545-550. 1977.

Hamilton, W.D. and R.M. May, Dispersal in stable habitats. Nature 269:578-581, 1977.

Harrison, R., Dispersal polymorphisms in insects. Ann.Rev.Ecol.Syst. (to appear).

Karlin, S., Models of multifactorial inheritance: I, multivariate formulations and basic convergence results. Theor.Pop.Biol. 15:308-356, 1979.

Kimura, M., Some recent advances in the theory of population genetics. Jap. J. Hum. Genet. 10:43-48., 1965.

Kingman, J.F.C., A matrix inequality. Quart. J. Math 12:78-80, 1961a.

Kingman, J.F.C., A mathematical problem in population genetics. Proc. Cambridge Phil. Soc. 57:574-582, 1961b.

Lande, R., The maintenance of genetic variability by mutation in a polygenic character with linked loci. Genet. Res. 26: 221-235, 1976.

Levin, S.A., On the evolution of ecological parameters. Pages 3-26 in P.F.Brussard, ed., Ecological Genetics: The Interface. Springer Verlag, Heidelberg, 1978.

Levin, S.A. and R.T. Paine, Disturbance, patch formation, and community structure. Proc. Nat. Acad.Sci.USA 72:2744-2747, 1974.

Levin, S.A. and L.A. Segel, A model for the influence of predator pressure on aspect diversity in prey populations. (In preparation, 1980).

Levin, S.A. and J.D. Udovic, A mathematical model of coevolving populations. Amer. Natur. 111:657-675, 1977.

Levin, S.A., D. Cohen, and A. Hastings, Optimal strategies in patchy environments. (In preparation, 1980).

Lewontin, R.C., Adaptation. In Enciclopedia Einaudi Turin 1:198-214, 1977.

Maynard Smith, J., Evolution and the theory of games. Amer.Sci. 64:41-45, 1976.

Maynard Smith, J., Evolution and the theory of games. In: W. Matthews (ed.), Mathematics in the Life Sciences. Lecture Notes in Biomathematics. Springer Verlag, Berlin-New York. 1977.

Motro, U., Optimal rates of dispersion and migration in biological populations: I. Haploid models. (ms) 1979a.

Motro, U., Optimal rates of dispersion and migration in biological populations: II Diploid models. (ms) 1979b.

Mulholland, H.P. and C.A.B. Smith, An inequality arising in genetical theory. Amer. Math.Monthly 66:673-683, 1959.

Nagylaki, T., The evolution of one- and two-locus systems. Genetics 83:583-600, 1976.

Orzack, S.H., J.S. Sohn, K.D. Kallman, S.A. Levin and R. Johnston, Maintenance of the three sex chromosome polymorphism in the platyfish, *Xiphophorus maculatus*. Evolution, in press.

Paine, R.T., Disaster, catastrophe, and local persistence of the sea palm *Postelsia palmaeformis*. Science 205:685-687, 1979.

Paine, R.T. and S.A. Levin, Intertidal landscapes: disturbance and the dynamics of pattern. Ecological Monographs, to appear 1980.

Rand, A.S., Predator-prey interactions and the evolution of aspect diversity. Atlas do Simposio Sobra a Biota Amazonica 5 (Zoologia):73-83, 1967.

Ricklefs, R.E. and K.E. O'Rourke, Aspect diversity in moths: a temperate-tropical comparison. Evolution 29:313-324.

Rocklin, S. and G. Oster, Competition between phenotypes. J. Math.Biol. $\underline{3}$:225-262, 1976.

Roff, D.A., Population stability and the evolution of dispersal in a heterogeneous environment. Oecologia $\underline{19}$:217-237, 1975.

Roughgarden, J., Resource partitioning among competing species. A coevolutionary approach. Theor.Pop.Biol. $\underline{9}$: 388-424, 1976.

Roughgarden, J., Coevolution in ecological systems II. Results from "loop analysis" for purely density-dependent coevolution. In F.B. Christiansen and T. Fenchel (eds.), Symposium on the Measurement of Selection in Natural Populations. Lecture Notes in Biomathematics. Springer Verlag, Heidelberg, 1977.

Scheuer, P.A.G. and S.P.H. Mandel, An inequality in population genetics. Heredity $\underline{13}$:519-524, 1959.

Strathman, R., The spread of sibling larvae of sedentary marine invertebrates. Amer.Natur. $\underline{108}$:29-44, 1974.

Slatkin, M., Selection and polygenic characters. Proc.Nat.Acad.Sci. $\underline{66}$:87-93, 1970.

Slatkin, M., Frequency- and density-dependent selection on a quantitative parameter. Genetics (to appear, 1979b).

Slatkin, M. and R. Lande, Niche width in a fluctuating environment-density dependent model. Amer.Natur. $\underline{110}$:31-55. 1976.

Slatkin, M. and J. Maynard Smith, Models of coevolution. Q.Rev.Biol. (to appear, 1979).

Slatkin, M. and M.J. Wade, Group selection on a quantitative character. Proc. Nat. Acad. Sci. $\underline{75}$:3531-3534. 1978.

Wade, M.J., A critical review of the models of group selection. Quarterly Review of Biology $\underline{53}$:101-114. 1978.

Wright, S., Adaptation and selection. pp. 365-389 in G.L. Jepson, G.G. Simpson, and E. Mayr (eds.), Genetics, Paleontology, and Evolution. Princeton University Press, Princeton, N.J. 1949.

EVOLUTIONARY GAME THEORY

J. Maynard Smith
University of Sussex
England.

Evolutionary game theory is a method of analysing the evolution of phenotypes when fitnesses are frequency-dependent. The assumption made about inheritance is the simplest possible one, that individuals produce offspring identical to themselves - i.e. parthenogenetic inheritance. Hence the method is not well suited for analysing the genetic structure of populations, or the way in which evolution depends on breeding systems. Essentially, it is concerned with deciding which phenotypes will win in competition in an evolving population. If the fitnesses of phenotypes are constant and independent of their frequencies, it is simply a matter of deciding which is the fittest; if this is difficult, optimisation methods may be useful. Game theory is relevant only when fitnesses vary with frequency. This paper presents a formal account of evolutionary game theory; applications to field and laboratory data are discussed by Maynard Smith (1979).

The method was first developed (Maynard Smith & Price, 1973) to analyse contests between animals, because in a contest the most effective behaviour depends on the behaviour of one's opponent. It is still easiest to introduce the method in terms of a simple model of an animal contest - the "Hawk-Dove Game". It is supposed that two animals are contesting a resource of value V, "value" here meaning that if an animal obtains the resource, its fitness (= expected number of offspring) is increased by V units. An individual can adopt one of two "strategies", Hawk or Dove. A Hawk fights all out or "escalates", until either it is injured and must retreat, or its opponent retreats; in the former case its fitness is reduced by D units and in the latter is increased by V. A Dove displays, and retreats at once before it is hurt if its opponent escalates. If two Hawks meet, each has a ½ chance of winning, and ½ of being injured. If two Doves meet, they divide the resource between them, obtaining V/2. The full payoff matrix for the contest is then

	H	D
H	½(V–D)	V
D	O	V/2

where the payoffs are to an individual adopting the strategy on the
left against one adopting the strategy above. "Pay off" is taken to
mean the <u>change</u> in the fitness of an individual resulting from a contest.

This matrix can be analysed by the methods of classical game theory;
for example, if $V > D$ it is equivalent to the "Prisoner's Dilemma".
However, in an evolutionary contest we want to know what would happen
to a population of individuals playing this game, and reproducing in
proportion to their payoffs. There is no need to confine ourselves to
a game in which only two strategies are possible, so we will suppose
that strategies A,B,C.... are possible, and will use $E(A,B)$ to mean
the expected payoff to an individual adopting strategy A, if his opponent adopts strategy B.

We seek a strategy I which is "evolutionarily stable", in the sense
that if almost all the members of a population adopt I, the population
cannot be invaded by individuals adopting any mutant strategy M. Such
a strategy will be called an "evolutionarily stable strategy" or ESS.
It is easy to write down the conditions which must be satisfied by I.
Thus suppose a fraction p of the population adopt the mutant strategy
M, where $p \ll 1$, and (1-p) adopt I. Then if each individual starts
life with a fitness C, and fights r contests, then the fitnesses of I
and M individuals are

$$W(I) = C + r \left\{ (1-p) \, E(I,I) + pE(I,M) \right\}$$

$$W(M) = C + r \left\{ (1-p) \, E(M,I) + pE(M,M) \right\} .$$

If I is to be an ESS, then $W(I) > W(M)$ for all mutants. Since p is small,
this will be the case provided that, for all $M \neq I$,

<u>either</u>	$E(I,I) > E(M,I)$	(1a)
<u>or</u>	$E(I,I) = E(M,I)$ <u>and</u> $E(I,M) > E(M,M)$	(1b)

Conditions (1) will be referred to as the "standard conditions" for
I to be an ESS. A game may have one or several ESS's, or it may have
no ESS. If there are several ESS's, the final state of a population
will depend on the initial frequencies of the various strategies.

Let us now return to the Hawk-Dove game, and suppose that individuals
either always play Hawk, or always play Dove; that is they are "pure
strategists". If $V > D$ (i.e. the Prisoner's Dilemma) then the strategy

Hawk satisfies 1a. Hawk is the only ESS, and a mixed population will evolve until it consists entirely of Hawks. If V < D, neither Hawk nor Dove satisfies conditions 1. A mixed population of Hawks and Doves will evolve until it consists of a stable mixture of P Hawks and (1-P) Doves, where P = V/D. This would be a "stable polymorphism" in the population geneticist's sense, maintained by frequency-dependent selection.

Suppose now, however, that in addition to "pure Hawks" are "pure Doves", individuals can exist which, in each contest, adopt the strategy "Play Hawk with probability P and Dove with probability 1-P". Such individuals produce offspring like themselves. In game theory terms, they adopt a "mixed" as opposed to a "pure" strategy, the essential feature of a mixed strategy being that it contains a stochastic element. It is then easy to see that the mixed strategy with P = V/D satisfies conditions 1.

For a game such as the Hawk-Dove game with only two pure strategies, if both pure and mixed strategies can exist and reproduce, it is easy to show two things:

    i) at least one ESS, pure or mixed, exists.

    ii) if a mixed ESS exists, playing P Hawk: (1-P)Dove, then the corresponding polymorphic mixture of pure Hawk and pure Dove is also stable.

Unhappily, neither of these statements is true if more than two pure strategies are possible. There may be no ESS, pure or mixed. Further, if A,B,C... are possible pure strategies, and $\tilde{P}$ a vector of probabilities or frequencies over these strategies, then the mixed strategy $\tilde{P}$ may be an ESS but the polymorphism $\tilde{P}$ be unstable, or vice versa; examples of both situations will be given.

Consider first the children's game "Rock-Scissors-Paper". In this game Rock beats Scissors, Scissors beats Paper, and Paper beats Rock. If we give both players a small negative score -e if they adopt the same strategy, we can write the payoff matrix:

	R	S	P
R	-e	+1	-1
S	-1	-e	+1
P	+1	-1	-e

Clearly no pure strategy is an ESS. The mixed strategy $I = \frac{1}{3}R + \frac{1}{3}S + \frac{1}{3}P$ does satisfy conditions 1. In fact, if a population contains mixed strategists I and pure strategists in any proportions, then I always increases in frequency (except when the frequencies of R,S and P are exactly equal, when the population is stationary). However, if only pure strategists exist, the polymorphic population $\frac{1}{3}$R, $\frac{1}{3}$S, $\frac{1}{3}$P is at an unstable equilibrium, and if disturbed cycles with increasing amplitude. In this case, then, the mixed strategy is stable but the polymorphism is not.

Consider now the following matrix, shown to me by Professor C.Zeeman.

	A	B	C
A	0	5	-4
B	-7	0	8
C	-1	2	0

In this case, the polymorphism $\frac{1}{3}$A, $\frac{1}{3}$B, $\frac{1}{3}$C is stable, although it is not the only stable state for a population in which only pure stategists can exist. The dynamics of such a population are shown in figure 1.

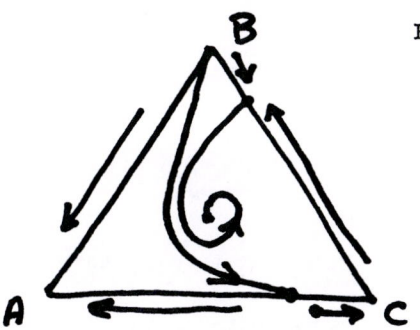

Figure 1.

Trajectories for the matrix above, if only pure strategists exist.

However, the mixed strategy $I = \frac{1}{3}A + \frac{1}{3}B + \frac{1}{3}C$ is not an ESS. It does not meet conditions 1, because it can be invaded by strategy A. The polymorphism is stable, but not the corresponding mixed ESS.

These two cases illustrate the fact that, if there are more than two pure strategies, the conditions for a stable polymorphism and for a mixed strategy to be an ESS are not identical. However, this does not alter the fact that conditions 1 are necessary and sufficient to ensure that a strategy I is stable against invasion, provided that, if I is a mixture of strategies, it is interpreted as a mixed strategy and not a polymorphism. (Difficulties arise in the degenerate case when all four expectations appearing in the standard conditions are equal.)

Despite these difficulties, it is very often the case that a probability vector giving a mixed ESS also gives a stable polymorphism, and this is

always so for games with two pure strategies. Consequently, in applying these ideas in practice, it may often turn out that a predicted
mixed ESS is actually realised as a genetic polymorphism; as we shall
see later, it may also be realised as a mixture of learnt strategies.

In formulating the concept of an ESS, I had in mind the population
geneticist's model of a series of non-overlapping generations. More
formally, let p_i, p_i' be the frequency strategy i in successive generation,

$$W_i = C + \sum_j p_i \, E(i,j) \text{ is the fitness of strategy i}$$

and $\quad \bar{W} = \sum_i p_i \, W_i$ is the mean fitness of the population.

Then $\quad p_i' = p_i \, W_i / \bar{W}$. $\hspace{3cm}$ (2)

It is natural for mathematicians to replace this recurrence relation
by a differential equation. Since (2) is equivalent to $p_i' - p_i = p_i \, (W_i - \bar{W})/\bar{W}$, the natural differential equations are

$$\frac{dp_i}{dt} = \frac{p_i(W_i - \bar{W})}{\bar{W}}. \hspace{2cm} (3)$$

However, both Taylor & Jonker (1978) and Zeeman (1979) have understand-
ably preferred

$$\frac{dp_i}{dt} = p_i(W_i - \bar{W}). \hspace{2cm} (4)$$

In fact, (3) and (4) give identical trajectories and stationary points.

The interest of equations (4) is that Eigen & Schuster (1977, 1978)
have reached identical equations in their models of the origin of life.
This is not surprising, since they also are concerned with populations
of asexually reproducing entities. Further investigation of these
equations may have more relevance for the origin of life than for the
evolution of behaviour, because the assumption of asexual reproduction
may well be correct for the former problem, whereas it is an approximation made for convenience for the latter.
Returning for a moment to the problem of stability, if the strategies
i, j.... of equations (4) are treated as pure strategies, it turns out
that conditions (1) are sufficient but not necessary to ensure stability of a polymorphism. Thus figure 1 is an example of a stable polymorphism in which the conditions are not satisfied. In contrast, the
instability of the polymorphism $\frac{1}{3}$ Rock, $\frac{1}{3}$ Scissors, $\frac{1}{3}$ Paper arose from
the discrete, generations-separate nature of the model.

So far, I have supposed that there is no "role differentiation" between the contestants; that is, prior to the contest they have identical information. In most animal contests there is a clear role differentiation. For example, one may be a male and one a female; one may be old and the other young; one may be large and the other small; one may be the owner of a resource and the other an interloper. Before such an asymmetry can influence the strategy adopted, it must be known to the contestants. Thus one may be bigger than the other, but if neither know this it cannot affect their behaviour, although it may affect the outcome of an escalated fight. Considerable theoretical difficulties arise if information about asymmetries is imperfect (Maynard Smith & Parker 1976). Thus if both contestants estimate the difference in size, but do so inaccurately, they may both conclude that they are the larger. In what follows, I assume that there is an asymmetry associated with the contest, and that this is known certainly to both contestants.

Consider the Hawk-Dove game, but suppose that every contest is between the "owner" of that resource and an interloper. I assume that the strategy type to which an individual belongs does not influence its likelihood of being an owner or an interloper in a particular contest. In addition to pure Hawk and pure Dove, we introduce a third strategy, "Bourgeois", i.e. "if owner, play Hawk; if interloper, play Dove". The payoff matrix then becomes

	Hawk	Dove	Bourgeois
Hawk	$\frac{1}{2}(V-D)$	V	$\frac{3}{4}V - \frac{D}{4}$
Dove	0	$\frac{V}{2}$	$\frac{V}{4}$
Bourgeois	$\frac{1}{4}(V-D)$	$\frac{3V}{4}$	$\frac{V}{2}$

In estimating these payoffs, the important point is that a contest between two Bourgeois strategists never leads to injury, since it is always between an owner who plays Hawk and an interloper who plays Dove. As before, if $V > D$ pure Hawk is the only ESS. Now, however, if $V < D$ the only ESS is pure Bourgeois. The role asymmetry is used to settle the contest.

The analysis of asymmetric games has been made much simpler by a theorem of Selten's (in press), stating that in an asymmetric game there cannot be a mixed ESS. Thus an ESS for an asymmetric game must specify what an individual will do in each role. Selton shows that such a specification involving a mixed strategy cannot satisfy conditions (1).

Asymmetries of size and/or weapons can also be used to settle contests. Strategies involving a relatively cheap assessment phase are likely to evolve. Many contests involve asymmetries both of ownership and of size. Such contests are complex, but Selten's theorem makes it possible to analyse them into a series of simpler contests (Hammerstein, in press).

If an individual engages in a series of contests during its life, it is likely to modify its behaviour in the light of experience. I want here to consider only one very simple model of learning. I suppose that a population of individuals play a certain game - for example the Hawk-Dove game - repeatedly, each individual playing a different randomly selected opponent in successive games. An individual is supposed not to know the payoff matrix, nor the strategies adopted or payoffs achieved by its opponents. It does know its own strategy choices in each successive contest and the payoffs associated with them. Given a particular learning rule, to what state will the population tend?

An obvious type of learning rule would be as follows. Start with some probability P of playing Hawk (P might not be $\frac{1}{2}$ because of evolutionary "experience" in previous generations). Record strategies played, and payoffs; if the average payoff when playing Hawk is greater than when playing Dove, increase P, and vice-versa. Averaging could be from the start of the series, or recent games could be weighted more heavily.

I have not tried to treat this problem analytically. Computer simulation suggests that such learning rules rather easily give rise to a population of individuals playing pure Hawk and pure Dove in the predicted ESS proportions. An analytical proof of this would be valuable, but may not be easy. This conclusion has two morals - one for the animal and one for the investigator. For the animal, learning would adjust the strategy frequencies to payoffs which changed from place to place or generation to generation. For the investigator, it does not follow from the fact that animals are adopting strategies in the appropriate ESS proportions that they are genetically programmed to do so.

The standard conditions (1) for an ESS are based on the assumption of asexual inheritance. In what circumstances will a sexual population evolve to an ESS? If the ESS is a pure strategy, or if it is a mixed strategy which can be produced by a genetic homozygote, then the stability of a sexual population is identical to that of a sexual one.

Difficulties arise, however, if there is a mixed ESS which does not correspond to any genetic homozygote. I have analysed (Maynard Smith, in press) the case of the two-pure-strategy game (e.g. the Hawk-Dove game), when the choice of strategy is determined by two alleles at a locus. Let the three genotypes, 11,12 and 22, have probability P_0, P_1 and P_2 of playing Hawk, and let P^* be the ESS frequency given by conditions (1). Then if there is no overdominance ($P_0 \leqslant P_1 \leqslant P_2$), the population will evolve to P^* if this is genetically possible ($P_0 \leqslant P^* \leqslant P_2$). If P^* lies outside the range P_0 to P_2, the population will become homozygous for the allele bringing it closest to P^*. If there is overdominance, matters are more complex. However, it remains true that if P^* lies in the genetically possible range, it will be stable, and that if it lies outside that range, the genetic state bringing the population closest to P^* will be stable.

However, it is not always true that a sexual population will evolve to an ESS if this requires genetic polymorphism. If the ESS is relatively simple (few pure strategies involved) and the genetic system complex (many loci, or many alleles), the population is likely to reach the ESS. If the ESS is complex and the genetic system simple, genetic constraints are likely to prevent it from doing so.

Although it is not the purpose of this article to describe actual applications of game theory in biology, I will finish by listing some of the problems which have been treated in this way:

i)   Animal contests (Maynard Smith & Price, 1973; Maynard Smith,1979).

ii)   Inter-species competition (Lawlor & Maynard Smith, 1976).

iii)   Animal dispersal (Hamilton & May, 1977).

iv)   Parental care (Maynard Smith, 1977).

v)   Resource allocation in plants (Mirmirani & Oster, 1978).

vi)   Hermaphroditism (Charnov et al., 1976).

vii)   The sex ratio (Hamilton, 1967).

viii) Anisogamy (Maynard Smith, 1978).

REFERENCES

Charnov, E. L., Maynard Smith, J., Bull, J. J.: Nature, 263(1976) 125.
Eigen, M., Schuster, P. Naturwissenschaften, 64 (1977) 541, 65 (1978) 7, 65 (1978) 341.
Hamilton, W. D.: Science, 156 (1967) 477.
Hamilton, W. D., May, R. M.: Nature, 269 (1977) 578.
Hammerstein, P.: Anim. Behav. (in the press).
Lawlor, L. R., Maynard Smith, J.: Am. Nat. 110 (1976) 79.
Maynard Smith, J.: Anim. Behav. 25 (1977) 1.
Maynard Smith, J.: The Evolution of Sex. Cambridge University Press (1978).
Maynard Smith, J.: Proc. Roy. Soc. B. 205 (1979) 475.
Maynard Smith, J., Parker, G.A.: Anim. Behav. 24 (1976) 159.
Maynard Smith, J., Price, G.R.: Nature, 246 (1973) 15.
Mirmirani, M., Oster, G.: Theor. Pop. Biol. 13 (1978) 304
Selten, R.: J. Theor. Biol. (in the press).
Taylor, R.D., Jonker, L.B.: Math. Biosc. 40 (1978) 145.
Zeeman, E.C.: Proc. Int. Conf. Global theory of dynamical systems. Northwestern, Evanston (1979).

VARIABILITY AND PERMANENCE IN MOLECULAR GENETICS

G. MALECOT

Université Claude Bernard

Mathématique appliquées

Villurbane (France)

Introduction

The problem of "stability versus variability" of living creatures is a very old problem; indeed it was already a problem for primitive man.

The problem of general resemblance among all individuals of a certain kind - and also of resemblance between parents and children -leads to the concept of "species" as a reproductive community keeping some common characters through its dispersion in space and the replacement of generations in time.

Mendelian genetics, and its modern daughter molecular genetics, explained the stability of each species by the permanence of "genes" distributed all along a linear chain of DNA (broken into several chromosomes in the cells of the higher organism), which selfreplicates through each mitosis in the embryonic or adult individual and is transmitted from parent to child by the peculiar sexual cells (sperm and eggs resulting from meiosis).

This meiosis or "chromatic reduction" enabling to pass from the double (diploid) set of chromosomes of adult individuals to a simple (haploid) set of chromosomes in each gamete, and anew to a diploid set when gametes fuse to give eggs, is accompanied by an interchange of parts of chromosomes ("crossing over") which ensures that, in many positions along the chromosomes, in many "loci", paternal and maternal genes of every adult are independently transmitted to his children.

So, we shall neglect the case of several genes strongly linked (because of too small crossing over) on a small part of the same chromosome; and we shall study the genes occupying the same chromosomic locus over the individuals of a population of the same vegetal or animal species, population extended over some geographic space, and followed during its successive generations.

It is a matter of experience that the genes occupying the same locus in different individuals, or in different gametes, in the same generation or in different generations, are not all identical.

The different genes occupying the same locus may belong to few or many "allelic classes" which ensure polymorphism among individuals (and naturally also among generations). Their polymorphism, for an important number among perhaps 10^6 loci or "cistrons" distributed all along the chromosomes, ensures that no two individuals (in a sexually reproducing species) may be identical. The genetic polymorphism is the basis of individual differences (indeed amplified afterwards by environment or culture which "selects" peculiar genetic complexes).

The "statistical genetics" is interested, not in individual differences, but in the overall frequencies of the alleles occupying each given locus (for instance q and p = 1-q for alleles a and A in case of diallelism, or when all alleles other than a are grouped under the notation A).

If the population were very large (in total number of contemporaneous individuals) and if it were "panmictic" (i.e. if each individual were able to choose as mate for reproduction with equal probability any individual of the required sex) then, by Hardy-Weinberg theorem, q and p would be constant over space and time.

Causes of Randomness

For many reasons (random drift due to finite number, mutation, selection, etc.), the constancy of frequencies is not realized in many natural populations. For sake of clarity, we shall consider each population in a gametic stage, i.e. as a set of gametes considered just before they unite two by two to give birth to diploid individuals. To distinguish the really uniting gametes from the much more numerous produced gametes (among which are many wasted sperm and eggs), we shall call them useful gametes (in number 2N if there are N diploid individuals in the adult stage).

Each useful gamete Γ (*figure 1*) bears, in the given locus (solid dot in figure) a gene which is a copy of the gene which had previously occupied the same locus

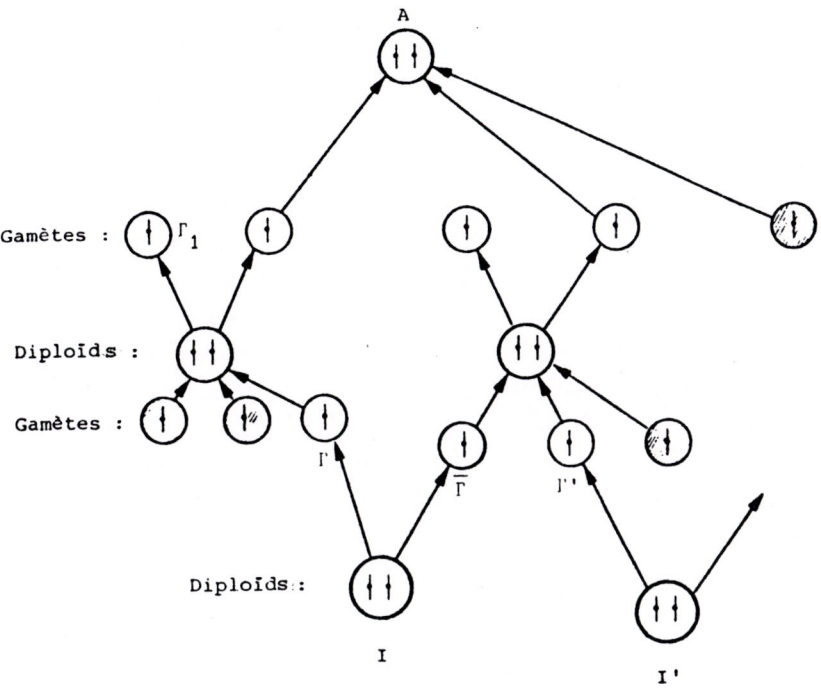

Figure 1

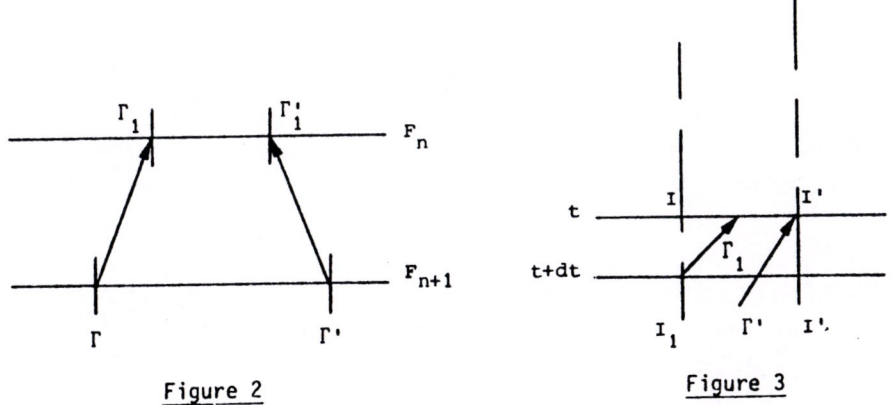

Figure 2   Figure 3

in one useful gamete Γ_1 (belonging to the previous generation). The random drift due to 2N independent "samplings with replacement" among gametes Γ_1 of diploids would define a Markoff process with absorbing states (extinction, at length, of all alleles except one). If no population may become and remain monomorphic, it is because of the unavoidable occurrence of new mutations.

The copy of Γ_1 by Γ, which corresponds to the DNA selfreplicating mechanism, is not always an identical copy: it may be a mutated copy owing to a random chemical change (random mutation) occurring during replication in one among the nearly 10^3 nucleotides constituting the segment of DNA which defines a given locus or "cistron" indeed, not all these point mutations are immediately discernible, owing to the redundancy of the translation of the triplets of nucleotides ("codons") into the amino-acids of the protein expressing the gene.

Let us call k ("mutation rate") the probability of some mutational change in a cistron when it is copied in the cellular transition from gamete Γ_1 to gamete Γ; k is not larger than 10^{-6}, since each nucleotide has only a probability around 10^{-9} of point mutation and at most 10^3 nucleotides code for the protein.

A small number of these mutations act on the protein by changing an amino-acid which is at a key position for the structure and enzymatic activity of the protein; but most of the mutations are translated into a trifling change of structure and may be considered of negligible selective value; they are called "(selectively) neutral".

So the picture of the population, with respect to the given locus, consists in a partition of all useful gametes into allelic classes of "identical gametes", each class bearing identical genes (a fortiori coding for identical proteins) because all are unmutated copies of the same gene originated by one mutation in some gamete of some previous generation.

Non-identical genes ("allelic genes") in the same locus come from different mutations, which practically cannot have exactly the same set of nucleotides; the result of each mutation is a "new" gene (even if it is not easy to distinguish from the preceding gene). But each new gene may give, when its descendants are prolific (which may be the case owing to the large variance of progeny number), many copies constituting a large allelic class, which may become the entire population: the gene is then fixed (and all other allelic genes are eliminated) up to the appearance of a new mutation.

The fixation of some alleles is, as time passes, a transitory state: from time to time some new genes appear by mutation while others disappear; so no gene is definitively established. There is, in a given locus studied for a very long time, a statistical flux of genes, an ever-changing partition of the population into variable allelic classes. This is far from the "classical" model of only 2 allelic classes, a and A, with "reversible" mutations (a $\rightarrow$ A with probability u, A $\rightarrow$ a with

probability v), and 3 "zygotic" frequencies q^2, $2pq$, p^2, for diploids aa, Aa, AA.
Nevertheless we may retain for every non inbred random diploid individual I, the
notion of heterozygosity H (probability that I bears two different alleles) or

homozygosity $1-H = \sum_{i=1}^{2} q_i$ when there are n allelic classes of respective gametic

frequencies q_i. For many species 1-H is between 85 % and 95 %; so each individual
is in the mean heterozygous in approximately 10 % of his loci. Gametes in nearby
individuals are different in 10 % and identical in 90 % of their loci; this seems
to be a sort of optimum value for diversity among individuals of the same species.

The proportion of identical loci is naturally smaller between two geographically
distant individuals belonging to the same species, or between individuals belonging
to different subspecies or related species (provided it is possible to define ho-
mologous loci in spite of the absence of fertile intercrossing). In many populations,
heterozygosity is seen to be a stable characteristic of the flux of transient allelic
classes; this is explained by the stability of the coefficient of kinship (which I
defined in 1948; KIMURA and CROW used it for heterozygosity in 1964); indeed I first
used it to calculate the variances and correlations of local frequencies and it was
afterwards used by MORTON to compare the frequencies of some polyallelic loci in
local populations; all the mentioned properties are easy consequences of the following definitions.

Coefficient of Kinship

The coefficient of kinship (a function of time and geographical place) is defined
as the a priori probability φ that 2 gametes randomly chosen at given dates and
places bear (in the given locus) 2 "identical genes", i.e. 2 genes descending without any mutation from the same gene of some common ancestor (such as A in *figure 1*).
Clearly non-identical genes can arise only from different and independent mutations.
So the concept of "identity by descent", and of probability of identity by descent,
is related to two sorts of random events, the random ancestry of each gamete (among
its 2^p ancestors of each order p) and the random arrival of new mutations along
each line of descent. The a priori probability φ depends on time, i.e. on a parameter t if we consider only contemporaneous individuals, and also of place if all
produced gametes are not equally probable as genitors of each individual (non-
panmictic case or "structured population"). This, for individuals I and I' (*figure
1*) at date t, $\bar{\varphi}_{II'}(t)$ will be the notation for the probability of identity by
descent of two genes randomly chosen (in the given locus) in I and I', or equiva-
lently, chosen at random among the set of gametes (gametic pool) which may give
birth to I and I'. $\varphi_I(t)$ will be the "coefficient of inbreeding", probability of
identity of two uniting gametes Γ and $\bar{\Gamma}$. It is also the coefficient of kinship of

the parents, independently chosen if rules of mating are not dictated by kinship;
I is then said to be "non inbred".

For instance, if $\sum_i q_i^2 = 1-H$ is the realised homozygosity at date t, calculated from
the realized frequencies q_i of all alleles, $\varphi_I(t)$ for a non inbred is the a priori
expectation of $\sum_i q_i^2$ and so may be statistically estimated over individuals.

Calculation in a Structured Population

What we said about random factors amounts to stressing the essential role of the
finite number of individuals constituting the whole population; this finiteness
ensures that no genes persist indefinitely without being modified by mutations, and
that some genes may, for a time, gain large frequencies even without selection in
their favour. When a gene has a large frequency, it is explained by the very large
progeny descending from an unique common ancestor (the first individual where this
gene appeared by mutation). So the inequality of progenies is an important feature
of population genetics. The older model supposed that the distribution of the number
of adult descendants of each individual was poissonian. A somewhat different (and
better) formulation is that the relevant gametes at the origin of each child are
randomly copied among those constituting the population of its possible parents,
this random choice bearing a sample with replacement, each parental gamete being,
during its life, liable to an indefinite number of independent copies (Wright's
correction may be made if the variance of progeny is larger than in the usual model).

In a stable population, the constancy of carrying capacity sets a negative correlation between the numbers of deaths and births; if the coefficient of variation
along time of the total number of individuals is small, this number may, with sufficient approximation, be considered as constant over time. This implies that the
random death of one individual is immediately balanced by a birth; the death of an
individual (and of its two gametes) is a sampling without replacement, in contrast
with the sampling of the new gametes. We shall use φ to denote the probability of
identity for a random choice of 2 gametes with replacement, and $\bar{\varphi}$ for a random choice
without replacement.

We have to study the variation of φ or of $\bar{\varphi}$ from date t to date t+dt, in the
"time-continuous" case where deaths (and immediate replacements by birth) take place
one by one, with constant probability μdt for each individual alive at date t to
die between t and t+dt (independently of other individuals).

It would be too restrictive to suppose that each newly born gamete is sampled
among the whole population of the considered species. It is more realistic to suppose that each new gamete is sampled among a "geographical neighbourhood", which
is called either "parental neighbourhood" or "gametic pool" defined in the following
manner:

Each gamete used to replace an individual dying (between t and t+dt) in geographical place i has probabilities $g_{i\ell}$ of being sampled in geographical place ℓ, with $\sum_{\ell} g_{i\ell} = 1$, the summation being over the "range" R_i of the "parental neighborhood", or "gametic pool" for gametes used in place i. It is theoretically general to suppose that we allot a place i to each of the 2 gametes of a living diploid. But it is more realistic to suppose that each place i is the "territory" of N_i living diploids ($2N_i$ gametes) each of which may independently die and be replaced by gametes drawn in the gametic pool R_i with probability $g_{i\ell}$ of coming from place ℓ. All the $2N\ell$ gametes existing in place ℓ are considered equally probable ("local panmixy").

We shall call $\overline{\varphi_{ij}(t)}$ the a priori probability of identity in 2 distinct randomly chosen gametes in places i and j at date t; $\varphi_{ij}(t)$ changes only when one of these tow gametes appears to die and to be replaced by a copy sampled with replacement over the corresponding gametic pool. Between t and t+dt, a death changing the value of $\varphi_{ij}(t)$ may occur in place i (with probability μdt, see *figures 4 and 5a*) or, independently, in place j (with probability μdt). So we have:

$$\overline{\varphi_{ij}(t+dt)} = (1-2\mu dt)\overline{\varphi_{ij}(t)}+[\sum_{\ell} g_{i\ell} \; \varphi_{\ell j}](1-k)\mu dt+[\sum_{m} g_{jm} \; \varphi_{im}](1-k)\mu dt \qquad (1)$$

1-k being the probability of persistency of identity (non mutation) through each copying of a parental gamete.

Figure 4

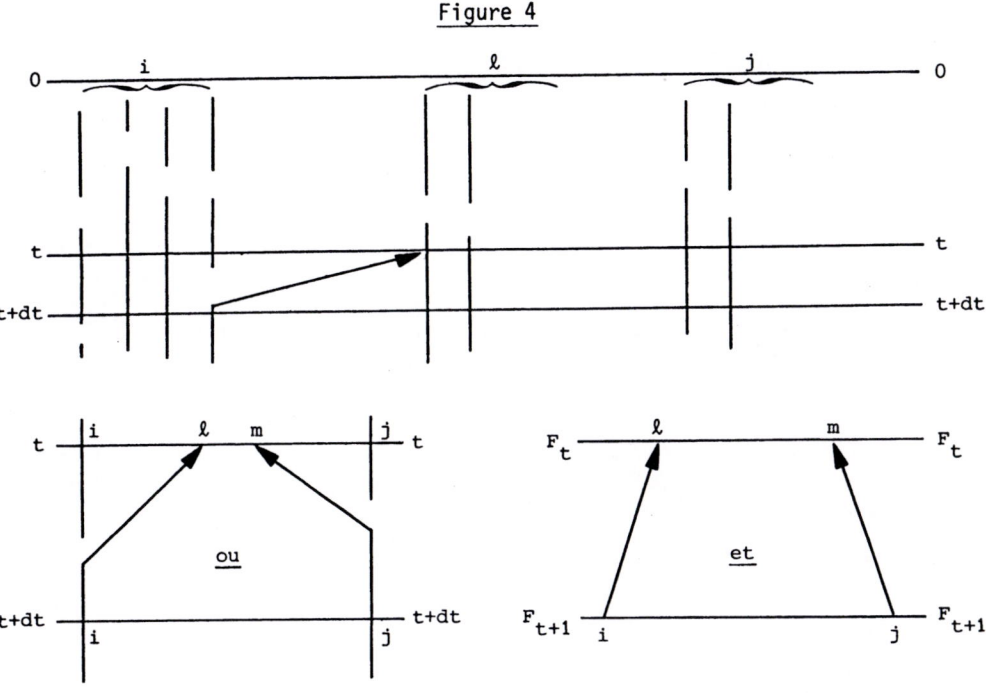

Figure 5a

Figure 5b

This model is somewhat different from the model (*figure 5b*) of separate generations with simultaneous deaths and replacements (at every integer date t) of all gametes; but the asymptotic results are analogous, except that now the life-length of every gamete is stochastic instead of being a fixed constant, and the number of copies successively made of each gamete is negative binomial instead of poisson.

Even if each range R_i (set of values of ℓ such as $g_{i\ell} > 0$) is finite, the number of geographic places (the cardinal of the set of places i, j, etc.) has been supposed to be infinite in many models of "infinite habitats". I was the first to introduce such an habitat in 1948. I now think that it is better, and as easy, to have a finite habitat (and a finite total population) as in the unidimensional circular case of my 1951 paper, taken again by MARUYAMA (1970). I shall emphasize in what circumstances the infinite habitat is really a good approximation for a large but finite one when considering only asymptotic values $\varphi_{ij}(+\infty)$; nevertheless the speed towards these asymptotic values when k = 0 is very different (MARUYAMA, 1970; MALECOT, 1971-1975) for finite and infinite habitats. The unreal problem of infinite habitat has indeed a mathematical interest (SAWYER, 1976-1979).

When the $g_{i\ell}$'s are constants over time, (1) is a linear differential system with constant coefficients which we first solve in terms of Laplace transforms

$$\Phi_{ij}(\lambda) = \int_o^{+\infty} e^{-\lambda t} \varphi_{ij}(t) \, dt \cdot \qquad (\lambda > 0)$$

The asymptotic limit is given by $\varphi_{ij}(\infty) = \lim\limits_{\lambda \to o} \lambda\Phi(\lambda)$, and the Laplace transform of $\overline{\dfrac{d\varphi}{dt}}$ is $\overline{\lambda\Phi} - \overline{\varphi_{ij}}(o)$, $\overline{\lambda\Phi}$ being related to $\lambda\Phi$ as $\overline{\varphi}$ is related to φ, so we have :

$$\overline{\lambda\Phi}_{ij} - \lambda\Phi_{ij} = \delta_{ij}(\lambda\Phi_{ii}-1)/M \qquad (M_j = 2N_j-1)$$

thus transforming (1) into :

$$(\lambda+2\mu)\Phi_{ij}(\lambda) - \overline{\varphi_{ij}}(o) = \mu(1-k)[\sum_\ell g_{i\ell} \Phi_{\ell j}(\lambda) + \sum_m g_{jm} \Phi_{im}(\lambda)]$$

$$+ \delta_{ij}[1/\lambda - \Phi_{ij}(\lambda)](\lambda+2\mu)/M_j \qquad (1')$$

We may put $2\mu(1-k)/(\lambda+2\mu) = \beta < 1$ if $\lambda > 0$, and see that there is then a unique solution of (1').

Homogeneous Case

We now suppose that all N_j are equal ($N_j = N$, $M_j = M$) and that the probabilities g_{ij} are invariant in every translation over the periodic

(torus-like) lattice of geographical places, i.e. that $g_{ij} = g(y)$, y being

the bidimensional vector j-i, of components y_1 and y_2 . Putting $\alpha_1^{y_1} \alpha_2^{y_2} = \alpha^y$,

we introduce the bidimensional Fourier transform $L(\alpha) = \sum_y g(y)\alpha^y$, the

summation being defined over $r_1 r_2$ values of y_1 and y_2 (the addition to y_1

and y_2 of arbitrary multiples of r_1 and r_2 leaving the vector unchanged).

α_1 and α_2 have to be arbitrary roots of equations :

$$\alpha_1^{r_1} = 1 \quad ; \quad \alpha_2^{r_2} = 1 \qquad (2)$$

We also may put :

$$\begin{cases} \alpha_1 = e^{i\theta_1} \quad , \quad \theta_1 = 2h\pi/r_1 \in]-\pi \ , \ +\pi] \\ \\ \alpha_2 = e^{i\theta_2} \quad , \quad \theta_2 = 2g\pi/r_2 \in]-\pi \ , \ +\pi] \end{cases} \qquad (2')$$

Then (1') gives the Fourier transform $R(\alpha,\lambda) = \sum_j \Phi_{ij}(\lambda) \ \alpha^{j-i}$ (we have

to suppose that the $\overline{\varphi_{ij}}(o)$ are invariant in every translation and to put

$\sum_j \varphi_{ij}(o) \ \alpha^{j-i} = p(\alpha)$). $\Phi_{ii}(\lambda)$ will be called Φ_o. The convolutions in the

second member of (1') give ordinary products of Laplace transform :

$$(\lambda+2\mu)[R(\alpha,\lambda)-(1/\lambda-\Phi_o)/M]-p(\alpha) = \mu(1-k)[L(\alpha)+L(1/\alpha)] \ R(\alpha,\lambda)$$

introducing the symmetrised Fourier transform of migration $[L(\alpha)+L(1/\alpha)]/2 = H(\alpha)$:

$$[1-\beta H(\alpha)] \ R(\alpha,\lambda) = (1/\lambda-\Phi_o)/M + p(\alpha)/(\lambda+2\mu) = P(\lambda) \qquad (3)$$

The study of $\varphi_{ij}(t)$ when $t \to +\infty$ is related by Tauberian theorems to the

behaviour, when $\lambda \to 0$, of the inverse Fourier transform $\Phi_{ij}(\lambda)$ of $R(\alpha,\lambda)$;

it is easy to see that when $\lambda \to 0$, $p(\alpha)$ is negligible with respect to infinite

terms, so we shall reduce $P(\lambda)$ to $(1/\lambda-\Phi_o)/M$.

The inversion of $R(\alpha,\lambda)$ gives :

$$\phi_{ij}(\lambda) = (1/r_1 r_2) \sum_{\alpha_1} \sum_{\alpha_2} \alpha_1^{y_1} \alpha_2^{y_2} R(\alpha,\lambda) = [P(\lambda)/r_1 r_2] \sum_{\theta_1} \sum_{\theta_2} e^{i(\theta_1 y_1 + \theta_2 y_2)} /[1-\beta H(\alpha)] \quad (4)$$

The first summation, over the r_1 values of θ_1 defined in (2'), may be made

as was shown [in G. MALECOT, 1975, p. 227] , by use of the roots (for θ_2 fixed)

of equation $1-\beta H(\alpha) = 0$: one of them is generally the most important if we are

interested only in the asymptotic results when $\beta \to 1$; this explains why a good approximation of the general results is given by the "stepping stone case" when $g_{i\ell}$ is > 0 only for nearest neighbours ($\sigma_1^2/2$ for each of the 2 neighbours along the first axis, $\sigma_2^2/2$ for the two along the second axis), i.e. when :

$$H(\alpha) = 1 + \sigma_1^2(u_1-2)/2 + \sigma_2^2(u_2-2)/2 \tag{5}$$

with $u_j = \alpha_j + 1/\alpha_j = e^{i\theta_j} + e^{-i\theta_j} = 2\cos\theta_j$.

The summation over θ_1 in (4) may be exactly calculated, owing to the linearity of $1-\beta H(\alpha)$ with respect to u_1 :

$$(1/r_1)\sum_{\alpha_1} \alpha_1^{y_1}[1-\beta H(\alpha)]^{-1} = 2(a_1^{y_1} + a_1^{r_1-y_1})/(1-a_1^{r_1})\beta\sigma_1^2(1/a_1-a_1) \tag{6}$$

$$(0 \le y_1 < r_1) \ ;$$

a_1 being the smallest of the two values of α_1 which (for $\theta_2 = 2g\pi/r_2$ fixed) are zeros of the denominator $1-\beta H(\alpha)$. If we put $a_1 = e^{-\psi_g}$ and $1/a_1 = e^{\psi_g}$ ($\psi_g > 0$), equation $1-\beta H(\alpha) = 0$ gives [by (5)]:

$$\sigma_1^2(\text{ch } \psi_g-1) = 1/\beta - 1 + \sigma_2^2(1 - \cos\theta_2)$$
$$= 2\,\sigma_1^2\,D' + 2\,\sigma_2^2\,\sin^2(g\pi/r_2) \tag{7}$$

when putting $\quad D' = \dfrac{1-\beta}{2\beta\sigma_1^2} = \dfrac{\lambda+2\mu k}{4\mu(1-k)\sigma_1^2} = \dfrac{D}{4\sigma_1^2}$

From the unique value $\psi_g > 0$ given by (7), the sum (6) may be written

$T_g(y_1) + T_g(r_1-y_1)$, $T_g(y)$ being given by :

$$T_g(y) = e^{-\psi_g y}/(1-e^{-\psi_g r_1})\text{sh }\psi_g \qquad (y \ge 0) \tag{8}$$

Limit Case   (infinite population)

The formula for an infinite population ($r_1 = r_2 = \infty$) that I had directly established may also be obtained by putting $a_1^{r_1} = 0$ and replacing sums by integrals in (4) and (6) ; thus giving (in the isotropic case where $\sigma_2 = \sigma_1$) :

$$\Phi_{ij}(\lambda)/P(\lambda) = (1/2\pi\beta\sigma_1^2) \int_{-\pi}^{+\pi} e^{i\theta_2 y_2} e^{-\psi y_1} (\text{sh }\psi)^{-1} d\theta_2$$

ψ being defined, as a function of θ_2 , by (7) ; its value for $\theta_2 = 0$ will be called $\psi_0 \sim 2\sqrt{D'}$.

The evident symmetry due to isotropy allows the equating of the two values obtained either by putting $y_2 = 0$ and $y = y$, or $y_1 = 0$ and $y_2 = y$, thus expressing :

$$I(y) = \int_o^\pi e^{-y\psi} (\text{sh } \psi)^{-1} d\theta_2 \qquad (9)$$

by the following elliptic integral ($\alpha_2 = e^{i\theta_2}$ along the unit circle C)

$$I(y) = (1/2i) \int_C \alpha_2^{y-1} (\text{sh } \psi)^{-1} d\alpha_2 \; ; \qquad (9')$$

these elliptic integrals may be expressed recursively for $y \in \mathbb{N}$ (G. MALECOT, 1950, 1971) and decrease asymptotically as $y^{-1/2} e^{-\psi_o y}$ when $y \to +\infty$ ("quasi exponential decrease", i.e. reduction by a factor $\# e^{-1}$ when the increase of y is $1/\psi_o \backsim 1/2 \sqrt{D'} = \sigma_1/\sqrt{D}$).

General case (finite)

Returning now to the finite (non isotropic) case, only when $y_2 = 0$, we get the coefficients of kinship for distance y_1 along the first axis, their Laplace transforms given by summations (4) and (6) being called :

$$\beta\sigma_1^2 \Phi(y_1,\lambda)/P(\lambda) = \sum_{\theta_2} [T_g(y_1) + T_g(r_1-y_1)]/r_2 \qquad (10)$$

$T_g(y)$ being defined by (8).

The 2 sums $\sum_{\theta_2 \geq 2\pi/r_2} T_g(y)$ and $\sum_{\theta_2 \leq -2\pi/r_2} T_g(y)$ may be approximated by an integral (the integrand being a decreasing function of θ_2) ; let us put :

$$J(y,\delta) = \int_\delta^\pi e^{-\psi y} (\text{sh } \psi)^{-1} d\theta_2 \qquad (11)$$

If we now suppose $r_1/\sigma_1 \geq r_2/\sigma_2$ i.e. that the first axis is "the axis of smallest exploration", the function $(1-e^{-\psi r_1})$ in (8) differs from 1, when $|\theta_2| \geq 2\pi/r_2$ and in virtue of (7), by less than $e^{-2\pi} \# 2.10^{-3}$; so, with less than 2 ‰ error over the integral :

$$\sum_{\theta_2 \neq 0} T_g(y) = J(y,2\pi/r_2) \, r_2/\pi + 2\gamma \, e^{-\psi_1 y}/\text{sh } \psi_1 \qquad (12)$$

γ being between 0 and 1, and near 0,5 if the trapezoïd approximation of the integrand in (11) is good between its values $e^{-\psi_1 y}/\text{sh } \psi_1$ and $e^{-\psi_2 y}/\text{sh } \psi_2$.

The complete sum $\sum\limits_{\theta_2} T_g(y)$ is naturally deduced by adding

$$e^{-\psi_o y}/(1-e^{-\psi_o r_1}) \, \text{sh} \, \psi_o \, .$$

All this amounts to inserting in (10), instead of $T_g(y)$, the integral J of

(12) augmented by the values of (8) for ψ_o and ψ_1 (we shall, when needed,

approximate ψ_o by $\sqrt{D}/\sigma_1$ and ψ_1 by $2\sqrt{D'+\pi^2\sigma_2^2/r_2^2\sigma_1^2}$, which is larger than $2\pi/r_1$).

(10) may now be written :

$$\beta\sigma_1^2 \phi(y_1,\lambda)/P(\lambda) = \sum_{g=o}^{g=1} [T_g(y_1)+T_g(r_1-y_1)]/r_2 + J(y_1,\frac{2\pi}{r_2})/\pi + J(r_1-y_1,\frac{2\pi}{r_2})/\pi \qquad (13)$$

The principal part of (13) when $\lambda \to 0$, i.e. when $D \sim 2k$, is given either

by terms T_o or by terms J ; the following discussion uses the non-dimensional

parameters :

$$a = r_2 \, \sqrt{2k}/\sigma_2 \qquad \text{and} \qquad a_1 = r_1 \, \sqrt{2k}/\sigma_1$$

a and a_1 small   (quasi panmictic case)

$J(y,\delta)$ is bounded by $J(0,\delta)$ which is, owing to (7), an incomplete elliptic

integral $\sim (\sigma_1/\sigma_2) \, F(v_1|m)$

with $F(v_1|m) = \int_o^{v_1} (1-m \sin^2 v)^{-1/2} \, dv$

$1-m \sim (\sigma_1^2 + \sigma_2^2) \, D/4 \, \sigma_1^2 \, \sigma_2^2$

$\text{tg} \, v_1 \sim \text{cotg} \, (\delta/2) \, \sigma_1(\sigma_1^2 + \sigma_2^2)^{-1/2}$

a) The special value $\delta \doteq 0$ gives $v_1 = \pi/2$, $F(v_1|m) = K(m)$.
$K(m)$ is approximated, when $1-m$ is small, by $\Pi^{-1} K(1-m) \, \text{Log} \, [16/(1-m)]$.

b) For δ small, it is easy to see that

$$\int_o^\delta (\text{sh} \, \psi_g)^{-1} \, d\theta_2 \sim (\sigma_1/\sigma_2) \, \text{Arg sh} \, (\delta\sigma_2/\sqrt{D}), \text{ so:}$$

$$|J(y,\delta)| \leq (\sigma_1/\sigma_2) \, [K(m)-\text{Arg sh}(\delta\sigma_2/\sqrt{D})] = -\text{Log} \, \delta+0(D \, \text{Log} \, D)+0(D/\delta^2) \qquad (14)$$

c) Putting $\delta \doteq 2\pi/r_2$, we may replace the 2 last terms of (13) by

$\text{Log} \, r_2 + 0(1)$:

for $g = 1$, $\text{sh} \, \psi_1 \sim \psi_1 \sim \sqrt{D + 4\pi^2\sigma_2^2/r^2} /\sigma_1 = 0(1/r_2)$;

for $g = 0$, $\psi_0 \sim \sqrt{D}/\sigma_1$, $e^{-\psi_0 y}$ /sh $\psi_0 (1-e^{-\psi_0 r_1}) r_2 \sim 1/\psi_0^2 r_1 r_2 \sim \sigma_1^2 / D r_1 r_2$;

So (13) gives:

$$(1-k) \lim[\Phi(y_1,\lambda)/P(\lambda)] = 2(Dr_1 r_2)^{-1} + O(\text{Log } r_2) + O(D\text{Log}D) + O(Dr_2^2) \qquad (15)$$

When $\lambda \to 0$, $D \to 2k/(1-k)$; $kr_1 r_2$ has been (as the product aa_1) supposed small ; kr_2^2 also ; but Log r_2 may be large (if r_2 is large).

(15) shows that the principal part of $\Phi(y_1,\lambda)$ is Φ_0 , given [(14) being an equality when $y = 0$] from Eq. (15) by :

$$k\, r_1 r_2\, M\, \lambda\Phi_0/(1-\lambda\Phi_0) \underset{(\lambda\to 0)}{\sim} 1 + kr_1 r_2 \text{ Log } r_2/\pi\sigma_1\sigma_2 + O(kr_1 r_2) = 1+\epsilon$$

Hence the limit of $\varphi_{jj}(t)$ when $t \to +\infty$:

$$\varphi_{jj}(+\infty) = \lim_{\lambda\to 0} \lambda\Phi_0 = (1+\epsilon)(1+Mr_1 r_2 k+\epsilon)^{-1}$$

which is somewhat larger (except when $kr_1 r_2$ Log r_2 is small ; for instance, when r_1 and r_2 are finite) than the known value $(1+Mr_1 r_2 k)^{-1}$ of the stationary coefficient of kinship in a wholly panmictic population gathering all the $2Nr_1 r_2$ useful gametes.

a and a_1 large   (occupied over larger than "panmictic neighbourhood")
_____

(which includes the case of an infinite population, with $r_1 = r_2 = +\infty$)

$$\left| J(y , o) - J(y,2\pi/r_2) \right| \leq \int_0^{2\pi/r_2} (\text{sh } \psi_g)^{-1} d\theta_2 \sim 2\pi/a$$

$$\sim (\sigma_1/\sigma_2) \text{ Arg sh}(2\pi\sigma_2/r_2\sqrt{D}) \sim (\sigma_1/\sigma_2) 2\pi/a$$

We now apply this formula to (13) [where $\psi_1 \sim \psi_0 \sim \sqrt{D}/\sigma_1$, and, by (8) :

$$T_g(y)/r_2 \sim e^{-y\sqrt{D}/\sigma_1} \sigma_1/r_2\sqrt{D} \text{ when } g = 0 \text{ or } 1] :$$

$$\pi\beta\sigma_1^2 \Phi_{ij}(\lambda)/P(\lambda) = J(y_1,o) + J(r_1-y_1,o) + O(1/a) + O(1/a_1) \qquad (16)$$

If the population were infinite, the second member would be reduced to

$$J(y_1,o) = \int_o^\pi e^{-\psi y} (sh\ \psi)^{-1}\ d\theta_2 \text{ , which is (see V) the same elliptic integral as :}$$

$$I(y) = (1/2i) \int_{|\alpha_2|=1} \alpha_2^{y-1} (sh\psi)^{-1} d\alpha_2\ ;$$

the asymptotic decrease of $I(y)$ is the same as $y^{-1/2} e^{-y\sqrt{D}/\sigma_1}$. In the present finite case where $0 \le y_1 < r_1$, formula (16) shows that $\Phi_{ij}(\lambda)$ decreases from $J(0,0)$ [for $y_1 = 0$] , to $2J(r_1/2,0)$ [for $y_1 = r_1/2$] which is small.

$\Phi_{ij}(\lambda)$, and its inverse Laplace transform $\varphi_{ij}(t)$, are, for λ small (for t large) quasi-exponentially decreasing functions of distance y (quasi-reduced by a factor e^{-1} when the increase of y_1 is $\sigma_1/\sqrt{2k}$).

For $y_1 = 0$, $\varphi_{jj}(\lambda) = \Phi_o$, the principal part of the second member of (16) is $J(0,0) = (\sigma_1/\sigma_2)\ K(m) = (\sigma_1/\sigma_2)\ Log[8\sigma_1\sigma_2/D^{1/2} \sqrt{\sigma_1^2+\sigma_2^2}][1+0(D)][\text{by VII - a}]$ which gives :

$$2\pi M\sigma_1\sigma_2\lambda\Phi_o/(1-\lambda\Phi_o)\{Log(1/k)+Log[32\sigma_1^2\sigma_2^2/[\sigma_1^2+\sigma_2^2]]\} =$$

$$= 1+0(k)+0(1/a\ log\ k)+0(1/a_1\ log\ k) = 1+\varepsilon$$

Hence, as in VII, the asymptotic formula :

$$\varphi_{jj}(+\infty) = \frac{1+\varepsilon}{1+2\pi M\sigma_1\sigma_2/\{log(1/k)+Log[32\sigma_1^2\sigma_2^2/(\sigma_1^2+\sigma_2^2)]\}+\varepsilon}$$

which is of the same form as the formula given by G. MALECOT (1967) in the continuous isotropic infinite case.

Conclusion

When $r_1\sqrt{2k}/\sigma_1$ and $r_2\sqrt{2k}/\sigma_2$ are large, all the formulas for an infinite population are valid : the quasi-exponential decrease with distance, and the local coefficient of kinship, which depend essentially of the largeness of $4\pi N\sigma_1\sigma_2/log(1/k)$; practically, to obtain a value of φ_{jj} near 0,9, the product $N\sigma_1\sigma_2$ must have a numerical value of 1/9, if $2k = 10^{-6}$, or of 1/7, if $2k = 10^{-8}$; the dependence on the smallness of k is weak : the homozygosity φ_{jj} in the bidimensional case with large values of $r_1\sqrt{2k}/\sigma_1$ and $r_2\sqrt{2k}/\sigma_2$ depends practically on the value of $4N\sigma_1\sigma_2$, which is the number of diploid individuals in a rectangle of sides equal to $2\sigma_1$ and $2\sigma_2$, a rectangle which might be called the "area of parental neighbourhood"; this number must be about 0,5 when φ is about 0,9; so, when φ is calculated from the fine molecular structure of neutral genes, it gives a simple relation between the density of an adult reproducing population and its propensity to migration.

It is easy to see that the above value of φ_{jj}, even if r_1 and r_2 are infinite, is the same as in a panmictic population which number would be the number of individuals in a rectangle ("panmictic neighbourhood") of sides $\sigma_1/\sqrt{2k}$ and $\sigma_2/\sqrt{2k}$; the total number of individuals does not matter, provided a and a_1 are large, i.e. provided that the occupied area is large with respect to the "panmictic neighbourhood" (the same result in the unidimensional case was given by G. MALECOT, 1951, p. 116).

REFERENCES

[1] G. MALECOT, La consanguinité dans une population limitée. C.R. Acad. Sci.
     Paris, 222, 841-843, 1946.

[2] G. MALECOT, Les processus stochastiques de la génétique dans "Le Calcul des
     Probabilités et ses applications". Lyon 28 juin au 3 juillet 1948. Colloque
     International du C.N.R.S., 13, 121-126, 1949.

[3] G. MALECOT, Quelques schémas probabilistes sur la variabilité des populations
     naturelles. Ann. Univ. Lyon, Sciences, Section A, 13, 37-60, 1950.

[4] G. MALECOT, Un traitement stochastique des problèmes linéaires (mutation,
     linkage, migration) en génétique de populations. Ann. Univ. Lyon, Sciences,
     section A, 14, 79-117, 1951.

[5] G. MALECOT, Les processus stochastiques et la méthode des fonctions généra-
     trices ou caractéristiques. Publ. Inst. Statist. Paris, 1, F 3, 1-16, 1952.

[6] G. MALECOT, Probabilités et hérédité, Travaux et Documents de l'I.N.E.D.,
     cahier n° 47 - P.U.F. Paris, 1966.

[7] G. MALECOT, The Mathematics of heredity, W.H. FREEMAN & Co, San Francisco, 1969.

[8] G. MALECOT, Heterozygosity and relationship in regularly subdivided popu-
     lations, Theor. Pop. Biol., Vol. 8, n° 2, 1975.

[9] G. MALECOT, Kinship in the birth and death process of a population subdivided
     in finite panmictic groups. Recent Developments in statistics, North-Holland
     Publishing Company, 1977.

[10] G. MALECOT, Evolution, Parentés, Migrations, 1978, to appear in Lecture Notes
     in Mathematics.

EVOLUTION IN HUMAN POPULATIONS:

DATA AND MODELS

A. Piazza

Istituto di Genetica Medica, Università di Torino

Torino, Italy

and

Department of Genetics, Stanford University

Stanford, California 94305

Introduction

Differences between human populations are usually overestimated by our
cultural attitude of dividing the world into a group of "us" and a remainder of "them". However the reconstruction of the historical proces
ses that have led to the present differentiation among individuals within populations, and among populations within our species, continues
to be of intense interest not only for assessing the relative rôles of
different biological pressures on human evolution, but also for provid
ing models and analogies to other, not necessarily biological, mechanisms of evolution.

Blood types detected by immunological techniques, electrophoretic variants reflecting variations in electrophoretic mobility by enzymes or
proteins, and anthropometric or anthroposcopic traits as morphological
measurements, skin and hair colour, body shape, etc., are the major

source of data for measuring variations in extant human populations. While blood and electrophoretic types are monofactorial mendelian characters, anthropometric traits are usually defined only at the phenotype level. As pointed out by Lewontin [1] also in this Symposium, the population genetic theory shows a paradoxical situation in this respect by having two parallel systems of evolutionary descriptions, one operating in the space of genotypes and bypassing the phenotypic space through models with almost constant genotypic fitness, and the other one - the quantitative or biometrical approach - operating entirely in the phenotype domain with little or no reference to the genetic determination of the phenotype.

When human population data are analyzed in the genotype space as they usually do, we are faced by the problem of distinguishing a similarity by common origin, from a similarity by common environment or common culture. Differentiation by origin and differentiation by environment or culture are evolutionary processes which obviously affect and are affected by the genetic component of the human populations.

Can samples of now living populations provide some insight into the final assessment of either process of differentiation?

Some tentative answers to this problem have been recently advanced and some results, mostly by Cavalli-Sforza, Menozzi and myself at the Genetics Department of the Stanford University are here presented.

2. Human evolution described by trees

A very popular representation of human evolution uses trees of descent.

Relationships among populations can be always represented by trees, as they are one of the possible modes of showing similarities among taxo-nomic units. Trees have been also a tool for the analysis of the human evolutionary process which is likely to be meaningful only when there have been neither major hybridizations nor evolutionary convergence [2,3,4]. The problem is: can human evolution be reconstructed in terms of "phylogenetic" trees?, or, in other words, how can we test whether real data are well or poorly represented by tree-like structures? Until recently there existed no direct way for testing the validity of this mode of representing a specific set of populations. A method has been introduced for this purpose [5,6] and validated by simulations [7]: it has been called the "treeness" test. The procedure developes a likelihood-ratio test which compares an observed variance-covariance (dispersion) matrix between extant populations (each tested for the same set of quantitative traits, for instance gene frequencies) with a theoretical dispersion matrix computed according to a specified evo-lutionary hypothesis. It should be noted that for this approach, a di-spersion matrix with elements V_{ij} - and not a distance matrix with elements D_{ij} - is required; using Euclidean distances the latter could be obtained from the former because $D_{ij} = V_{ii} + V_{jj} - 2V_{ij}$, but the inverse operation can be done only approximately because the loss of the diagonals in the distance matrix involves a loss of information. Some evolutionary models predict a peculiar pattern in the dispersion matrix of gene frequencies among populations. It is this pattern which is at the basis of the test of the validity of the tree model. If evo-lution is assumed to be independent in the various branches of the tree (e.g., there are no migratory exchanges, no major hybridization, no convergence, etc.) the covariance between two populations is expected to be equal to the variance accumulated by their most recent common ancestor. The result is that the expected covariance matrix has a special pattern, all population pairs which have the same last common ancestors having the same covariance. The test for measuring the agreement with this pattern is the test for evolutionary independence. The variances of extant populations (the diagonal elements of the dispersion matrix) are expected to be a simple function of the difference between the gene frequency in the extant populations and that in the ancestor common to all populations (the root of the tree), so that, if evolutionary rates are constant, the diagonal elements of the matrix are expected to be equal. The test for constancy of evolutionary rates (CER) will thus depend on testing for equality of the diagonal values of the dispersion matrix. When on the contrary the diagonal elements of the dispersion matrix are unequal, evolutionary rates in the divergence of human ethnic groups differ. Also this hypothesis of variable evolutionary rates (VER) can be tested.

The pattern of the expected dispersion matrix corresponding to a tree of seven populations is shown in Fig. 1. The value of the covariances in each block corresponds to the node shown in the tree. Covariances that are expected to be equal among themselves are those that span populations across the split specified by a node. In a VER model, $V_1, V_2, \ldots, V_7$ may differ; in a CER model $V_1 = V_2 = \ldots = V_7$.

The treeness method above (for more details see the original publications [5,6]) provides also a theorical criterion for choosing the

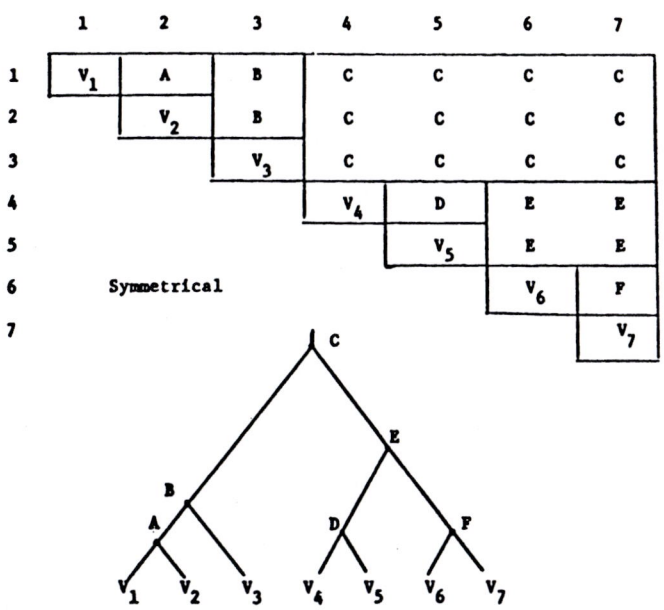

Fig.1. The pattern of a dispersion matrix expected for a tree of 7 populations.

"best" among all possible trees: all topologies arising from a given number of populations could be tested and the one showing the best goodness of fit with the evolutionary hypothesis could be eventually chosen. However this criterion, as all explicit ones (least square, maximum likelihood, minimum length, etc.) is made practically impossible when dealing with many populations, by the number of possible different topologies (for istance with 12 populations they are 13, 749, 310, 575 !). Some compromise is therefore necessary and our attitude is to look for a concordant support from a variety of clustering methods such as single linkage, average linkage, etc. [8]. Obviously, by using this strategy it is possible that there exist topologies fitting a set of data better than any method employed. However it may added that with as many topologies as in practical cases, (i) there is a high density of topologies per unit of likelihood and therefore there will exist many topologies which are practically equally acceptable by any criterion; (ii) in any case the probability of identifying the "right" topology when examining trees generated by a known probability model depends on the number of populations and of characters [7].

2.1. Gene frequency data

When Edwards and Cavalli-Sforza made the first reconstruction of human evolution by trees of descent based on gene frequencies, their analysis grouped together populations known to be related: Africans with Africans, Europeans with Europeans, and so also for American natives and Orientals including Australian aborigenes. These four population groups were further clustered by placing Europeans with Africans and American natives with Orientals.

The study of further genetic markers (mostly blood types) confirmed this original classification [5,9,10,11]. The analysis reported in [11] includes also the treeness test and it makes available some human data for discussion. A sample of 35 human populations has been selected and an attempt was made in making this sample as close representation as possible of the world's aborigenes (in practice, descendants of the populations inhabiting the world before 1492). 18 genetic loci (including the two loci HLA-A and HLA-B which control the human histocompatibility antigens) for a total of 58 independent gene frequencies have been collected for each population. The resulting 35x35 dispersion matrix is synthesized in fig. 2 in a way to bring out also the peculiarity of some populations. Variances and covariances are averaged within the following blocks of populations:

Group	Populations
America (Amer)	Makiritare,Maya,Papago,Yanomama,Zuni
Oriental (Orient)	Chinese,Japanese,Korean,Tibetan
Oceanian (Ocean)	Australia West,North; New Guinea Highlands,Karkar
Caucasian (Cauc)	Basque,English,French,German,Icelandic,Italy,Sardinia,Norwegian,Scots,Lebanese,Turk,Punjabi
Arab	Arab,Yemenite
African (Afr)	Khoi San (Bushmen),Ila Tonga,Babinga (Pygmies).

The rectangles indicated as A,B,C in fig. 2 include covariances that should be equal under perfect treeness (independent evolution) for the major splits of the tree shown on the left. The biggest rectangle, B, is subdivided into a left part including two populations (Indian,Lapp) which may have special relationships with Easterners, and a right part, not expected to have such relationships. Covariances of Indians with Easteners are always higher than those of other Caucasians. This and the low variance of India indicate a hybridization with Easteners,especially the nearest ones, the Oriental groups. A Caucasian group with a unique position is that of Lapps. Their covariances with Easteners are only slightly and inconsistently above those of other Caucasians, but that with Eskimos (2.50) stands out as the highest of those in rectangle B. This can hardly be a coincidence, and may indicate either convergent selection between Lapps and Eskimos due to life in a similar

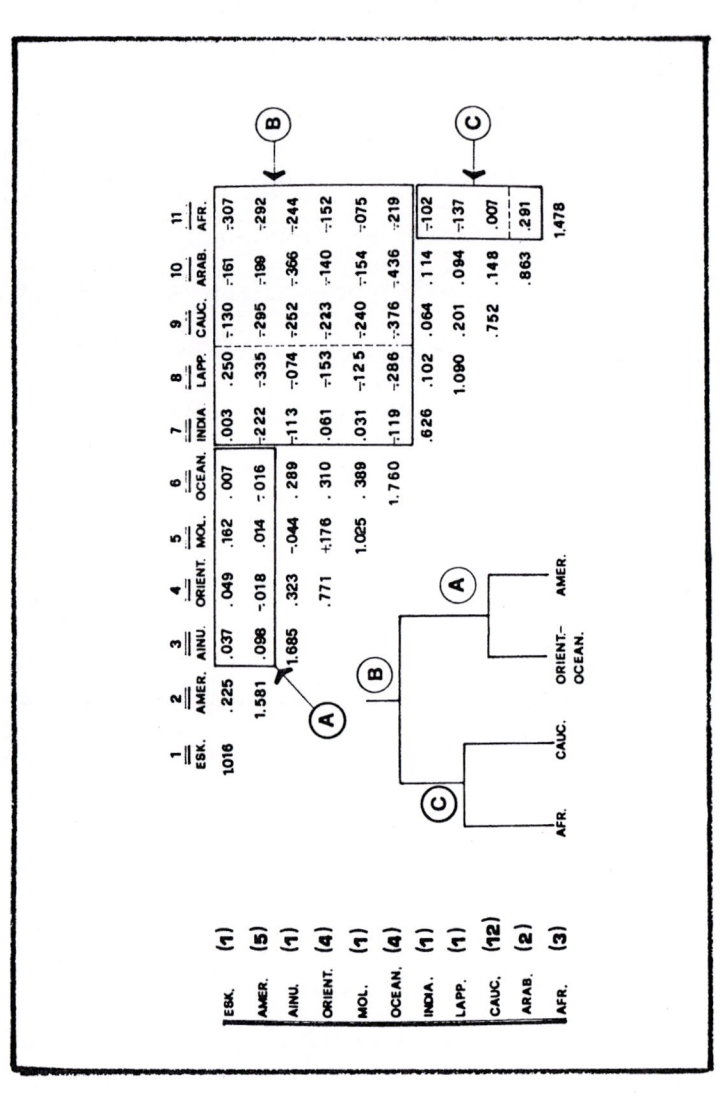

Fig. 2. Average variances and covariances for block of populations, synthesizing the 35 x 35 dispersion matrix (see text). The number in parentheses after population symbols in the rows indi̱
cate the number of populations averaged. Esk = Eskimo, Mol = Moluccan.

environment, or hybridization from one of the following mechanisms: a) an ancient stock of Northern Asians common to Eskimos and Lapps may have hybridized with Easteners in Near East Asia and with Caucasians in North East Europe; b) there may have been hybridization between a preneolithic stock of North East Europe (from which Lapps may have arisen) and paleosyberians, from which Eskimos may have arisen; c) a recent and not direct hybridization between Lapps and Eskimos, but of both groups with Scandinavians. Arabs show only a slightly higher similarity with East Asian populations than other Caucasians; their high covariance (.291) with Africans which is higher than that of any other Caucasian group, is presumably the result of hybridization. The association of Moluccans with Orientals (3.98) seems higher than that with Oceanians (.176), indicating a larger proportion of Orientals than of Oceanians in this ethnic group. Ainus have always been a puzzle for anthropologists. They have some characters to some extent in common with Caucasians (fingerprints, hairiness), while genetic markers have shown them to be Orientals [12]. Our analysis agrees entirely with the latter conclusion in showing no trace of association with Caucasians. Ainus differ from other Orientals in having a much higher variance (see fig. 2) in agreement with their smaller population size (they have been hunters and gatherers until recently). Their highest association is with their closest neighbours, the Japanese (covariance .566), probably because of recent gene flow. Eskimos associate with the five other American native samples, but they show a relatively lower variance in spite of being a small population (still hunters in contemporary times). Prevalence of social customs determining strict avoidance of inbreeding may be the main cause; but possible small hybridization with Caucasians is indicated by their significantly higher covariance with them (-.13) compared with that of other American natives (-.296). The similarity of Eskimos and Lapps, however, seems too high to be explained entirely in terms of Caucasian admixture. It may thus reflect also convergent selection, or ancient common origin as already discussed.

As explained above, variances are affected by evolutionary rates, increasing with them, but they decrease with increasing admixture between remotely related populations The distribution of variances shown in figure 2 shows that 1) the variances are significantly different; 2) aboriginal populations who are still hunters and gatherers or who have abandoned this condition most recently are those having the highest variances. This rule may be justified considering that a) the tran sition to agriculture increases population densities and thus decreases the variability due to the effect of drift; and also b) the increased means of communication, that accompany the increase of technological level and social complexity, probably determined increased admixture.

The test of treeness on all 35 world populations summarized in fig. 2 was impossible because of the too high number of parameters to be esti mated. A subsample of 10 populations, two from each continent (Pygmy, Bushmen, English, Italian, Eskimo, Maya, Chinese, Japanese,Australian, New Guinean) has already been analyzed in [5], showing an excellent agreement (x^2_{36} = 38.2) of the data with a model of independ evolution and variable evolutionary rates (VER). Figure 8 in [11] and fig. 3 below are other trees, representing world human evolution, which agree (good treeness) with a VER model.

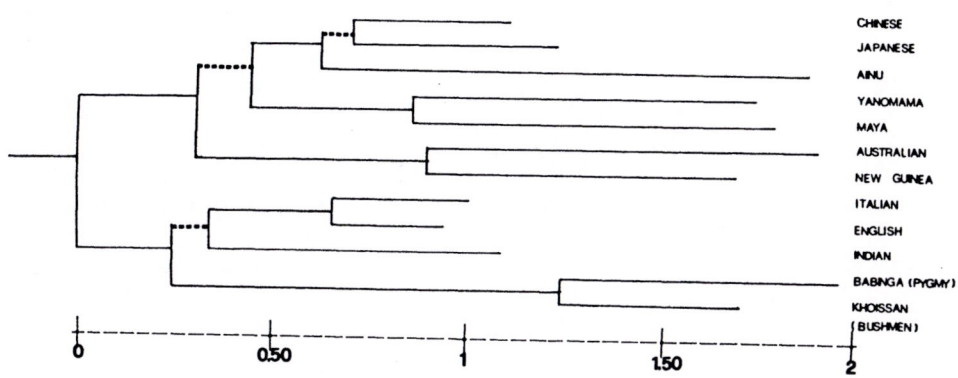

Fig. 3. Treeness analysis for a world sample of 12 populations. $x^2_{55} = 70.77$ (P > 0.05). Dotted lines are segments whose length is not statistically different from zero.

One clear finding in the analysis of human data [5,11] is that in the divergence of human ethnic groups, evolutionary rates are not constant. The populations showing shorter branches are mostly Europeans and Orientals (fig. 2 and 3). As it will be discussed below (section 3), we hypothesize that admixture which accompanied extensive radiations of people at the time of the development and spread of agriculture may be responsible for this phenomenon independently for Europeans and for

Orientals. Another possibility is that markers chosen for their poly-morphism among certain ethnic groups may tend to put these groups at the center of the map, and thus give them shorter branches. Almost all genetic markers have been developed as polymorphisms first detected in Caucasians. This does not explain why Orientals also have shorter bran-ches, and thus cannot be the correct, or the only correct, reason.Other possible causes responsible for the inequality of the length of the tree branches are true differences in evolutionary rates, due to major differences in population sizes when drift is the major cause of diffe-rentiation, or to differences in overall intensities of selection. The finding that the branches of human phylogenetic trees have different lengths - whichever real or apparent variation in evolutionary rates may be the cause - casts serious doubts on the validity of attempts at dating the separation times of the various human ethnic groups.

If the evolution of humans can be represented by a tree of splitting populations, the split which is most interesting and most difficult to determine is the root of the tree. Results with our data, put Africans and Caucasians on one side of the first split, and all "Easterners" (Orientals, American natives, Australians and Melanesians) on the other side. This pattern differs from those proposed by Imaizumi et al. [13] and Nei [14] who put Africans on one side of the first split, and all remaining major ethnic groups on the other side. However they did not introduce any statistical test for goodness of fit and the data used by Nei are compatible with either model of evolution when our treeness test is applied [15].

2.2 Anthropometric data

Along with the first attempts based on blood group data, similar efforts were made to reconstruct human evolution by using anthroposcopic
(skin colour, hair shape, etc.) and anthropometric (including cranio-
metric) traits [2]. Results obtained from anthropometric data disagree
with those from genetic markers. The former type of analysis associates Africans with Australians and Melanesians, while Europeans are
grouped with Orientals and American natives (figure 4).

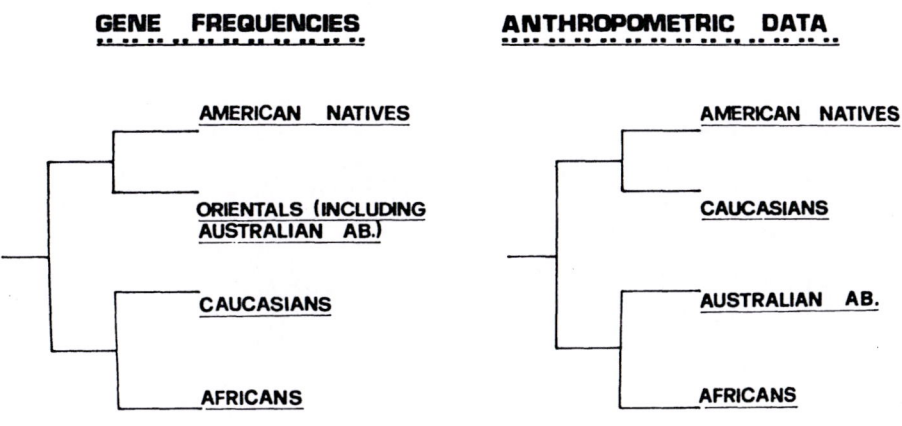

The analysis of 70 skull measurements belonging to 17 ancient populations carried out by Howells [16] and recently completed with climate
data by Guglielmino-Matessi et al. [17] fully confirmed the "anthropometric" type of tree (fig. 4). It is remarkable that the populations
which associate together when "external" morphology, i.e. anthropo-

metric or anthroscopic traits are considered, have had a similar climatic pattern for most of their evolution. Thus it is not surprising to see Africans associate with Australian aborigenes and Malanesians. American natives have undergone in the period spent in the Americas exposure to different climates; but those investigated mostly come from temperate or cold climatic areas. Thus it is again not surprising to see American natives associate with Europeans.

There seems to be no major exception to the rule that the main separation suggested by external morphology is into a branch with populations that experienced for most of their life a tropical climate, and another

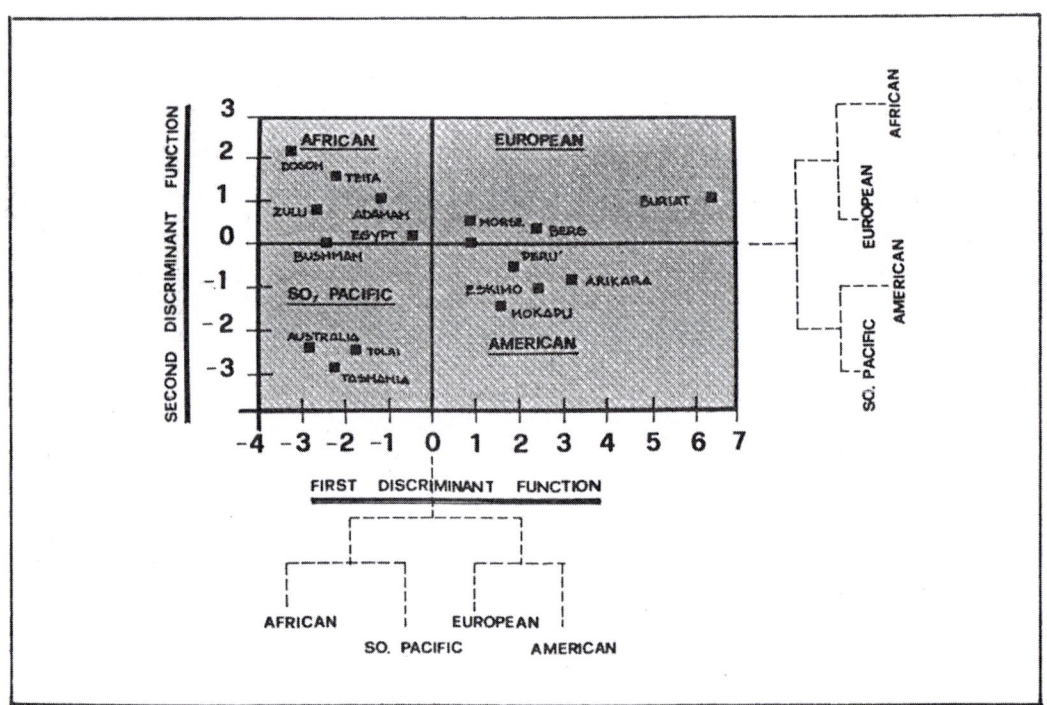

Fig. 5. Reanalysis of Howells' data on skull variation (from [17]).

branch of populations exposed mostly to temperate and cold climate.The
Howells' 70 skull measurements were condensed into fewer (16) functions
by using discriminant analysis. The first discriminant function accoun
ted for over 25% of all the variations and the second for about 15%:
both functions are represented in fig. 5.
The first discriminant separates populations according to the "anthro-
poietic" tree and the second to the "genetic" tree. (For the relationships of trees and spectral representation as in discriminant analysis,
see [5] and [6]). But Table 1 below shows that the first discriminant
function is highly correlated with climate,in particular temperatures,
while the second (and all other) discriminant function is not.

Table 1

Correlation of Howells' first two discriminant functions for
skull measurements with climatic variables (from [17])

Climatic variables	Function 1		Function 2	
	Male	Female	Male	Female
Average temperature/year	-.78***	-.72***	.04	.23
Absolute max temperature	-.51*	-.40	.15	.10
Absolute min temperature	-.77***	-.76***	-.19	-.21
Mean relative humidity	.46	.41	-.17	-.21
Rainfall in a year	-.22	-.21	-.13	.04

*   significant at 5%
*** significant at 0.1%

Once the regression on climate indicators is eliminated from the discriminant functions, the first discriminant can be shown to be unimportant in comparison with the second one, the "genetic" tree becoming the more informative. Therefore removal of climate effects from cranio metric data may well lead to our former "genetic" tree.

2.3 "Selective" or "migrational" tree of evolution

It is well known that external morphology is under close control of na tural selection in response to climatic conditions. The rules of Bergmann and of Allen are approximately valid also for Man [18,19]. The correlation of skin colour and climate is too well known, even if only partially explained, to require further stressing. External morphology, because it is external, expresses the interface between the outside en vironment and the organism. Such interface is most likely to respond adaptively to climatic conditions. Natural selection has very probably promoted traits that favor the homeostasis of internal body temperature. Furthermore traits of external morphology are likely to be polygenic and polygenic traits are expected to have been more influenced by natural selection than monofactorial traits as genetic markers. All these considerations make it likely that the phylogenetic tree derived from morphological traits (figure 4, right) does describe a history of adaptive responses to climate, i.e. it may represent a "selective" pat tern of evolution.

On the other side, one relevant aspect which emerges from the gene fre quency analyses summarized in fig. 4 (left) is the genetic centrality of South and East Asia.

Let's assume that <u>Homo sapiens sapiens</u> developed in some part of Asia and, whatever was the cause, soon proved such a very successful organism, that shortly after 50,000 to 40,000 years B.P. he is found all over the world. It may be hypothesized that <u>Homo sapiens sapiens</u> spread first towards both West and East, so to originate the two branches of the first split in the genetic tree. The western branch subdivided further when Europe and Africa were occupied. The eastern branch also differentiated. One evolutionary line went south through South East Asia to Australia and Melanesia, the other went north and eventually reached America across the Bering Strait. The major weakness of interpretations of phylogenetic history like this one is, of

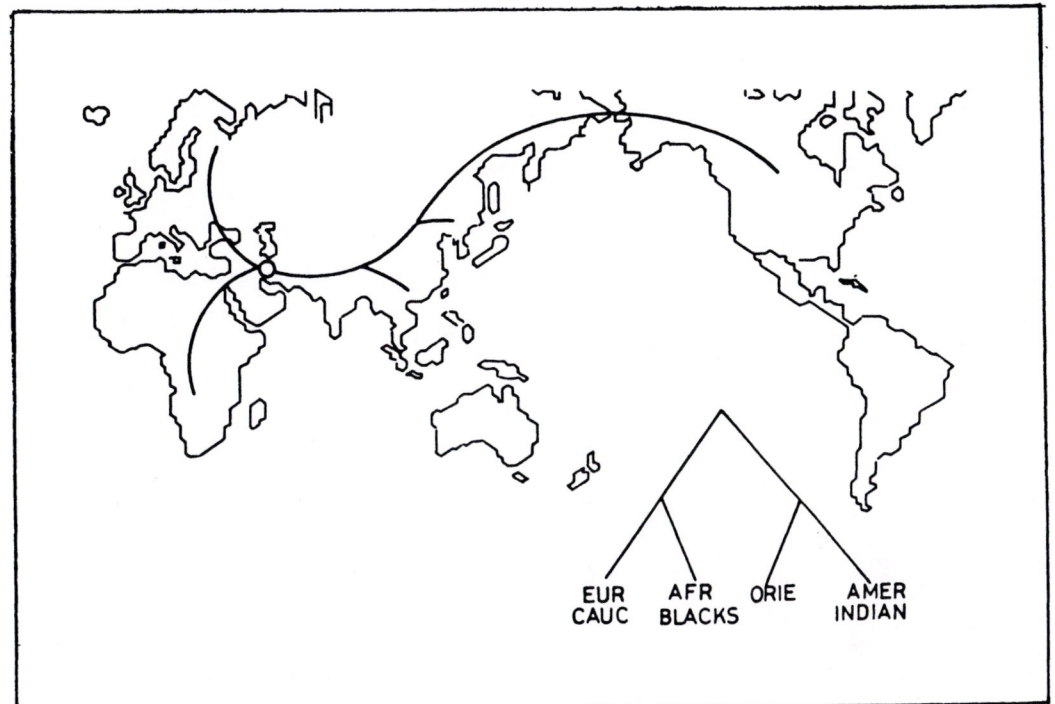

map reproduces possible routes of migration. Adapted from [21] fig.11.4.

course, the lack of fossil evidence, but if the mass migrations in the late Pleistocene which have contributed or indeed determined modern ethnic variation started mostly from Asia [20], the "genetic" tree discussed above may represent a mostly "migrational" evolutive pattern as shown in fig. 6.

3. The evolution of Caucasians and the spread of agriculture

Caucasians offer some interesting peculiarity from an evolutionary point of view which can be explained on the basis of their history. Starting from the age of the great geographic discoveries (the XV century), Caucasians, under demographic pressure, colonized the rediscovered continents which were at the time relatively underpopulated: the Americas and Australia. But even before that time Caucasians already occupied a very large territory, shaped like a rough ellipsoid with extremes in Iceland and India, spanning a continent and a half. In spite of the wide territory occupied, they were fairly homogeneous. We can get an idea of the genetic variation between Caucasians, as compared with that in other population clusters, by looking at the map of the two first principal components of the 35 world population gene frequency data of reference [11] discussed above. Figure 7 is such a map. Some Caucasian groups, like Indians, depart somewhat from the cluster (in the expected direction, e.g. towards Orientals with whom they are likely to have had some admixture). But most Caucasians cluster closely together, especially if compared with natives of America or Oceania.

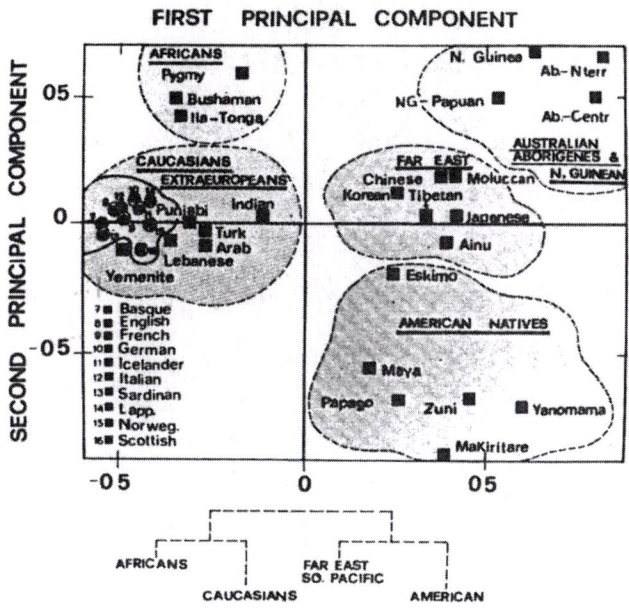

Fig. 7. 35 world populations grouped according to 58 independent

alleles blood markers (adapted from [11]).

In a representation of the same data by trees (see [5], [11], and Ita-

lian, English and Indian populations in fig. 3 of this paper) Cauca-

sians show a) very short branches, mostly not significantly different

from zero, when compared to the non Caucasian populations; and b) a

very poor fit of all the 15 Caucasian populations to the model of in-

dependent evolution. Both these peculiar features would be expected

if admixtures of earlier groups had an important part in their origin

[5]. Although the actual observations are not so extreme for all Cau-

casian populations, it is a fact that both Caucasian, and some Oriental populations (in particular Chinese, see fig. 3) show this pattern. An explanation for it is probably to be found in one important reason for admixture: at the center of the area inhabitated by Caucasians (and also in China and in South East Asia) we find the beginnings of plant and animal breeding. Concentrating on Caucasians, of whom more is known both from an archeological and a genetic point of view, it has been ascertained that the domestication of many cereals and also of animals such as cattle, pigs, sheep and goats, took place in the Middle East in a period about 10,000-9,000 years ago. From there the farming economy spread slowly, but at a regular rate in all directions.The spread towards Europe is far better known than that in other directions,given the more extensive archeological knowledge available in Europe. Ammerman and Cavalli-Sforza have mapped the progress of agriculture in Europe on the basis of existing archeological records and radiocarbon [22]. As shown in fig. 8, this progress was found to take place fairly regularly at an average rate of one Km per year. Thus, it took for instance 3000 years for agriculture to diffuse over the approximately 3000 Kilometers separating the Middle East from England.

Diffusion of agriculture may have occurred in two different ways:

1) By diffusion of the farmers themselves (demic diffusion). This would be expected if the transition to farming were accompanied by population growth. A farming economy is very likely to do that a) by increasing the carrying capacity of the land over that prevailing in previous economies (hunting and gathering), b) by increasing the motivation for breeding larger families (hunters-gatherers have usually

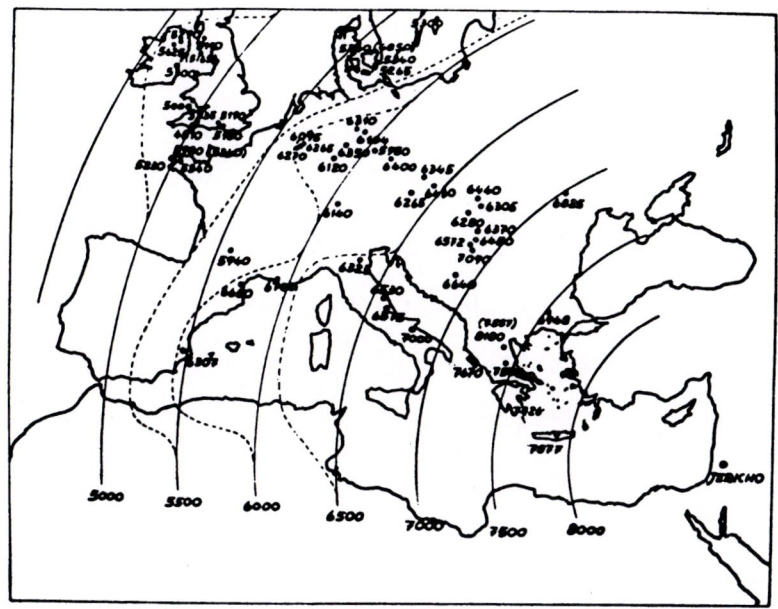

Fig. 8. Map showing the spread of early farming in Europe. Dates are

in years B.P. The broken lines take into account some regional

variation in the rate of spread. From [22].

smaller families than farmers) and c) by decreasing mortality with a

decrease in the likelihood of famine, food being more easily stored up.

2) The technology might have spread to preexisting populations of hun-

ters or gatherers living in these areas (cultural diffusion).

The two mechanisms are not mutually exclusive, but the genetic conse-

quences of the two modes of diffusion are quite different. The migra-

tion of farmers from the Near East toward Europe should spread the far

mers' genes to all of Europe. By contrast, with purely cultural diffu-

sion no direct effect on genes is expected, except for possible selec-

tion due to a changed way of life. Finally if farmers spread and also mixed with preexisting hunter-gatherers, one should observe clines, that is gradients of gene frequencies originating in the Near East and expanding radially to all Europe. Data from single genes (for example the Rh-negative allele [23]) are in agreement with the idea of an earlier, largely Rh-negative population occupying mostly the west of Europe (hunterers-gatherers) with which a slow wave of farmers coming from the east intermingled gradually. Other genes, especially some HLA-B alleles show a similar northwest-southeast gradient across Europe [24]. Is the gradient shown by these genes confirmed when all the information from all other available genetic markers is accumulated, or is it a peculiarity of these genes alone?

Just to test the hypothesis that the spread of early farming from Near East in the neolithic period was largely determined by the spread of farmers, we developed ways of studying jointly the spatial distribution of many genes by preparing geographic maps of synthetic variables which represent many genes with the least possible loss of information [25]. Synthetic variables used were linear functions of gene frequencies generated by standard multivariate techniques, such as analysis by principal components or discriminant functions. The evaluation of these canonical variates to human gene frequencies is complicated, however, by the incompleteness of the data. Very few population samples have been tested for all or even a majority of the many different genes known. Multivariate analysis usually cannot be applied to such incomplete data. We have faced this problem by developing automatic techniques for making and testing geographic maps of gene frequencies [26] with which one can interpolate gene frequency values at suitably

chosen locations. This can be done for all genes for which sufficiently detailed maps can be drawn. Values of gene frequencies interpolated
at fixed locations for all genes under study can then be subjected to
multivariate analysis.

This technique has been successfully applied to a total of 10 loci and
38 independent alleles [25]. The geographic distribution of their first
canonical variate in Europe is mapped in fig. 9. It summarizes close
to 30 percent of the information from all genes and shows clines in
remarkable agreement with those expected on the basis of early farming
in Europe, thus supporting the hypothesis that this spread was a demic
spread rather than a cultural diffusion of farming technology.

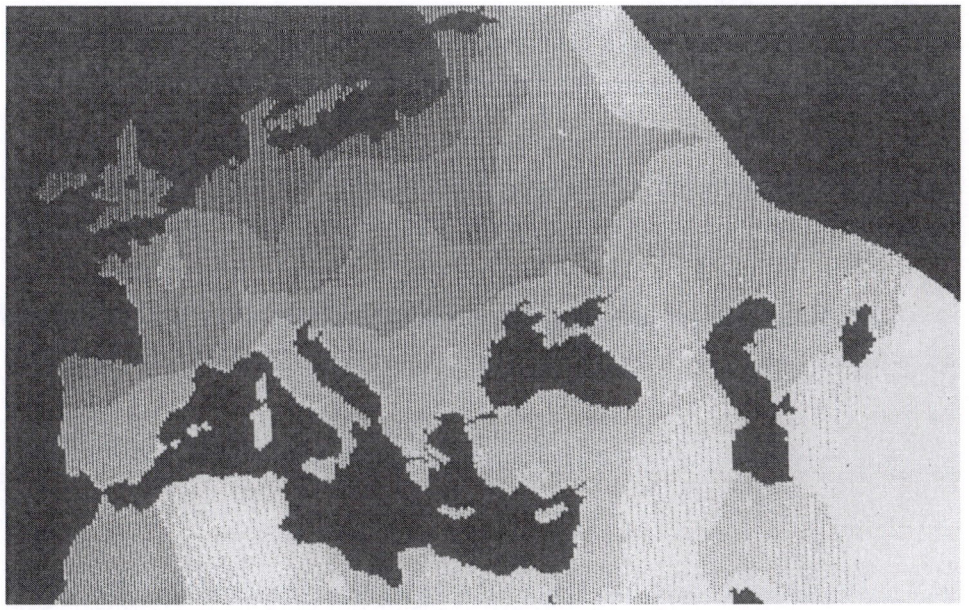

dependent alleles at the human loci: ABO,Rh, MNS, Le, Fy, Hp,
PGM$_1$, HLA-A, HLA-B. Shades indicate different values of the
principal component. From [25].

If the spread of farmers associated with the first canonical variate has been shown to be the major contributor to the geography of Caucasian genes, also the next two canonical variates (fig. 2 and 3 of reference [25]) could be explained as independent migratory fluxes. The second principal component is probably representative of prehistoric and historic migrations from northern and central Asia into Europe, and the third principal component of barbarian migrations at the end of the Roman empire. As with most reconstructions of historical events, these associations are inevitably tentative, at least without archeological and/or anthropological evidence. We are confirmed, however, in our relying on the heuristic value of this "synthetic mapping" technique for reconstructing migration patterns on the basis of genetic data.

4. The world distribution of human gene frequencies: isolation by distance and selective effects by climate.

Using the technique summarized in the previous section (for more details see [25] and [26]), we have also built the geographic maps of principal components for the whole world [27]). 39 independent alleles from 10 loci (ABO, MNS, Rh, Lewis, Duffy, Haptoglobin, Acid Phosphatase, Phosphoglucomutase, HLA-A and HLA-B) have been used. The non-HLA data were obtained from Mourant et al. [23], while the HLA data were taken from a world data bank collected by the author.
Extreme values of principal components are found in Africa, Australia or America, but not in the southern (central or eastern) part of Asia,

which has always intermediate values of the first and second principal components. This is also true when using the HLA data (21 independent alleles) [28]. The genetic centrality of Asia, shown by synthetic variables, can be explained also by the geographic centrality of Asia with respect to both the New and the Old World, a centrality that disappeared when the crossing of the Atlantic Ocean became easy. As already discussed, the two major, early areas of origin of agriculture postulated so far for the Old World, the Near East and the Far East, both correspond to intermediate values in the case of a principal component representation and to short branches in the case of a tree representation.

In order to show the relative effects of longitude and latitude, the values of principal components were subjected to a two-way analysis of variance. The results shown in the following table 2 were obtained.

It is apparent immediately that the variation by longitude is much more important than that by latitude for the first and third component, but somewhat less important for the second component.

Both latitude and longitude show effects because of isolation by distance. Longitude is expected to show the greater effect, as there is a wider range in the East-West then in the North-South directions. The variance due to latitude, however, may also include effects due to climate, and hence natural selection, which are partially confounded with those of distance. Therefore, the lack of a major effect of latitudes in this analysis gives a first qualitative indication that climate does not play a major rôle in determining the total genetic variation, since climate is associated with latitude rather than with

Table 2

Variation by longitude and latitude of the three leading principal components summarizing 39 allele frequencies distributed in the world (from [27]).

Source of variation	d.f.	First principal component		Second principal component		Third principal component	
		Mean Squares	F	Mean Squares	F	Mean Squares	F
between longitudes	11	4.431	227	1.090	35	2.115	53
between latitudes	11	0.201	10	2.011	65	0.583	15
interaction	78	0.099	5	0.100	3	0.183	3
residual	58	0.020		0.031		0.040	

longitude.

To further clarify the effect of latitude, the first discriminant function between latitudes of the 39 independent world gene frequencies was also correlated with the distance from the equator. In both northern and southern hemispheres, the discriminant function rises with latitude as it can be seen in fig. 10. As discrimination has been carried out between latitudes irrespective of whether they were northern or southern and therefore irrespective of distance from the equator, the association of the first discriminant with distance from the equator (and therefore presumably with climate) is truly striking.

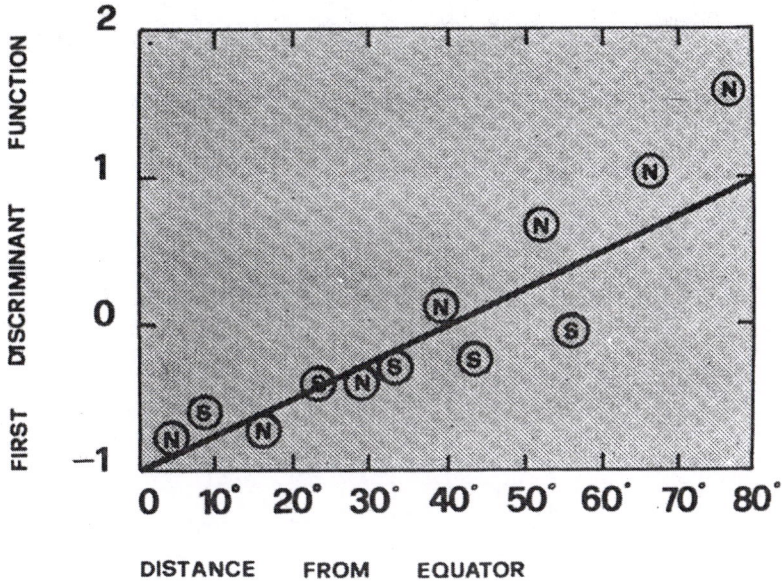

Fig.10. The first discriminant function between latitudes is plotted against the distance from the equator (in degrees) on the abscissa. Northern (N) and southern (S) latitudes are indicated and fitted with a common regression line. (From [27]).

An indication of which genes are most sensitive to the effect of climate is of some interest and it has been obtained by correlating directly the frequencies of each allele with the distance from the equator of the corresponding populations. It should be noted, however, that the data are usually highly clustered in space because some areas have been tested much more extensively than others and thus are more dense with data points. This kind of clustering is especially true of Europe and is likely to generate spurious correlations with geogra-

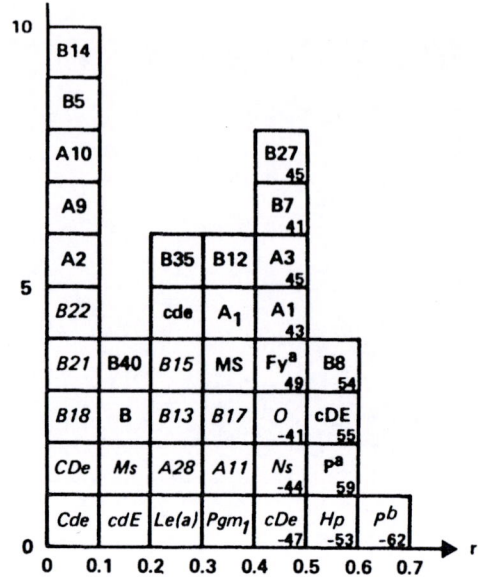

Fig. 11. Distribution of the "corrected" correlation coefficients between distance from equator and gene frequencies for 39 alleles.
The negative correlations are pointed in italics. (From [28]).

phic variables such as latitude. Moreover, as most variation in gene

frequencies is associated with longitude, correlations of distance

from the equator with gene frequency values have also to be corrected

for this longitude effect.

Correlation coefficients which accounted for these corrections are

summarized in the distribution of fig. 11.

The highest correlation with distance from the equator is for the red

cell acid phosphatase polymorphism (r = 0.59 for P^a). A possible se-

lective rôle of acid phosphatase alleles has been reported by Bottini et al. [29], who observed that among Sardinian males with clinically manifest favism due to G6PD deficiency, the frequency of P^a and P^c carriers was significantly higher than in the general population of the same area. Other alleles showing high correlations (above 0.4) are Fy^a, haptoglobin, Rh (cDE, cDe), O, Ns. It has been shown that the Fy antigen has receptor-like properties for malarial parasites which could explain the correlations with climate [30]. The positive, about equally high, correlations of the HLA alleles (A1, A3, B8, B7) with distance from equator support the notion [31] that the linkage disequilibrium observed between the pairs of alleles (A1, B8) and (A3, B7) at loci HLA-A and HLA-B is not due to genetic drift and/or migration alone. It is worth mentioning that the allelic combination A3-B7-Dw2 is associated with multiple sclerosis whose prevalence seems to increase in colder climates [32]. The remaining HLA alleles correlating more than .4 with distance from the equator is B27 ($r = 0.45$) whose association with rheumatic diseases (mostly ankylosing spondylitis) is very well known.

Another interesting result of this kind of analysis is that two out of the three proteins studied electrophoretically included in our data, show significant associations with climate, throwing doubts on their selective neutrality [14].

5. Summary

1. Blood types, electrophoretic variants, and anthropometric and/or

anthroposcopic traits are the major source of data for measuring varia
tions in extant human populations. A major problem is that of distinguishing the differentiation of humans by origin from their differentiation by environment or culture. Both are evolutionary processes
which interplay with the genetic component of the human populations.

2. A very popular representation of human evolution uses trees of
descent. Evolutionary independence is defined as the absence of correlation between changes in traits of isolated populations. The variance-
covariance matrices of extant populations are expected to have, under
evolutionary independence, a specific block pattern. It is possible to
measure how close the observed pattern is to its expectation. We called
this testing the treeness of the variance-covariance matrix. Good tree
ness is a necessary condition of evolutionary independence and allows
one to conclude whether real data are well represented by tree models.

3. Reconstruction of the human differentiation on the basis of gene
frequencies shows that between that the major separation among human
groups was that between Africans and Europeans on one side, and peop-
les from Australia. East Asia and Americas on the other. Anthropometric data disagree with the analysis based on genetic markers by showing the major separation between Africans and Australians on one branch
of the first split of the tree and Europeans, Asians and Americans on
the other. Analyses using gene frequency data show the genetic centrality of South and East Asia, and are consistent with the idea that the
latest mass migrations in the late Pleistocene, which might have contributed or indeed determined modern ethnic variation, started mostly
from Asia and follow the four major routes exemplified in fig.6 above.

Analyses using anthropometric measurements show high correlations with climatic indicators, so they are likely to be confounded by the adaptive effects of natural selection. The finding that the branches of human phylogenetic trees have different lengths - evolutionary rates being <u>not</u> constant - casts doubts on the validity of attempts at determining separation times between different ethnic groups.

4. The differentiation among Caucasian is the consequence of the spread from a center of origin in the Middle East of farmers who migra ted slowly in all directions into a variety of areas.They were already inhabited by hunterers-gatherers with whom farmers mixed to varying de grees. Multivariate techniques have been used to construct "synthetic" genetic maps for Europe and the Near East, which condense the information of many loci. These maps show clines in remarkable agreement with those expected on the basis of the spread of early farming in Europe, thus supporting the hypothesis that this spread was a spread of people rather than a cultural diffusion of farming technology.

5. The world distribution of 39 independent gene frequencies in human populations has been analyzed elsewhere by using the technique of synthetic geographic maps.The main results reported here indicate that most genetic variation is associated with longitude, with Asia showing a tendency to be genetically central. Also, latitude and, more particularly, distance from the equator play a significant rôle in a way which suggests that climatic factors exercise selective pressures,espe cially for certain genes.

Acknowledgments

Research supported by CNR, Centro per l'Immunogenetica e l'Istocompati bilità, Torino, Italy and by Grant NIH GM 20467, 20832, ERDA EY 76 S 03 0326.

References

1. LEWONTIN,R.C.: *The Genetic Basis of Evolutionary change*, Columbia University Press, New York,   12-16, 1974.

2. CAVALLI-SFORZA, L.L. and EDWARDS, A.W.F.: Analysis of human evolution. In: *Genetics Today*, Proc. XI Internat. Cong. Genet.,   923-933, Pergamon, Oxford, 1965.

3. CAVALLI-SFORZA,L.L. and EDWARDS, A.W.F.: Phylogenetic analysis. Models and estimation procedures. *Amer. J. Hum. Genet. 19*, 233-257, 1967.

4. EDWARDS, A.W.F. and CAVALLI-SFORZA, L.L.: Reconstruction of evolutionary trees. *Systematic Assoc. Pub. No. 6*, 67-76, 1964.

5. CAVALLI-SFORZA, L.L. and PIAZZA, A.: Analysis of evolution: Evolutionary rates, independence and treeness. *Theoret. Pop. Biol. 8*, 127-165, 1975.

6. PIAZZA, A. and CAVALLI-SFORZA, L.L.: Spectral analysis of patterned covariance matrices and evolutionary relationships. In: *Proceedings of the Eighth International Conference on Numerical Taxonomy*, Freeman, San Francisco,   76-105, 1975.

7. ASTOLFI, P., PIAZZA, A., KIDD, K.K.: Testing of evolutionary independence in simulated phylogenetic trees. *System. Zool. 27*, 371-400, 1978.

8. SNEATH, P.H.A. and SOKAL, R.R.: *Numerical Taxonomy*, Freeman, San Francisco, 1973.

9. CAVALLI-SFORZA, L.L.: Population structure and human evolution. *Proceedings Royal Society of London 164*, 362-379, 1966.

10. KIDD, K.K.: Genetic approaches to human evolution. In: *L'origine dell'Uomo*, Accademia Nazionale dei Lincei n. 182, 148-174, Rome, 1973.

11. PIAZZA, A., SGARAMELLA-ZONTA, L., GLUCKMANN, P. and CAVALLI-SFORZA, L.L.: The Fifth Histocompatibility Workshop gene frequency data. A phylogenetic analysis. *Tissue Antigens 5*, 445-463, 1975.

12. OMOTO, K.: The Ainu: A racial isolate? *Israel J. Med. Sciences 9*, 1285-1290, 1973.

13. IMAIZUMI, Y., MORTON, N.E., and LALOUEL, J.M.: Kinship and Race. In: *Genetic Structure of populations*, vol. III, Morton, N.E. ed. University Press of Hawaii, 228-233, 1973.

14. NEI, M.: The theory of genetic distance and evolution of human races. *Japan. J. Hum. Genet. 23*, 341-367, 1978.

15. CAVALLI-SFORZA,L.L. and PIAZZA,A.: Alternative Trees Describing Human Evolution and the Problem of Variable Evolutionary Rates. Submitted, 1980.

16. HOWELLS, W.: Cranial variation in Man. *Papers of the Peabody Museum of Archeology and Ethnology*, Harvard University, vol. 67, 1973.

17. GUGLIELMINO-MATESSI, C.R., GLUCKMAN, P. and CAVALLI-SFORZA L.L.: Climate and the evolution of skull metrics in Man. *Am. J. Phys. Anthrop. 50*, 549-564, 1979.

18. ROBERTS, D.F.: Climate and Human Variability. *Benjamin-Cummings Coll. 1956*, 12, 615-618, 1978.

19. SCHREIDER, E.: Ecological rules, body-heat regulation, and human evolution. *Evolution 18*, 1-9, 1964.

20. CLARK, G.: *World Prehistory in New Perspective.* Cambridge University Press, 1977.

21. CAVALLI-SFORZA, L.L. and BODMER, W.F.: *The Genetics of Human Populations*, Freeman, San Francisco, 1971.

22. AMMERMAN, A. and CAVALLI-SFORZA, L.L.: Measuring the rate of spread of early farming in Europe. *Man 6*, 674-688, 1971.

23. MOURANT, A.E., KOPEC, A.C. and DOMANYIEWSKA-SOBCZAK: *The distribution of the Human Blood Groups.* Oxford University Press, Oxford 1976.

24. RYDER, L.P., ANDERSON,E. and SVEJGAARD, A.: An HLA map of Europe. *Hum. Hered. 28*, 171-200, 1978.

25. MENOZZI, P., PIAZZA, A. and CAVALLI-SFORZA, L.L.: Synthetic Maps of Human Gene Frequencies in Europeans. *Science 201*, 786-792,1978.

26. PIAZZA, A., MENOZZI, P. and CAVALLI-SFORZA, L.L.: The making and testing of geographic gene frequency maps. Submitted to *Biometrics*, 1980.

27. PIAZZA, A., MENOZZI, P. and CAVALLI-SFORZA, L.L.: Synthetic gene frequency maps of Man and selective effects of climate. Submitted to *Proc. Nat. Acad. Sci.*, USA, 1980.

28. PIAZZA, A., MENOZZI, P. and CAVALLI-SFORZA, L.L.: The HLA-A,B gene frequencies in the world: migration or selection? Submitted to *Human Immunology*, 1980.

29. BOTTINI, E., LUCARELLI, P., AGOSTONI, R., PALMARINO, R., BUSINCO, L., ANTOGNONI, G.: Favism: Association with Erythrocyte Acid Phosphayase Phenotype. *Science 171*, 409-411, 1971.

30. MILLER, H.L., MASON, S.J., DVORAK, J.A., Mc GINNIS, M.H., ROTHMAN, I.K.: Erithrocyte Receptors for Malaria: Duffy Blood Determinants. *Science 189*, 561-563, 1975.

31. BODMER, W.F., CANN, H. and PIAZZA, A.: Differential genetic variability among polymorphisms as an indicator of natural selection. In: *Histocompatibility Testing 1972*, eds. Dausset, J. and Colombani, J., Williams and Wilkins, Baltimore, pp. 753-768, 1973.

32. KURTZKE, J.F.: The epidemiology of multiple sclerosis. *J. Neurol. 215*, 1-26, 1977.

MODELS OF DENSITY- AND FREQUENCY- DEPENDENT SELECTION FOR THE EXPLOITA-
TION OF RESOURCES. II. COEVOLUTION OF SPECIES IN COMPETITION.

C. Matessi and S.D. Jayakar
Laboratorio di Genetica Biochimica
ed Evoluzionistica. CNR.

Via S. Epifanio 14, Pavia, Italy.

INTRODUCTION

Whereas naturalists have surmised for a long time the intuitive
results of competition between species, theoretical models for dealing
with this problem are relatively recent. Classical population dynamics
dealt with constant competition parameters. The introduction of models
which allowed for genetic adaptation within a species according to the
pressures exerted on it by the presence of competing species had to wait
for a union between population dynamics and population genetics.

Most competition models use the Lotka-Volterra equations to describe interaction between phenotypes, and one of the most important
concepts which have emerged from this theory is that of "limiting similarity". The question one is interested in is: How similar can two species be with respect to a given character relevant to competition and
still coexist? These theories were developed with respect to the utilisation of a single common resource which was assumed to vary with respect to a property which varied along a "resource axis", different
phenotypes utilising this resource with different patterns along this
axis.

Mac Arthur, in his papers on interspecific competition (see e.g.
Mac Arthur, 1969, 1970), without considering genetic variation, studied
a Lotka-Volterra model of competition between many species. In that analysis, he showed that there is a function which is maximised at equilibrium, and interpreted it as an evolution towards maximum utilisation
of resources. In the present paper, we present a more general model
which includes genetic variability at one locus within each species, and
show that even in this more general situation, coevolution is still

in the direction of such a maximum, and that a certain function (analogous to the Mac Arthur function) is maximised during this process.

In a previous paper (Matessi and Jayakar, 1975), we have used the
Lotka-Volterra model to study the effects of competition within a single
species between phenotypes determined by a single Mendelian locus. The
present model is an extension of that model to several species. Similar
models have been proposed by other authors. Fenchel and Christiansen
(1977) examined the consequences of such selection on the niche position
along a resource axis and on the niche width, and showed that it led to
changes in both. In particular they showed that ecological character
displacement took place - in other words, that species with an overlap
in their utilisation of the resource tended to diverge in their niche
position. Roughgarden (1976), also using a similar model, showed that
such niche separation increases with the variability of available resources and decreases when the number of species increases.

On the contrary, Slatkin (1979), using a different genetic determination, namely the Lande (1976) model for a continuous character,
found that character displacement occurs only in very particular situations.

Here we limit ourselves to developing certain general principles
of coevolution and to applying them to resources varying along a single
dimension, and discuss these contrasting results.

THE MODEL

We will consider models in discrete time only. The single species
density- and frequency-dependent model proposed by Matessi and Jayakar
(1975) used the Lotka-Volterra equations to decribe the competition
between phenotypes. The transition from one generation to the next can
be expressed, using the parametrisation introduced by Mac Arthur, (1969,
1970), by the following equations:

$$\nu_\alpha = N_\alpha \left\{ \frac{1}{r} + K - \sum_\beta A_{\alpha\beta} N_\beta \right\},$$

describing competition and

$$N^1 = r\nu = N + r\{KN - \sum_{\alpha}\sum_{\beta} A_{\alpha\beta} N_\alpha N_\beta\}$$

$$p_s^1 = p_s \{\frac{1}{r} + K - V_s(p)\}/ \{\frac{1}{r} + K - V(p)\} ,$$

describing reproduction with random mating, where N_α, ν_α are the densities of genotype α before and after competition has occurred, $\sum N_\alpha = N$ and $\sum \nu_\alpha = \nu$; N^1 is the total density in the successive generation; r is the average number of offspring produced by an individual. The K and A parameters are not the usual carrying capacity and competition coefficients of the Lotka-Volterra model but are proportional to them, differing by a factor $A_{\alpha\alpha}$. The vector $\{p_s\}$ is the vector of allele frequencies at the locus being considered, and $V_s(p)$ and $V(p)$ are functions of allele frequencies and of the A (interaction) parameters.

The multi-species extension of this model is immediate. Let $N_\alpha^{(i)}$ be the density of the genotype α of species i. Then using the Lotka-Volterra dynamics

$$\nu_\alpha^{(i)} = N_\alpha^{(i)} \{\frac{1}{r} + K_\alpha^{(i)} - \sum_j\sum_\beta A_{\alpha\beta}^{(ij)} N_\beta^{(j)}\} , \qquad (1.1)$$

where $\nu_\alpha^{(i)}$ are the post-competition densities, and $K_\alpha^{(i)}$ and $A_{\alpha\beta}^{(ij)}$ are Lotka-Volterra parameters standardised as before. $N^{(i)1}$, the densities in the next generation, are given by

$$N^{(i)1} = \sum_\alpha N_\alpha^{(i)1} = N^{(i)} + r\{\sum_\alpha K_\alpha^{(i)} N_\alpha^{(i)} - \sum_j\sum_\alpha\sum_\beta A_{\alpha\beta}^{(ij)} N_\alpha^{(i)} N_\beta^{(j)}\} . \qquad (1.2)$$

An assumption crucial to our analysis is that of symmetry of the matrix of interaction parameters (A s), namely that

$$A_{\alpha\beta}^{(ij)} = A_{\beta\alpha}^{(ji)} .$$

Though Slatkin and Maynard Smith (1979) criticise the use of a symmetric matrix in this context, most theoretical models of limiting similarity include such an assumption. Further, if exploitative competition is measured from niche overlap, a symmetric A matrix is a logical consequence.

Once again, we assume that the phenotypes are genotypes (within species) controlled by a single Mendelian locus; α, β etc. can then be written as (st), (uv), etc., where s, t, u, v denote the alleles at that locus. Since $N_\alpha^{(i)}$ etc. are counted immediately after random mating, they will be in Hardy-Weinberg proportions. Thus

$$N^1 = \sum_i N^{(i)^1} = N + rN\{ \sum_i \sum_s \sum_t K_{st}^{(i)} w^{(i)} p_s^{(i)} p_t^{(i)} -$$

$$- N \sum_i \sum_j \sum_s \sum_t \sum_u \sum_v A_{stuv}^{(ij)} w^{(i)} w^{(j)} p_s^{(i)} p_t^{(i)} p_u^{(j)} p_v^{(j)} \} ,$$

where $w^{(i)} = N^{(i)}/N$, are the relative species densities, $i = 1, \ldots, I$, I being the total number of species present.

Although, for convenience, the genotypes (st) and (uv) are considered distinct in these equations, with s, $t = 1, \ldots, S_i$, S_i being the number of alleles present at the locus in the ith species, the genetic hypothesis imposes further symmetries on the parameters, namely,

$$K_{st}^{(i)} = K_{ts}^{(i)} \; ; \; A_{stuv}^{(ij)} = A_{tsuv}^{(ij)} = A_{stvu}^{(ij)} = A_{tsvu}^{(ij)} .$$

We now define certain average Ks and As as follows:

$$K_s^{(i)} = \sum_t K_{st}^{(i)} p_t^{(i)} , \quad K^{(i)} = \sum_s K_s^{(i)} p_s^{(i)} , \quad K = \sum_i K^{(i)} w^{(i)} ; \quad (1.3)$$

$$A_{st}^{(i)} = \sum_j \sum_u \sum_v A_{stuv}^{(ij)} w^{(j)} p_u^{(j)} p_v^{(j)} , \quad A_s^{(i)} = \sum_t A_{st}^{(i)} p_t^{(i)} ,$$

$$A^{(i)} = \sum_s A_s^{(i)} p_s^{(i)} , \quad A = \sum_i A^{(i)} w^{(i)} . \quad (1.4)$$

This permits us to write down the dynamics of the system as follows:

$$N^1 = N + rN\{K - AN\} , \quad (1.5.1)$$

$$w^{(i)^1} = w^{(i)} \left\{ \frac{1/r + K^{(i)} - NA^{(i)}}{1/r + K - NA} \right\} , \quad i = 1, \ldots, I , \quad (1.5.2)$$

$$p_s^{(i)^1} = p_s^{(i)} \left\{ \frac{1/r + K_s^{(i)} - NA_s^{(i)}}{1/r + K^{(i)} - NA^{(i)}} \right\} , \quad i = 1, \ldots, I , \quad s = 1, \ldots, S_i . \quad (1.5.3)$$

The expressions (1.5) are in terms of the dynamics of the total population density (1.5.1), the relative density of species i (1.5.2), and
the frequency of allele s of species i (1.5.3). This is then the complete multispecies system.

EQUILIBRIA, STABILITY AND A MAXIMUM PRINCIPLE

From (1.5), one can directly write down the conditions for an
equilibrium, namely

$$K = AN , \tag{2.1.1}$$

$$K^{(i)} = NA^{(i)} , \quad i=1,\ldots,I , \tag{2.1.2}$$

$$K_s^{(i)} = NA_s^{(i)}, \quad s = 1,\ldots,S_i , \quad i = 1,\ldots,I, \tag{2.1.3}$$

or, written in a slightly different form,

$$N = \frac{K}{A} = \frac{K^{(i)}}{A^{(i)}} = \frac{K_s^{(i)}}{A_s^{(i)}} .$$

The function which Mac Arthur (1969, 1970) showed to attain a maximum
at equilibrium in his multispecies competition model can be written in
our notation as

$$\Psi = 2KN - AN^2 .$$

Let us find the stationary points of Ψ under the constraints

$$\sum_i w^{(i)} = 1; \quad \sum_s p_s^{(i)} = 1 , \quad i=1,\ldots,I .$$

By the method of Langrange multipliers the conditions for them can be
written as follows:

$$\frac{\partial \Psi}{\partial N} = 0 , \tag{2.2.1}$$

$$\frac{\partial \Psi}{\partial w^{(i)}} - \sum_i w^{(i)} \frac{\partial \Psi}{\partial w^{(i)}} = 0, \quad i = 1,\ldots,I , \tag{2.2.2}$$

$$\frac{\partial \Psi}{\partial p_s^{(i)}} - \sum_s p_s^{(i)} \frac{\partial \Psi}{\partial p_s^{(i)}} = 0, \quad s = 1,\ldots,S_i , \quad i = 1,\ldots, I. \tag{2.2.3}$$

But: $\dfrac{\partial \Psi}{\partial N} = 2K - 2AN ,$

and from (1.3) and (1.4), making use of symmetries:

$$\frac{\partial K}{\partial w^{(i)}} = K^{(i)}; \quad \frac{\partial K}{\partial p_s^{(i)}} = 2K_s^{(i)}; \quad \frac{\partial A}{\partial w^{(i)}} = 2A^{(i)}; \quad \frac{\partial A}{\partial p_s^{(i)}} = 4A_s^{(i)} .$$

Substituting these values into (2.2) gives us the same system as (2.1). Thus any interior equilibrium of the system is a stationary point of Ψ in the appropriate space. To examine whether this is a maximum, we resort to an approximation near the equilibrium. Since in this neighbourhood (with r small), all changes are of small magnitude, we can approximate the recursion system by a system of differential equations:

$$\dot{N} = rN(K-NA) , \qquad\qquad\qquad (2.3.1)$$

$$\dot{w}^{(i)} = rw^{(i)}\{K^{(i)}-NA^{(i)}-K+NA\} , \qquad\qquad (2.3.2)$$

$$\dot{p}_s^{(i)} = rp_s^{(i)}\{K_s^{(i)}-NA_s^{(i)}-K^{(i)}+NA^{(i)}\} . \qquad\qquad (2.3.3)$$

Hence,

$$\dot{\Psi} = 2\dot{K}N+2\dot{N}K-\dot{A}N^2-2\dot{N}NA$$

$$= 2rN(K-AN)^2+2rN\sum_i w^{(i)}\{K^{(i)}-NA^{(i)}-K+NA\}^2$$

$$+ 4rN\sum_{is}w^{(i)}p_s^{(i)}\{K_s^{(i)}-NA_s^{(i)}-K^{(i)}+NA^{(i)}\}^2 . \qquad (2.4)$$

Thus, in the immediate neighbourhood of an interior equilibrium of the system, $\dot{\Psi} > 0$, i.e. Ψ increases, which demonstrates that Ψ is maximised at a stable equilibrium. In other words, Ψ is a Ljapunov function for the system. This result is a generalisation of Mac Arthur's result. There may, of course, be more than one stable equilibrium, but Ψ has necessarily a local maximum at every stable equilibrium.

Mac Artur's (1969) interpretation of his results was that at a stable equilibrium the resources are utilised to the maximum possible. Matessi and Jayakar (1975) on the other hand showed that at their stable equilibria the average competition between genotypes was minimised. Here we obtain at once a generalisation of both these results.

If we fix the relative densities $w = \{w^{(1)},...,w^{(I)}\}$ and the gene frequencies $p^{(i)} = \{p_1^{(i)},...,p_s^{(i)}\}$ for $i = 1,...,I$, a maximisation of Ψ with respect to N gives $N = K/A$, and Ψ takes the values

$$\Gamma\{w,p^{(1)},...,p^{(I)}\} = K^2/A .$$

Thus at the stable equilibrium, Γ is also maximised with respect to w and the $p^{(i)}$s. Now if the $K_{st}^{(i)}$ are all equal, then coevolution is towards a minimisation of A. This is a generalisation of the Matessi--Jayakar principle for one species to the multispecies case. Thus the whole community behaves as a single species in coevolution with competition. Secondly, if we consider a single species with the Ks being different for the different phenotypes, then the result obtained here, namely the maximisation of Γ, is another kind of generalisation of the Matessi-Jayakar result. Further, if the As are equal for all species, while the Ks are different, coevolution proceeds so as to maximise the average K, namely the average carrying capacity of the community. When both Ks and As depend on the phenotype, a compromise solution must be reached and this compromise is the maximisation of Γ.

APPLICATION TO A CONTINUOUS RESOURCE AXIS

Mac Arthur (1969, 1970) has shown that if one analyses a model with prey whose dynamics is according to a Lotka-Volterra model, and several predators which depend on these prey, then the dynamics of the predators is given by the Lotka-Volterra competition equations. When one assumes that the prey (resource) are classified along a continuous axis (z), the parameters of the Lotka-Volterra competition model among predators are given by

$$K_i = \int \alpha_i(z)\gamma_i(z)k(z)dz - \varepsilon_i \; ,$$

$$A_{ij} = \int \alpha_i(z)\alpha_j(z)\gamma_j(z)\frac{k(z)}{\rho(z)}dz \; ,$$

where $\alpha_i(z)$ = rate at which predator i preys on the resource at point z of the axis, given a certain abundance of the resource (the utilisation function);

$\gamma_i(z)$ = the conversion efficiency of resource at z by predator i;

$k(z)$ = abundance of resource at z in the absence of predators;

$\rho(z)$ = rate of growth of resource at z;

ε_i = mortality rate of predator i in the absence of resources. If we now assume $\gamma_i(z) = \gamma$ for each predator and resource type, $k(z)$ proportional to $\rho(z)$, and if we incorporate γ into $k(z)$, then we have

$$K_i \propto \int \alpha_i(z)k(z)dz - \varepsilon_i \ ,$$

$$A_{ij} \propto \int \alpha_i(z)\alpha_j(z)dz \ .$$

The term ε_i needs to be handled with some care. If, as is usual, we incorporate it into $k(z)$ so as to define $k_i(z) = k(z) - \varepsilon_i$, and if we assume that $\int k(z)dz = \bar{k} < \infty$ (as is reasonable), then for $|z|$ sufficiently large, $k(z) - \varepsilon_i$ becomes negative, and $\int k_i(z)dz$ is unbounded. If, on the other hand, $k(z) \geq \varepsilon_i$ for all values of z, $\int k_i(z)dz$ can be finite but $\bar{k}$ must be infinite.

Let us consider now a community of several consumers (predators), each with its utilisation function $\alpha_i(z)$, then the total utilisation by the community of the resource at value z will be

$$\phi(z) = \sum_i w^{(i)} \alpha_i(z) \ .$$

Assuming $\varepsilon_i = \varepsilon$ for all i, and writing $k(z)$ for $k(z) - \varepsilon$,

$$K = \int k(z)\phi(z)dz \ ,$$

$$A = \int \phi^2(z)dz \ .$$

Thus coevolution would lead to the maximisation of

$$\Gamma(\phi) = (\int k\phi dz)^2 / \int \phi^2 dz,$$

with the conditions

$$\phi(z) \geq 0 \text{ for all } z, \tag{3.1.1}$$

$$\int \phi(z)dz = \Phi \text{, a costant } (>0) \ . \tag{3.1.2}$$

The latter condition implies that the total harvesting ability of the community is not allowed to change in coevolution.

Under these conditions, we now wish, by applying the maximisation result, to examine how ϕ changes in coevolution. We will let $\phi(z)$ change without any constraint other than those listed above. Let us consider the two possibilities discussed above.

__Case 1.__ $k(z)>0$, $\int k(z)dz =\bar{k} <\infty.$

We can maximise $\Gamma(\phi)$ over all $\phi(z)$ which satisfy (3.1). Consider $\phi^*(z) = ck(z)/\bar{k}$, where c is a constant.

$$\Gamma(\phi^*) = \int k^2(z)dz \ .$$

From the Schwarz inequality,

$$\int k^2 dz \ \int \phi^2 dz \ \geq \ (\int k\phi dz)^2 \ ,$$

and the equality holds only for $\phi(z)$ proportional to $k(z)$. Thus we have demonstrated that $\Gamma(\phi)$ is maximised when the community utilises the resources in such a way that

$$\phi(z) = ck(z)/\bar{k} \ ,$$

and in this situation, the size of the community achieves the value

$$N = \frac{K}{A} = \frac{\int k(z)\phi^*(z)dz}{\int \phi^{*2}(z)dz} = \frac{\bar{k}}{c} \ ,$$

which is proportional to the total abundance of the resource. Thus, a coevolving community of competing species changes its utilisation pattern so as to exactly match the utilisation function to the resource spectrum along the axis, which is also what the Mac Arthur principle predicts.

__Case 2.__ $k(z)>0$ for $|z|\leq z_0$; $k(z)<0$ otherwise.

For any ϕ, let us define $\tilde{\phi}(z)$ such that

$$\tilde{\phi}(z) \ \propto\phi(z) \text{ for } |z|\leq z_0,$$

and $\tilde{\phi}(z) = 0$ otherwise.

Now :

$$\Gamma(\tilde{\phi}) = \{\int_{-z_0}^{z_0} k(z)\phi(z)dz\}^2 \ / \ \{\int_{-z_0}^{z_0} \phi^2(z)dz\}.$$

But $0<\int k\phi dz<\infty$. The right hand inequality follows from the fact that k is bounded and $\int \phi dz$ is finite; the left hand inequality must be satisfied if the population is to persist (see eq. 3.1).
Since:

$$\Gamma(\phi) = \{\int_{-z_0}^{z_0} k(z)\phi(z)dz - a\}^2 / \{\int_{-z_0}^{z_0}\phi^2(z)dz + b\} \, ,$$

where

$$b \geq 0, \text{ and } \int_{-z_0}^{z_0} k(z)\phi(z)dz \geq a \geq 0,$$

then

$$\Gamma(\tilde{\phi}) \geq \Gamma(\phi) \, .$$

Defining $\tilde{\phi}(z)$ in this manner implies that the resource range utilised is confined to $|z| \leq z_0$, i.e.

$$\tilde{k}(z) = k(z) \text{ for } |z| \leq z_0$$

and $\tilde{k}(z) = 0$ otherwise.

We can then apply the result of case 1 and the ϕ^* which maximises Γ is proportional to $\tilde{k}$. We have thus demonstrated that if no constraints are placed on ϕ, then coevolution leads to a $\phi^*(z)$ which is exactly proportional to $\tilde{k}(z)$ over the whole range of the resource axis.

In general, however, a genetic determination of $\phi(z)$ would impose certain restrictions. We will now consider some of the implications of such constraints. First let us assume that there is a family of variants, the variant θ having a utilisation function denoted by $h_\theta(z)$ and the probability density function of θ is $f(\theta)$. Thus

$$\phi(z) = \int f(\theta)h_\theta(z)d\theta \, .$$

We assume that selection acts on $f(\theta)$, while the $h_\theta(z)$ are fixed. If θ determines the location of the utilisation function, while leaving all other properties unchanged, then

$$h_\theta(z) = h(z - \theta).$$

At a stable equilibrium, $f(\theta)$ should be such that

$$\int f(\theta)h(z - \theta)d\theta = ck(z).$$

This can be solved for $f(\theta)$ and hence the community will again evolve towards a proportional utilisation of the resource spectrum available independent of the form of $h_\theta(z)$.

Let us now consider the case of only two different phenotypes with utilisation functions respectively $g(z)$ and $h(z)$, and with relative densities w and $(1-w)$. If evolution can act without restrictions on the shapes of g and h, then they will evolve so that

$\phi(z)=wg(z)+(1-w)h(z)$

corresponds exactly to the shape of $k(z)$, the resource spectrum; in other words, both g and h will match k.

All these example show that if the constraints on the utilisation functions are sufficiently lax, then the community always succeeds in making $\phi(z)$ the same shape as $k(z)$, and in this situation, phenomena such as limiting similarity and character displacement will not evolve since these imply an imperfect fit between availability and utilisation of resources. In order for there to be a lack of fit, the number of phenotypes must be finite and their shape during evolution should also be incapable of evolving unrestrained.

Let us now consider cases where such constraints are imposed and explore the evolution of character displacement. Assume there are two species with utilisation functions

$$h\left\{\frac{z-m_1}{\sigma_1}\right\} \text{ and } h\left\{\frac{z-m_2}{\sigma_2}\right\} ,$$

where m_1 and m_2 are the respective niche locations and σ_1 and σ_2 are the niche widths (standard deviations), and assume that the resource spectrum is defined by $h(z)$. Notice that all the hs denote the same form of distribution. If now the ms and the σs are all allowed to evolve on a continuous scale, then both the ms will evolve towards 0 and both the σs towards 1, so that once again, ϕ evolves so as to match $h(z)$ perfectly. If, however, we impose a constraint so that only the niche locations can evolve while σ_1 and σ_2 are held constant, things are somewhat different. Consider the case of Gaussian distribution, i.e.

$$h(z)=exp\left(-\frac{1}{2}z^2\right) .$$

It can be shown in this situation that the interaction parameters (A) are proportional to

$$(V_1+V_2)^{-\frac{1}{2}}exp\left\{-\frac{(m_1-m_2)^2}{2(V_1+V_2)}\right\} = C , \text{ say,}$$

and the K parameter of species i to

$$(V_1+V_2)^{\frac{1}{2}}(1+V_i)^{-\frac{1}{2}}exp\left\{-\frac{m_i^2}{2(1+V_i)}\right\} = D_i(V_1+V_2)^{\frac{1}{2}} , \text{ say,}$$

where $V_i=\sigma_i^2$.

Let us put $(2V_i)^{-\frac{1}{2}}=E_i$. Then Γ can be written in the form

$$\Gamma = \frac{(V_1+V_2)\{wD_1+(1-w)D_2\}^2}{2w(1-w)C+w^2E_1+(1-w)^2E_2} \, ,$$

and in order to find the equilibrium conditions it suffices to maximise this expression with respect to w, m_1 and m_2. When one does this, the conditions turn out to be

$$\frac{w}{1-w} = \frac{CD_2-E_2D_1}{CD_1-E_1D_2} \, , \qquad\qquad (3.2.1)$$

$$\frac{wD_1m_1}{1+V_1} \{ w^2E_1+(1-w)^2E_2+2w(1-w)C \} =$$

$$= \{ wD_1+(1-w)D_2 \} \frac{Cw(1-w)(m_1-m_2)}{V_1+V_2} \, , \qquad\qquad (3.2.2)$$

$$-\frac{(1-w)D_2m_2}{1+V_2} \{ w^2E_1+(1-w)^2E_2+2w(1-w)C \} =$$

$$= \{ wD_1+(1-w)D_2 \} \frac{Cw(1-w)(m_1-m_2)}{V_1+V_2} \, . \qquad\qquad (3.2.3)$$

At equilibrium, then, either $\hat{m}_1=\hat{m}_2=0$, or $\hat{m}_1\neq\hat{m}_2$ and $\hat{m}_i\neq0$, $i=1,2$, and in the second case,

$$\frac{wD_1m_1}{(1-w)D_2m_2} \frac{1+V_2}{1+V_1} = -1 \, ,$$

and since all the quantities involved except $\hat{m}_1$ and $\hat{m}_2$ are positive, in (3.2.2) and (3.2.3), $\hat{m}_1$ and $\hat{m}_2$ must have opposite signs. We proceed now to examine whether both these equilibria exist, and if so, which of them is stable. We consider here various situations.

Case 1. $V_1 \neq V_2$.

Consider the equilibrium with $\hat{m}_1=\hat{m}_2=0$. Then, from (3.2.1),

$$\frac{\hat{w}}{1-\hat{w}} = \frac{\sigma_1}{\sigma_2} \frac{\{2V_2(1+V_1)\}^{\frac{1}{2}} - \{(V_1+V_2)(1+V_2)\}^{\frac{1}{2}}}{\{2V_1(1+V_2)\}^{\frac{1}{2}} - \{(V_1+V_2)(1+V_1)\}^{\frac{1}{2}}} \qquad\qquad (3.3)$$

Thus for an equilibrium to exist with $0<\hat{w}<1$, the numerator and denominator of (3.3) must have the same sign, i.e. either

$$\frac{2V_1}{V_1+V_2} > \frac{1+V_1}{1+V_2} > \frac{V_1+V_2}{2V_2} \; , \tag{3.4.1}$$

or

$$\frac{2V_1}{V_1+V_2} < \frac{1+V_1}{1+V_2} < \frac{V_1+V_2}{2V_2} \; . \tag{3.4.2}$$

The inequalities (3.4.1) are impossible to satisfy. Hence at such an equilibrium, (3.4.2) must be true, and this reduces to

$$V_1 < 1 < V_2 \quad \text{or} \quad V_2 < 1 < V_1 \; .$$

Thus an equilibrium with both species present with niche locations at $z=0$ is not possible unless one of the species has a niche wider than the width of the resource spectrum and the other has a niche narrower than the resource spectrum. We have here the rather interesting situation of a generalist and a specialist in coexistence.

If both species have niches wider than or narrower than the resource spectrum width, then one or the other of these species must go extinct and presumably the surviving species is the one which has a width closer to that of the resource spectrum, since it has the closest match with the available resource distribution. Alternatively, there could be character displacement towards the other kind of equilibrium, and the niche locations move towards $\hat{m}_1$ and $\hat{m}_2$ on opposite sides of the spectrum centre.

Case 2. $V_1 = V_2$.

In this case, if $\hat{m}_1 = \hat{m}_2 = 0$, then the two species have identical niches, and therefore w can take any value between 0 and 1 at equilibrium. If $\hat{m}_1 \neq \hat{m}_2$, then there is an equilibrium with

$$\hat{m}_1 = -\hat{m}_2 \; , \quad \text{and} \quad \hat{w} = 1/2 \; .$$

In other words, the two species take up symmetrical positions on either side of the spectrum centre. Whether there are also asymmetric equilibria, we have not been able to find out.

Let us examine the symmetric equilibrium more closely. Let

$$\hat{m}_1 = -\hat{m}_2 = \mu \; , \quad \text{and} \quad V_1 = V_2 = V \; .$$

Then

$$C = (2V)^{-\frac{1}{2}} exp(-\mu^2/V) \; ,$$

$$D_i = D = (1+V)^{-\frac{1}{2}} exp\{- \frac{\mu^2}{2(1+V)}\} \; , \; i=1,2 \; ,$$

$$E_i = E = (2V)^{-\frac{1}{2}} \; , \; i=1,2 \; .$$

Then, from (3.2),

$$\frac{w}{1-w} = 1 \; , \; \text{or} \; \hat{w} = \frac{1}{2} \; ,$$

$$\frac{E+C}{1+V} = \frac{C}{V} \; , \; \text{or} \; C = VE \; ,$$

which gives us the solution

$$\hat{m}_1^2 = \hat{m}_2^2 = \mu^2 = -V \; ln(V) \; . \tag{3.5}$$

Thus this equilibrium can exist only if $V{\le}1$. In other words, character displacement can take place only if the niches of the two species are narrower than the resource spectrum. The displacement is largest when the niche width is about 0.6 times the width of the resource spectrum. At this point it becomes twice the niche width or about 1.2 times the standard deviation of the resource.

We proceed now to examine the stability of these two equilibria. Since an equilibrium is stable if and only if it is a maximum of Γ, the necessary and sufficient condition for stability is that the $3{\times}3$ matrix of the second partial derivatives of Γ, evaluated at the equilibrium point, be negative definite. Let us refer the first row (column) of this matrix to w and the second and third to m_1 and m_2 respectively. For the "convergence" equilibrium, $\hat{m}_1 = \hat{m}_2 = 0$, this matrix is proportional, by a positive factor, to

$$\underline{\underline{H}}_C = \left\| \begin{matrix} 0 & 0 & 0 \\ 0 & a-b & -a \\ 0 & -a & a-c \end{matrix} \right\| \; ,$$

where

$$a = \frac{w(1-w)}{2V} \; , \; b = \frac{w}{1+V} \; , \; c = \frac{1-w}{1+V}$$

All partial derivatives with respect to w in $\underline{\underline{H}}_C$ are zero for the obvious reason that at this equilibrium the two species are identical and hence Γ is insensitive to w. When $V{>}1$ both remaining eigenvalues of $\underline{\underline{H}}_C$ are negative. When $V{<}1$, $\underline{\underline{H}}_C$ has one positive and one negative eigenvalue. We thus conclude that the convergence equilibrium is stable only when the two species have niches broader than the resource spectrum.

For the "displacement" equilibrium the relevant matrix is

$$\underline{H}_D = \begin{Vmatrix} -d & -e & -e \\ -e & f-g & f+g \\ -e & f+g & f-g \end{Vmatrix} ,$$

where

$$d = 16(1-V) \; , \;\; e = 4\mu \; , \;\; f = \frac{\mu^2}{1+V} -1 \; , \;\; g = \frac{2\mu^2}{V(1+V)} \; ,$$

and μ is as defined in (3.5). From the Hurwitz criterion one obtains the following conditions which are necessary and sufficient for $\underline{H}_D$ being negative definite

$$d+2(g-f) > 0 \; ,$$
$$(d+2g)(g-f)-e^2 > 0 \; ,$$
$$df+e^2 < 0 \; .$$

These conditions are satisfied for all $0<V<1$. We conclude therefore that the displacement equilibrium is stable whenever it exists. Ecological character displacement is the stable evolutionary outcome when two competing species have niches of equal width and narrower than the resource spectrum. Coexisting species of broad niche evolve towards convergence, while species of narrow niche evolve towards divergence.

CONCLUSIONS

This model for the coevolution of several genetically variable species in a purely competitive situation described by the Lotka-Volterra equations leads us to the result that a certain function is maximised during this process. This is a generalisation of the principle which Mac Arthur (1969,1970) demonstrated for competing species in the absence of any genetic variation. It is also a generalisation of the result of Matessi and Jayakar (1975) for the evolution of a single genetically variable species whose phenotypes are in competition with each other.

This very general maximisation principle can be interpreted in a more concrete fashion if the parameters of the Lotka-Volterra equations are calculated in terms of a production function and a utilisation function on a resource axis. The maximisation principle is then equivalent

to a tendency of the community utilisation function to converge towards
the resource production function. This is true independently of the number of species, and both when the species can evolve genetically and
when they can not.

This general principle is a powerful tool for studying particular
ecological problems. In any given situation, the behaviour of the function which is maximised gives us the information we need for predictions
regarding coevolution. Species packing and character displacement, for
example, can be examined in this way.

In the example of two competing species, the niche shapes of the
two competing species are crucial to the consequences of coevolution.
If the niches can vary without restraint, both species (in any proportion) can evolve towards the shape of the resource spectrum. However,
if only location of the niche can vary, while its variance remains
fixed, the values of these variances with respect to that of the resource spectrum determine the fates of the species. In particular, character displacement depends on the species having narrow enough niches.
Two species with niches both broader than or narrower than the resource
spectrum cannot coexist if their niches are both located at the centre of
the resource spectrum, except in the limiting situation where the niche
widths are identical. In the latter situation, convergence of the two
species will occur if the niches are wider than the resource spectrum.
On the other hand, if their niche widths are less than that of the resource spectrum, character displacement will take place. This delicate
dependence of character displacement on the niche widths explains the
controversy in the literature regarding this phenomenon (see e.g. Fenchel and Christiansen, 1977 and Slatkin, 1979).

We seem then to have found a unifying principle which ties together several apparently unrelated results of theoretical ecology.

SUMMARY

A Lotka-Volterra model for coevolution of several diploid species
in competition has been presented. The genetic variation within each

species is assumed to be controlled by a single multi-allelic Mendelian locus which influences the parameters of the competition equations. A function, analogous to that found by Mac Arthur (1969, 1970) in a situation of interspecific competition without genetic variation, is shown to be maximised at all stable equilibria of this system. When the ecological parameters are interpreted in terms of a continuous unidimensional resource spectrum and utilisation functions, it is found that the maximisation principle leads to the conclusion that the community utilisation tends in coevolution to match the resource spectrum as closely as possible. Hence, the final outcome is dependent on the constraints imposed by the available genetic variability. In particular, an analysis of character displacement shows that the latter can evolve only if the niche widths of the competing species are held narrower than the resource spectrum.

REFERENCES

FENCHEL, T.M. and CHRISTIANSEN, F.B. 1977. Selection and interspecific competition. In "Measuring Selection in Natural Populations", F.B. Christiansen and T.M. Fenchel (Eds). Lecture Notes in Biomathematics, 19. Springer-Verlag, Heidelberg.

LANDE, R. 1976. The maintenance of genetic variability by mutation in a polygenic character with linked loci. Genet. Res., 26:221-235.

MAC ARTHUR, R.H. 1969 Species packing and what interspecies competition minimises. Proc. Natl. Acad. Sc., USA, 64:1369-1371.

MAC ARTHUR, R.H. 1970. Species packing and competitive equilibrium for many species. Theor. Pop. Biol., 1:1-11.

MATESSI, C. and JAYAKAR, S.D. 1975. Models of density- and frequency-dependent selection for the exploitation of resources. I. Intraspecific competition. In "Population Genetics and Ecology", S. Karlin and E. Nevo (Eds). Academic Press, New York.

ROUGHGARDEN, J. 1976. Resource partitioning among competing species - a coevolutionary approach. Theor. Pop. Biol., 9:388-424.

SLATKIN, M. 1979. Ecological character displacement. Ecology, 60 (in press).

SLATKIN, M. and MAYNARD SMITH, J. 1979. Models of coevolution. Quart. Rev. Biol., 54:233-263.

INTRASPECIFIC COMPETITION AND EVOLUTION

Freddy Bugge Christiansen and Volker Loeschcke

Institute of Ecology and Genetics, University of Aarhus, Aarhus, Denmark.
Department of Biological Sciences, Stanford University, California 94305.
Institute of Genetics, Free University of Berlin, Arnimallee 5-7, Berlin.

Introduction

The formulation of ecological genetic models allows specific assumptions about the interaction between an individual and its environment to be translated into evolutionary forces in the population. An approach to this is the analysis of phenotypic characters related to competition coefficients through the use of the niche concept as formulated by Mac-Arthur and Levins (1967; Levins, 1968). This formulation has been used in the analysis of intraspecific competition by Roughgarden (1972), Matessi and Jayakar (1976), and Christiansen and Fenchel (1977; Fenchel and Christiansen, 1977). The models used in these investigations are classical population genetic models with discrete non-overlapping generations, where the individual fitnesses are considered as functions of the population density (Wright, 1960). Intraspecific competition for a common uniform food supply will allow the influence of competition on the growth rate to be described in terms of the total population size of the species (Volterra, 1927; Lotka, 1932) resulting in pure density dependent selection (Anderson, 1971; Charlesworth, 1971; Roughgarden, 1971; Clarke, 1972). On the other hand, intraspecific competition for a more varied supply of resources may make the competition experienced by an individual dependent on the genotypic composition of the population resulting in so-called density and frequency dependent selection. For pure density dependent selection evolution will increase the population size in a well behaved population (Roughgarden, 1976; Asmussen and Feldman, 1976), a result which parallels the fundamental theorem of natural selection (Fisher, 1930; MacArthur, 1962; Ginzburg, 1977). However, in discrete generation models the result is not universal (Asmussen and Feldman, 1976; Prout, 1980), and it seems to be a feature of the formulation in terms of genotypic fitness values rather than a more complicated full ecological description of the population (Poulsen, 1980; Christiansen and Fenchel, 1977). Matessi and Jayakar (1976) established a similar result for more general intraspecific competition, in that for symmetric competition coefficients, in the sence of Gause (1934), the average competition expecienced by an individual in the population will decline during evolution if the genotypes only differ with respect to competition. However, in their general model for intraspecific competition neither maximalization of population size nor minimalization of competition occurs.

The exploitative competition model of MacArthur and Levins (1964; MacArthur, 1972) is an excellent device for predicting the parameters of an ecological model in terms of individual phenotypic characteristics. The growth of the population is assumed to be proportional to the ammount of food available to the individual, and an individual sences the pressence of other individuals only through the decline in available resources. The model is formulated as a Lotka-Volterra predator-prey model, where the species of interest are predators and the prey species are the food resources. By assuming that the generation times of the resources are very short compared to that of the species of interest, and that the rates of exploitation of the resources are very high, the growth and competition of the species of interest can be formulated simply in terms of their choise of resources and the availabillity of those resources. This model produces a competition model, which is mathematically equivalent to the Lotka-Volterra competition model, and which shares important aspects of the parametrization with these models, in particular the proportionality between the carrying capacity parameter and the intrinsic growth rate (Christiansen and Fenchel, 1977).

The choice of food resources is often correlated to a measurable phenotypic trait of the individual, e.g. head size and prey size in Anolis lizzards (Schoener and Gorman, 1968; Roughgarden, 1972) and body size and food particle size in Hydrobia snails (Fenchel, 1975). The competition in Hydrobia is well described by the competition model of MacArthur and Levins (Fenchel and Kofoed, 1976). These kinds of characters is usually determined by many genes, and their mode of inheritance is described by the use of quantitative genetics. Thus, it is natural to use methods from quantitative genetics to study their evolution (Bulmer, 1974; Slatkin, 1979). However, it is equally important to study the evolution of these characters at the level of single gene loci or pairs of loci to determine the structure of genetic variation for characters involved in exploitative competition. This approach to the study of intraspecific exploitative competition has been developed by Christiansen and Fenchel (1977) and Christiansen and Loeschcke (1980), and we will in the following review and extend some of the results. The parameters of the model is defined in terms of individual phenotypes in an ecological context, and the growth equations used should be viewed as a discrete time approximation to the Lotka-Volterra competition equations using the exploitative competition model of MacArthur and Levins (1964, 1967; Levins, 1968; MacArthur, 1972).

THE MODEL

Consider a measurable phenotypic character with individual values M which is related to the choice of resources made by the individual. Let the individuals in the population compete for resources in a one dimensional continuum, and let the resource availability in the absence of exploitation be given by a Gaussian resource spectrum, $N(0, \sigma^2)$, i.e., the mode of the resource spectrum is arbitrarily set at zero and the variance in available resource qualities is σ^2. Let the individual choice of resources be given by a Gaussian utilization function $N(M+D,V_U)$, where D is an arbitrary constant chosen to align the scale of resource qualities and the scale of phenotypic values (assumed to be measured in comparable units), and where V_U (assumed independent of M) is the variance among resources chosen by the individual. These definitions and the phenotypic distribution of M in the population defines the ecological parameters up to a proportionality constant by using the exploitative competition model of MacArthur and Levins (1964; Christiansen and Fenchel, 1977).

Consider a locus with n alleles, A_1, A_2,..., A_n, which influences the character M. We assume that the character follows a Gaussian distribution for given genotype, i.e., $M|A_iA_j \sim N(g_{ij},V_E)$, where g_{ij} is the genotypic mean value and V_E is the environmental variance or residual phenotypic variance which is assumed equal among genotypes. The mean and genotypic variance in the population is, under the assumption that reproduction occurs by random mating, given by

$$m = \sum_i \sum_j g_{ij} \, p_i \, p_j \tag{1}$$

$$s^2 = \sum_i \sum_j (g_{ij} - m)^2 \, p_i \, p_j \tag{2}$$

where p_i is the gene frequency of allele A_i for $i = 1,2,...,n$. Thus the total variance of the character in the population is

$$V_P = V_E + s^2 \tag{3}$$

The utilization variance of the genotypes is

$$W^2 = V_E + V_U, \tag{4}$$

so the total utilization variance in the population can be partitioned in two ways:

$$V_P + V_U \ = \ s^2 + W^2 \ , \tag{5}$$

where the first partitioning is the ecologically observable components, viz., the between individual component and the within individual component (Roughgarden, 1972; Fenchel, 1975), and the second partitioning is the evolutionarily relevant components, viz., the genotypic variance and the within genotype variance.

Among adults let y_{ij} $(i \neq j)$ be half the number of heterozygotes $A_i A_j$ and let y_{ii} be the number of homozygotes $A_i A_i$, i and j = 1,2,...,n. The number of individuals in the population is then

$$y_{..} \ = \ \sum_i \sum_j y_{ij} \ , \tag{6}$$

and the number of alleles A_i is

$$y_{i.} \ = \ \sum_j y_{ij} \tag{7}$$

so the gene frequency is $p_i = y_{i.}/y_{..}$. We suppose that these adults reproduce by random union of gametes with equal fecundities, so the number of offspring of genotype $A_i A_j$ will be proportional to $p_i p_j y_{..}$. The number of adults of genotype $A_i A_j$ in the offspring generation is then given in terms of the numbers

$$y_{ij}' \ = \ p_i p_j y_{..} \{1 + V(K_{ij} - \overline{\gamma}_{ij} y_{..})\} \ , \tag{8}$$

where

$$\overline{\gamma}_{ij} \ = \ \sum_k \sum_\ell \gamma_{ij,k\ell} \, p_k p_\ell \tag{9}$$

(Christiansen and Loeschcke, 1980). The parameter V (assumed less than one for technical reasons) is a proportionality constant related to the conversion of resources into individuals,

$$K_{ij} = \exp\{-(D + g_{ij})^2/(2\sigma^2 + 2W^2)\} \tag{10}$$

is a measure of the amount of resources available to individuals of genotype $A_i A_j$, and

$$\gamma_{ij,k\ell} = \exp\{-(g_{ij} - g_{k\ell})^2/(4W^2)\} \tag{11}$$

is a measure of the overlap in resource utilization between the genotypes $A_i A_j$ and $A_k A_\ell$ (Christiansen and Fenchel, 1977; Christiansen and Loeschcke, 1980).

From equation (8) the recurrence equations in the population size and the gene frequencies are

$$y_{..}' = y_{..}\{1 + V(K_{oo} - \overline{\gamma}_{oo} y_{..})\} \quad \text{and} \tag{12}$$

$$p_i' = p_i\{1 + V(K_{io} - \overline{\gamma}_{io} y_{..})\}/\{1 + V(K_{oo} - \overline{\gamma}_{oo} y_{..})\}, \tag{13}$$

where

$$K_{io} = \sum_j K_{ij} p_j, \quad K_{oo} = \sum_i K_{io} p_i, \quad \overline{\gamma}_{io} = \sum_j \overline{\gamma}_{ij} p_j, \quad \overline{\gamma}_{oo} = \sum_i \overline{\gamma}_{io} p_i. \tag{14}$$

These equations correspond to a classical population genetic model with density and frequency dependent fitnesses, i.e., the fitness of genotype $A_i A_j$ is

$$w_{ij} = 1 + V(K_{ij} - \overline{\gamma}_{ij} y_{..}), \tag{15}$$

so the ecological model has primarily been used to provide the functional form of these fitnesses and their correspondence to the genotypic values through (10) and (11). Allthough the competition coefficients (11) are symmetric, the fitnesses (15) are not corresponding to symmetric competition in the sence of Matessi and Jayakar (1976).

We will be mainly concerned with the situation where the genotypic values are close together, i.e., we assume that the considered locus has a small effect on the character. We may assume that the genotypic values are all numerically small, as the origin of the scale of measurement of the phenotypic variable can be chosen at will by adjusting the constant D. When the genotypic values are small, the parameters (10) and (11) are approximately given by

$$K_{ij} = \exp(-D^2/b) \times \left(1 - 2Dg_{ij}/b - g_{ij}^2/b + 2D^2 g_{ij}^2/b^2\right) , \qquad (16)$$

where $b = 2\sigma^2 + 2W^2$, and by

$$\gamma_{ij,k\ell} = 1 - (g_{ij} - g_{k\ell})^2/(4W^2) , \qquad (17)$$

where thrid and higher order terms in the genotypic values have been neglected in (16) and (17).

Finally, we will limit attention to intermediate dominance, i.e., for all i and j we will assume that

$$\text{if } g_{jj} < g_{ii} \text{ then } g_{jj} \le g_{ij} \le g_{ii} , \qquad (18)$$

and for definiteness we assume $g_{11} < g_{22} < \ldots < g_{nn}$. Two specific models will be discussed: The additive model with

$$g_{ij} = d_i + d_j , \qquad (19)$$

where d_i, $i = 1,2,\ldots,n$, are numerically small allele contributions to the character with $d_1 < d_2 < \ldots < d_n$. Secondly, the constant dominance model with

$$g_{ij} = d_i + d_j + a|d_i - d_j| , \qquad (20)$$

where d_i is as in the additive model and a, $-1 \le a \le 1$, is a dominance constant.

RESULTS

The evolution of the population depends strongly on the value of D, i.e., on the position of the genotypes in relation to the resource optimum. If $|g_{ij}| \ll |D|$ for all i and j = 1,2,...,n, then the population will evolve to become monomorphic for the allele whose corresponding homozygote makes $|g_{ii} + D|$ minimal, i.e., the population will evolve to use resources as close to the resource optimum as possible. In this situation the genotypic fitnesses are mainly determined by the parameters K_{ij} since the competition coefficients $\gamma_{ij,k\ell}$ only deviates from one by second order terms in the genotypic values and K_{ij} varies with the genotypic values. Thus the variation is subject to directional selection towards the resource optimum, and it will be monomorphic A_1A_1 if D > 0 and A_nA_n if D < 0 as we assumed $g_{11} < g_{22} < \ldots < g_{nn}$.

If all the genotypes in the population utilize resources close to the resource optimum, then we may choose D = 0 and measure the genotypic values as deviations from the value corresponding to a coincidence of the utilization mode and the resource optimum. By assuming the genotypic values small we get from (16)

$$K_{ij} = 1 - g_{ij}^2/(2\sigma^2 + 2W^2) . \tag{21}$$

Forming the averages (9) and (14) of the competition coefficients (17) we get

$$\overline{\gamma}_{ij} = 1 - \{(g_{ij} - m)^2 + s^2\}/(4W^2) , \tag{22}$$

$$\overline{\gamma}_{io} = 1 - (\xi^2_i + \alpha_i^2 + s^2)/(4W^2) , \tag{23}$$

$$\overline{\gamma}_{oo} = 1 - 2 s^2/(4W^2) , \tag{24}$$

where s^2 is the genotypic variance given by (2), α_i is the average effect of allele A_i, i.e.,

$$\alpha_i = \sum_j (g_{ij} - m) p_j \quad , \quad \text{and} \tag{25}$$

$$\xi^2{}_i = \sum_j (g_{ij} - m - \alpha_i)^2 p_j \quad . \tag{26}$$

Further, the averages (14) of the parameters (21) are

$$K_{io} = 1 - \{\xi^2{}_i + (m + \alpha_i)^2\}/(2\sigma^2 + 2W^2) \quad , \tag{27}$$

$$K_{oo} = 1 - (s^2 + m^2)/(2\sigma^2 + 2W^2) \quad . \tag{28}$$

We assume that the changes in population size are rapid compared to the changes in gene frequencies mediated by the small differences in genotypic values. Thus, we assume that equation (12) has reached its equilibrium,

$$y_{..} = K_{oo}/\overline{\gamma}_{oo} \quad , \tag{29}$$

when we study the changes in the gene frequencies given by equation (13). The condition for increase of the gene frequency of allele A_i is then

$$K_{io}\,\overline{\gamma}_{oo} > K_{oo}\,\overline{\gamma}_{io} \quad , \tag{30}$$

which from (23), (24), (27) and (28) is approximately the same as

$$(\kappa^2 - 1)(\xi^2{}_i + \alpha_i{}^2 - s^2) > 4\,m\,\alpha_i \quad , \tag{31}$$

where $\kappa = \sigma/W$ is the ratio of the resource width to the genotypic utilization width. From condition (31) it immediately follows that different patterns of evolution are expected when $\sigma > W$ and when $\sigma < W$ (for $\sigma = W$ the analysis later degenerates, so assume $\sigma \neq W$). Thus the changes in gene frequencies from a given initial condition is in opposite directions dependent on whether the resource width is wide compared to the utilization width or whether the resource width is comparatively narrow.

Suppose the population is initially monomorphic $A_j A_j$, and suppose the allele A_i is introduced in a low frequency, then the introduced allele will increase in frequency, from (31), if

$$(\kappa^2 - 1)(g_{ij} - g_{jj})\{g_{ij} - g_{jj}(\kappa^2 + 3)/(\kappa^2 - 1)\} > 0 , \quad (32)$$

and it will decrease if the opposite is true. If condition (32) and the similar condition with i and j interchanged both holds, then A_i and A_j will be kept in a polymorphic state in the population. From the assumption of intermediate dominance (18) we can conclude from (32), that in a population where only alleles A_i and A_j are possible, either the two alleles will be kept in a protected polymorphism, i.e., both fixation equilibria are unstable, or only one of the fixation equilibria is stable and the other unstable.

If the alleles A_i and A_j ($g_{ii} > g_{jj}$, say) are maintained at a stable equilibrium in the population, then a rare allele A_k will increase in frequency, from (31), if

$$(\kappa^2 - 1)\{\xi^2_i(\alpha_j - \alpha_i) + \xi^2_j(\alpha_k - \alpha_i) + \xi^2_k(\alpha_i - \alpha_j) - (\alpha_j - \alpha_k)(\alpha_k - \alpha_i)(\alpha_i - \alpha_j)\}$$

$$> 0 \quad (33)$$

and decrease if the opposite is true; the quantities in the condition (33) are given by

$$\xi^2_i = p_i p_j (g_{ii} - g_{ij})^2 ,$$

$$\xi^2_j = p_i p_j (g_{ij} - g_{jj})^2 , \quad (34)$$

$$\xi^2_k = p_i p_j (g_{ik} - g_{jk})^2 ,$$

and

$$\alpha_i - \alpha_j = p_i (g_{ii} - g_{ij}) + p_j (g_{ij} - g_{jj}) ,$$

$$\alpha_k - \alpha_i = p_i (g_{ik} - g_{ii}) + p_j (g_{jk} - g_{ij}) , \quad (35)$$

$$\alpha_j - \alpha_k = p_i (g_{ij} - g_{ik}) + p_j (g_{jj} - g_{jk}) .$$

For the additive model (19) conditions (32) and (33) simplifies, and in addition all stationary points of the recurrence equations can be characterized (Christiansen and Loeschcke, 1980). The only equilibria are the n trivial monomorphic equilibria and, subject to existence conditions, polymorphic equilibria segregating exactly two alleles. For small genotypic values no equilibria segregating three or more alleles exist. A polymorphic equilibrium segregating the alleles A_i and A_j exists and is stable if and only if the alleles are maintained in a protected polymorphism conditioned on A_i and A_j being the only possible alleles. Thus, from (32), the equilibrium exists and is stable when

$$(\kappa^2 - 1)(d_i - d_j)\{d_i - d_j(\kappa^2 + 7)/(\kappa^2 - 1)\} \; > \; 0 \qquad (36)$$

and the similar condition with i and j interchanged hold. If this equilibrium exists, then allele A_k will increase if introduced, from (33), when

$$(\kappa^2 - 1)(d_k - d_i)(d_k - d_j) \; > \; 0 \; . \qquad (37)$$

If the resource is wide, i.e., $\sigma > W$, then the globally stable equilibrium will be monomorphic for A_1 or A_n, or it will be polymorphic segregating the alleles A_1 and A_n. Thus only the alleles with the most extreme contributions to the character may be maintained in the population. A sufficient condition for polymorphism is $d_1 < 0 < d_n$, and if d_1 and d_n are of the same sign, the condition for polymorphism is that they shall differ by at least a factor $(\kappa^2 + 7)/(\kappa^2 - 1)$. If the resource is narrow, i.e., $\sigma < W$, then the globally stable equilibrium will be monomorphic for A_i or A_{i+1}, or it will be polymorphic segregating the alleles A_i and A_{i+1}, where i is the index of the numerically smallest negative allele contribution, i.e., $d_1 < \ldots < d_i < 0 < d_{i+1} < \ldots < d_n$ with i = 0,1,2,..., or n and A_0 is a non-existing allele. Thus a necessary condition for polymorphism is that $d_1 < 0 < d_n$, and polymorphism obtains if d_i and d_{i+1} (as defined above) differ numerically by at most a factor $-(\kappa^2 + 7)/(\kappa^2 - 1)$. In both cases, if the globally stable equilibrium is monomorphic, it is the monomorphic equilibrium with the allele with the numerically smallest contribution to the character.

For the constant dominance model similar results hold. A polymorphic equilibrium segregating the alleles A_i and A_j exists and is stable if and only if the alleles are maintained in a protected polymorphism conditioned on A_i and A_j being the only possible alleles. Thus, from (32), the unique equilibrium segregating A_i and A_j exists and is stable when, for $d_i > d_j$,

$$(\kappa^2 - 1)(1 + a)(d_i - d_j) \quad > \quad 8\, d_j , \qquad (38i)$$

$$(\kappa^2 - 1)(1 - a)(d_i - d_j) \quad > \quad -8\, d_i , \qquad (38j)$$

where (38i) is the condition for increase of allele A_i in a population monomorphic for A_j, and (38j) is the condition for increase of A_j in a population of A_i. Therefore, the condition $d_i > 0 > d_j$ is sufficient for polymorphism when $\sigma > W$, and it is necessary for polymorphism when $\sigma < W$. The condition for increase of allele A_k when introduced into a population segregating A_i and A_j at a stable equilibrium is again condition (37). Thus, the dynamics in the constant dominance model seem very similar to that in the additive model. However, we have not been able to establish the result that no equilibria segregating three or more alleles exist, so the description of the evolution of the additive model is valid if we drop the qualification "globally stable" from the equilibrium description and replace it with "locally stable". Nevertheless, we maintain the result that in the n allele system a monomorphic or a two allele polymorphic equilibrium is stable, where the monomorphic equilibrium has the allele with the numerically smallest allele contribution, and the polymorphic equilibrium segregates A_1 and A_n when $\sigma > W$ and the two alleles with numerically smallest negative and positive allele contribution when σ < W. However, the two models seem sufficiently similar to conjecture that they indeed has the same dynamical properties.

DISCUSSION

The evolution of a trophic character related to exploitative competition can be viewed as consisting of two stages. The first stage occurs in a population, where the resource utilization is displaced away from the optimum location. The genetic variation for the trophic character will be subject to directional selection towards the resource mode, and in this respect it is equivalent to character displacement as a responce to interspecific exploitative competition, where the resource optimum is modified by the presence of a competitor (Roughgarden, 1976; Christiansen and Fenchel, 1977; Fenchel and Christiansen, 1977; Jayakar and Matessi, this symposium). The selective force at this stage of the evolution is determined mainly by the extra-populational environment, so the process is parallel to classical directional selection, and it would be unnatural to ascribe this feature of the model to intraspecific competition.

The second stage in the evolution of the population occurs when the resource utilization is close to the resource optimum, i.e., when the goal of the first stage is approached. The selection imposed by the extra-populational environment now becomes weaker and may be characterized as optimizing selection. Selection determined by the intra-populational environment now becomes of importance, and it takes the form of centripetal or disruptive selection, in that phenotypes which deviate the most from the population mean typically are favored with respect to intraspecific competition. Selection due to intraspecific competition becomes important whenever the population is close to the evolutionary equilibrium with respect to the extra-populational environment, whether

this environment is givem directly by the resource spectrum or whether
it is modified by competing species (Christiansen and Fenchel, 1977;
Fenchel and Christiansen, 1977).

The outcome of evolution in this second stage will predict the genetic structure of the variation at loci influencing a trophic character.
Our results for the additive model show, that in general one or two alleles will be maintained at such a locus. If the resource spectrum is
more narrow than the utilization function of the genotypes, the condition for polymorphism is, that the utilization modes of the two homozygotes should be on opposite sides of the resource mode, and their position should not differ too much from a symmetric location. The exact
condition for polymorphism is, however, more easily fullfilled than the
condition for overdominance in fitness with respect to the external environment (Christiansen and Loeschcke, 1980), but the evolutionary outcome resembles that of classical stabilizing selection, in that an allele, that places its genotypes closer to the resource optimum than preexisting genotypes, is always favored (Wright, 1935; Singh and Lewontin,
1966; Levene, 1967). If the resource spectrum is wider than the utilization function of the genotypes, then the condition for polymorphism is
rather easily fullfilled, and in case of polymorphism the two alleles,
where the homozygotes have the highest and the lowest genotypic value,
is maintained in the population. If these two genotypic values are on
opposite sides of the resource optimum, polymorphism will prevail, and
even if they are on the same side of the optimum, polymorphism is possible. So intraspecific exploitative competition is a powerful force to
maintain two allele polymorphisms.

This describtion of the evolutionary outcome of intraspecific competition related to a character influenced by a multiple allele locus
with additive gene effects largely generalizes to a locus with constant
dominance as defined by equation (20). We have not ruled out the possibility of multiple allele polymorphisms, but we conjecture that they

do not. In any case, the above describtion of the evolutionary outcome of intraspecific competition is robust to the assumption of additive gene effects as long as the assumption of intermediate dominance is fulfilled.

The results are obtained under the assumption, that the genotypic values are small, or that the locus in question has a small effect on the character. This assumption is not very crusial to the results. For the additive model three or more allele polymorphisms can exist only when $|d_i|/W$ is larger than about unity (Christiansen and Loeschcke, 1980; Loeschcke and Christiansen, in preparation).

We envisioned the trophic character as being determined by many loci with small effects, and the results has an interesting corollary for multiple loci with additive effects between loci and within loci. If the loci are absolutely linked, then the multiple allele result says, that a unique globally stable equilibrium exists, and at that equilibrium only one or two types of gametes are maintained in the population. Thus, if the equilibrium is polymorphic at more than one locus, then the maximally possible linkage disequilibrium exists among the varying loci. For a wide resource the result is even more extreme, in that all loci will be polymorphic and one of the gametes will carry the alleles with the highest contributions to the character and the other those with the lowest contributions. Thus, by using the perturbation theory of Karlin and McGregor (1972), a group of closely linked loci is expected to show a high degree of linkage disequilibrium. The contributions of the loci to the character are assumed small, so for this effect to be of importance the linkage between the loci should be tight. However, a more specific consideration of two locus models show, that the effect is not negligible (Loeschcke and Christiansen, in preparation), and for more than two loci there exist the possibility of highly organized genotypes even when the pairwize linkage disequilibria are small (Franklin and Lewontin, 1970; Feldman, Franklin and Thomson, 1874). Therefore

the study of a trophic character involved in intraspecific exploitative
competition by quantitative genetic methodology involving the assumption of loci in linkage equilibrium should be made with caution.

The selective forces are assumed weak by assuming small genotypic
values, so mutation may disturb the conclusions reached above. At a
two allele polymorphic equilibrium let μ be the mutation rate to the
alleles not present in the population, then all these alleles will be
at a very low frequency due to mutation selection balance provided

$$\mu \ll (1/4) \, V \, \{(\kappa^2 - 1)/(\kappa^2 + 1)\} \, (d_n - d_1)^2/W^2 \ . \qquad (39)$$

and provided that none of the quantities $(d_{i+1} - d_i)/W$ are exceedingly
small. This condition should be easily satisfied for $(d_n - d_1)/W$ of the
order of 0.01 and probably also for the order of 0.001. Thus, unless
the contribution of the locus to the character is exceedingly small,
the effect of mutation can be neglected.

The genetic structure of the variation for a trophic character will
depend strongly on the environment. For a set of absolutely linked loci
a population exploiting a wide spectrum of resource qualities will segregate two gametes, which may be visualized as a + + + ... + and a
- - - ... - gamete with + designating an allele with a positive contribution to the character and - an allele with a negative (or small) contribution. A similar population exploiting a narrow resource will at
the same loci segregate two gametes + - - + + ... and - + - + - ... as an
example, where the + and - alleles need not be the same as those in the
above population. If the loci are not absolutely linked, but closely
linked, then an excess of the mentioned gamete types occurs. These two
populations will respond differently to a change in the environment.
If the resource mode is changed, so directional selection on the variation is imposed, then the population exploiting the wide resource will
have a higher potential genetic responce. This change in the environment
can be produced by the invasion of a competing species in case of a wide

resource, so the resident species is expected to show rather rapid character displacement and may be pushed to a rather marginal position in the environment (Christiansen and Fenchel, 1977). On the other hand, if the spectrum of resource qualities becomes wider, the species allready living in a wide resource environment will only respond slowly, whereas the species in the narrow environment might release some variation by recombination, and thereby show a more rapid ecological release.

The results for genetic equilibria with intraspecific exploitative competition is dual to the limiting similarity result for species competing by exploitation (MacArthur and Levins, 1967). Thus, the results are expected to be robust with respect to the assumption of Gaussian utilization functions, as many other types of unimodal symmetric utilization functions provide a limiting similarity condition for species coexistence (May, 1974; Roughgarden, 1974). However, there are reasons to believe that the result is not valid for intraspecific competition which is not exploitative competition. Roughgarden (1972) considered a competition model, which for interspecific competition does not produce a limiting similarity condition, and he showed that there is no limit to the number of genotypes that can be maintained in the population. Therefore we must emphasize that our results on the genetic structure of variation for a trophic character are valid only if that character is involved in intraspecific exploitative competition.

ACKNOWLEDGEMENTS

We are indebted to Dr. M. W. Feldman for his helpful suggestions on the manuscribt. This research was supported in part by NSF grant DEB77-05742 and NIH grant 10452.

REFERENCES

Anderson, W. W. 1971. Genetic equilibrium and population growth under
density-regulated selection. Amer. Natur. 105: 489-498.

Asmussen, M. A., and Feldman, M. W. 1976. Density dependent selection
I. A stable feasible equilibrium may not be attainable. J. Theoret.
Biol. 64: 603-618.

Bulmer, M. G. 1974. Density dependent selection and character displacement. Amer. Natur. 108: 45-58.

Charlesworth, B. 1971. Selection in density regulated populations.
Ecology 52: 469-474.

Christiansen, F. B., and Fenchel, T. M. 1977. Theories of Populations
in Biological Communities. Springer Verlag, Berlin.

Christiansen, F. B., and Loeschcke, V. 1980. Evolution and intraspecific exploitative competition I. One locus theory for small additive gene effects. Theoret. Popul. Biol., to appear.

Clarke, B. C. 1972. Density dependent selection. Amer. Natur. 106: 1-13.

Feldman, M. W., Franklin, I. R., and Thomson, G. 1974. Selection in
complex genetic systems I. The symmetric equilibria of the three-
locus symmetric viability model. Genetics 76: 135-162.

Fenchel, T. 1975. Character displacement and coexistence in mud snails
(Hydrobiidae). Oecologia (Berl.) 20: 19-32.

Fenchel, T. M., and Christiansen, F. B. 1977. Selection and interspeci-
fic competition. In Measuring Selection in Natural Populations
(F. B. Christiansen and T. M. Fenchel, eds.). Lecture Notes in
Biomathematics 19, Springer Verlag, Berlin: 477-498.

Fenchel, T., and Kofoed, L. H. 1976. Evidence for exploitative interspecific competition in mud snails (Hydrobiidae). Oikos 27: 367-376.

Franklin. I. R., and Lewontin, R. C. 1970. Is the gene the unit of selection? Genetics 65: 707-734.

Gause, G. F. 1934. The Struggle for Existence. Hafner Publ. Co., New York (Reprinted in 1964).

Ginzburg, L. R. 1977. The equilibrium and stability for h alleles under the density-dependent selection. J. Theoret. Biol. 68: 545-550.

Karlin, S., and McGregor, I. 1972. Polymorphisms for genetic and ecological systems with weak coupling. Theoret. Popul. Biol. 3: 210-238.

Levene, H. 1967. Genetic diversity and diversity of environment: Mathematical aspects. Proc. 5th Berkeley Symp. Math. Stat. Prob.: 305-316.

Levins, R. 1968. Toward an evolutionary theory of the niche. In Evolution and Environment (E. T. Drake, ed.). Yale Univ. Press, Conn.: 325-340.

Lotka. A. J. 1932. The growth of mixed populations: Two species competing for a common food supply. J. Wash. Acad. Sci. 22: 461-469.

MacArthur, R. M. 1962. Some generalized theorems of natural selection. Proc. Nat. Acad. Sci. U. S. A. 48: 1893-1897.

MacArthur, R. M. 1972. Geographical Ecology. Harper and Row, New York.

MacArthur, R. M., and Levins, R. 1964. Competition, habitat selection and character displacement in a patchy environment. Proc. Nat. Acad. Sci. U. S. A. 51: 1207-1210.

MacArthur, R. M., and Levins, R. 1967. The limiting similarity, convergence and divergence of coexisting species. Amer. Natur. 101: 377-385.

Matessi, C. and Jayakar, S. D. 1976. Models of density-frequency dependent selection for the exploitation of resources I: Intraspecific competition. In Population Genetics and Ecology (S. Karlin and E. Nevo, eds.). Academic Press, New York: 707-721.

May, R. M. 1974. On the theory of niche overlap. Theoret. Popul. Biol. 5: 297-332.

Poulsen, E. T. 1980. A model for population regulation with density and frequency-dependent selection. J. Math. Biol., in press.

Prout, T. 1980. Some relationships between density independent selection and density dependent growth. Evolutionary Biology 13, in press.

Roughgarden, J. 1971. Density-dependent natural selection. Ecology 52: 453-468.

Roughgarden, J. 1972. Evolution of niche width. Amer. Natur. 106: 683-718.

Roughgarden, J. 1974. Species packing and the competition function with illustrations from coral reef fish. Theoret. Popul. Biol. 5: 163-186.

Roughgarden, J. 1976. Resource partitioning among competing species - A coevolutionary approach. Theoret. Popul. Biol. 9: 388-424.

Schoener, T., and Gorman, G. 1968. Some niche differences in three Lesser Antillean lizards of the genus Anolis. Ecology 49: 819-830.

Singh, M., and Lewontin, R. C. 1966. Stable equilibria under optimizing selection. Proc. Nat. Acad. Sci. U. S. A. 56: 1345-1348.

Slatkin, M. 1979. Ecological character displacement. Ecology, in press.

Volterra, V. 1927. Variazioni e fluttuazioni del numero d'individui in specie animali conviventi. R. Comitato Talassografico Italiano, Memoria 131: 1-142 (English translation in F. M. Scudo and J. R. Ziegler: The Golden Age of Theoretical Ecology: 1923-1940. Lecture Notes in Biomathematics 22, Springer Verlag, Berlin 1979)

Wright, S. 1935. The analysis of variance and the correlations between relatives with respect to deviations from an optimum. J. Genet. 30: 243-256.

Wright, S. 1959. Physiological genetics, ecology of populations and natural selection. Prespectives in Biology and Medicine 3: 107-151.

ECOLOGICAL IMPLICATIONS OF NATURAL SELECTION

Lev R. Ginzburg
Department of Ecology and Evolution
State University of New York at Stony Brook
Stony Brook, NY   11794/USA

I. INTRODUCTION

In 1967 my friend, Professor E. M. Polyshuk, a biographer and admirer of
Vito Volterra (Polyshuk, 1977), introduced me to the classical book "Lecons sur la
théorie mathématique de la lutte pour la vie" (1931), and its English version "The
struggle for existence" (D'Ancona, 1954). They were the first two books on mathematical biology I had read and, thanks to this introduction, I have worked on different aspects of population theory ever since. In 1976 I was fortunate to meet in
Rome Professor Eduardo Volterra who has shown me things and places related to the
memory of his great father. It was a very special feeling to walk into the study
room in Vito Volterra's house where he wrote most of his work on population theory
during the 1920's. All my professional life was directly influenced by the work of
Vito Volterra. It is, therefore, a particular pleasure for me to participate in
this memorial symposium.

I shall start by the trivial statement that the greatest problem of theoretical population biology now is the gap between the theory and experiment. The
common feeling is that the theory has gone too far. I am not sure I can say "too far
ahead". Multilocus population genetics analyses operating with astronomical size
fitness matrices, which are not only unknown but will never be known, are one example.
Ecosystem models containing n nonlinear differential equations, where every term in
every function is first unknown, then replaced by the linear approximation "as the
first step towards...", is another example.

The original idea was to say something meaningful about the dynamics of a
real population. Instead, our journals are full of stability conditions, often expressed in terms of the eigenvalues of unknown matrices, diversity and complexity
measures having very little to do with reality and a growing number of "theorems"
which, I suspect, appear in publications on theoretical biology because they are too
trivial for a mathematical journal.

I think, a careful reassessment of the basic principles is in order. I am
trying to contribute to such a reassessment in this lecture.

II. THE MALTHUS LAW

The founders of theoretical physics conceived an interesting approach: to relate complex and unknown phenomena to "initial conditions" and those that are accessible to study - to the laws of nature (Wigner 1970). Newtonian mechanics describes, for example, the Earth motion around the Sun in such a way that it is possible to calculate the further motion of the Earth according to the initial position and speed. "Why the Earth has (or ever had) its current position and speed" is outside of the scope of theoretical mechanics though it is not a priori nonsense. Everything is explained by Newton s laws which establish the invariance of the physical laws with respect to the uniform straight-line motion. We are so accustomed to this statement that sometimes we forget that it is no more than a generalization (and in some way, an extrapolation) of our experience but is not, a priori, truth (Mach 1893, Wigner 1970). The history of pre-Newtonian physics includes unsuccessful attempts to develop theoretical mechanics considering speed as the significant quantity which is influenced by the "external forces". The two thousand year experience of this unfruitful but quite natural approach shows that the transition to the invariance postulate of mechanical laws with respect to the Galileo transformation was difficult and revolutionary. The modern viewpoint was rather successful, but at the same time, it narrowed the subject of physics. In modern terminology, the Newtonian revolution was basically the change in the forms of the description of the dynamic state of the system from only "position" to the "position and speed".

From the point of view of this historical analogy, the models of population dynamics can be classified as Aristotelian. All known models of population dynamics are based on the population size as the complete descriptor of the dynamic state. We can write this central assumption of the theory as follows:

$$\frac{1}{N}\dot{N} = f(E), \qquad (1)$$

where N is the population size;

$\frac{1}{N}\dot{N}$ is the relative growth rate (average number of surviving offspring per parent per unit of time);

f(E) is a function of the environment with the understanding that population size itself might be one of the environmental parameters, as in the case of density-dependence.

The time intervals considered should be appreciably longer than the generation time in order to ignore the processes which occur on the order of one generation (age structure, for example).

To construct an ecosystem model we write such equations for each of the populations in the ecosystem. Environment E for a given population includes sizes of other populations and that is how we obtain the system of equations designed to describe the ecosystem dynamics. The differences between models are due to different assumptions concerning the forms of the function f. There is no doubt that the growth rate actually depends on the environment. Nevertheless, this dependence is so complex and multifaceted that I, naturally, wish to change the formulation of the problem.

Let me call constant all environments in which a given population increases (or decreases) exponentially. There is no external way to determine such a constancy. We cannot, for example, do it by enumerating: Food is enough. Oxygen is present in necessary quantities, temperature is constant, etc. But there is no need to enumerate the separate causes. Environmental invariability for a given population can be established by examining the population itself, since only if the population size is constant or changes exponentially is the environment invariable.

I will write down the Malthusian law $N(t)=N_o e^{rt}$ in a slightly unusual form:

$$(\ddot{\ell n N}) = 0. \qquad (2)$$

Paraphrasing Hutchinson (1975): "Populations preserve exponential growth unless they do not". Although sounding tautological, it bears, in my opinion, a meaning analogous to Newton's first law describing what happens when "nothing happens in the environment" In the suggested form (2), it has no parameters and requires two initial conditions; population size and the growth rate.

I would like to end this section noticing that the Malthus law is the only formula in population theory to which the word "law" has been unanimously applied, all the rest were "models". I completely agree with this usage of words stressing the exponential growth as an important background for all events happening in population dynamics. In the next section I will try to reconstruct the principles of population dynamics based on an extended notion of the dynamic state.

III. EVOLUTIONARY ADÁPTATION IN MODELS OF POPULATION DYNAMICS

Classical models in theoretical ecology do not take into account genetic heterogeneity of the population. From the point of view of population dynamics this means that population growth rates "immediately" respond to any environmental change on the accepted time scale of the model. One of the direct effects of genetic heterogeneity is that the population will respond to environmental change with some time-delay (i.e., the population will have some inertia). The amount of this inertia is related to the intensity of natural selection that occurs in a population after the environmental change. This effect might be of considerable importance. In reality, a certain amount of inertia to a changing environment might be more adaptive than a "direct tracking" of the environment. The existence of genetic heterogeneity could, therefore, by creating this delayed reaction, be an important factor in the population dynamics for populations experiencing changing environments. Genetic variation, in this sense, is important not as a direct adaptation to environmental heterogeneity, but by damping fluctuations in the population dynamics. Inertia works as a mechanism that averages out fluctuations and, thereby, produces more stable behavior in varying environment. Both the total absence of inertia and very high inertia would seem maladaptive. The amount of inertia a population possesses should ultimately be translated into the amount of natural selection (fitness variability) and genetic variability in population.

Most of the theoretical work which has been done on the interface of genetics and ecology was inclined towards the ecological effects on the genetical constitution of populations. It has been well summarized in the recent book by Roughgarden (1979) and a good review paper by Slatkin and Maynard-Smith (1979). I am going to concentrate here on the opposite influence. I am interested in the effects genetic variability have on population dynamics. The problems are certainly interrelated. Macroscopically, though, different genetical systems might produce the same or similar effects on population dynamics. In such cases, a macroscopic description will be approximately invariant with respect to a specific genetic scheme.

Suppose that the environment was constant E_1 up to the moment $t=t_1$, then changed to the better and also constant environment E_2 (up to the moment t_2) and finally changed to the worse environment E_3 at the moment t_2 (Fig. 1). If we accept the model (1) literally the dynamics of the growth rate should look as the broken line on the Fig. 1. Taking into account adaptation effects we would expect the process to look like a solid line on the same figure. Remember that we do not consider effects on the order of the generation time and this includes possible physiological, demographic and other adaptations to the new environment which would change the character of the curves around the points t_1 and t_2 (see the classification of adaptation mechanisms with respect to their characteristic time of action in Slobodkin and Rapoport, 1974).

Since a constant natural selection regime is assumed here as the only cause of adaptation, the growth rate in a constant environment can only increase. This, certainly, is true for a haploid population and it is basically the content of the Fisher fundamental theorem of Natural Selection (1930) for a diploid population. It is well-known that recombination could act against this effect and cause sometimes a decrease in the overall population growth rate (average fitness). We have recently shown, however, (Ginzburg and Braumann, 1980), that in a multilocus context this influence is in most cases insignificant when a large number of loci is involved. We will accept, therefore, the Fisher theorem as a basis for our macroscopic consideration.

Of course, in the case of frequency-dependent selection the growth rate can

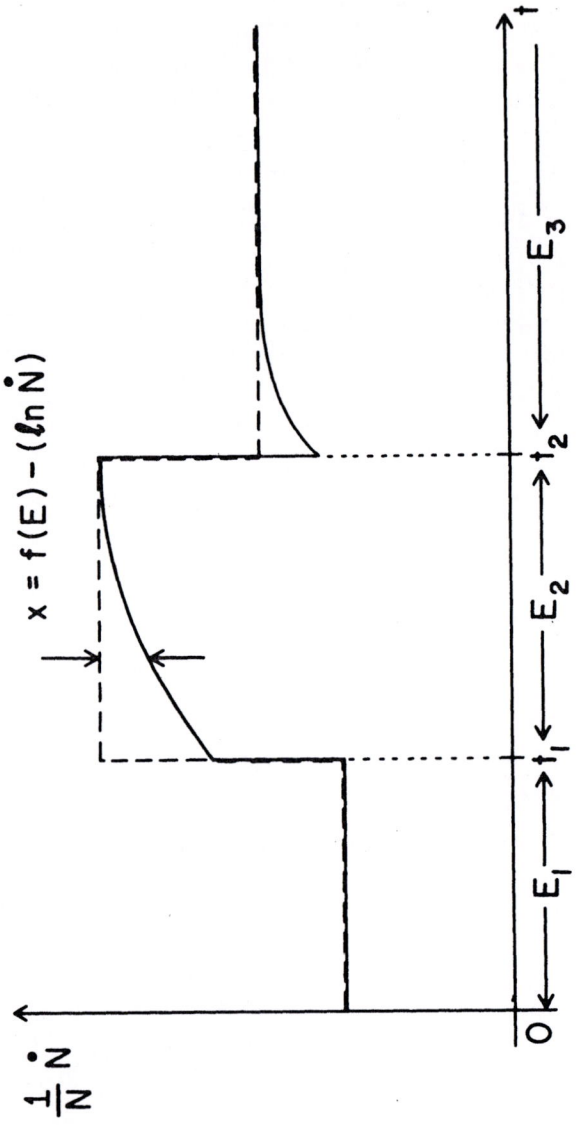

Fig. 1. Reflective growth rate of a population as a function of time in the thought experiment described in the text.

decrease during the adaptation process. We have assumed here a constant fitness selection only for the definiteness; appropriate generalization does not present a problem in our context.

In an attempt to include the adaptation process in the description of population dynamics I will postulate the basic equation in a new form:

$$(\ln N)^{..} = F(E, \dot{E}, (\ln N)^{.}) \qquad (3)$$

which describes the rate of change of the growth rate as a function of the environment, its rate of change and the growth rate. I remind, again, that population size is considered, if necessary, as one of the components of the environment. This equation, as well as the Malthusian law in the form (2), requires two initial conditions: population size and growth rate. In other words, in the suggested model the dynamic state of a population is described by two numbers instead of one as in the traditional approach.

In the fixed environment any population should eventually be able to reach its equilibrium (post-selected) growth rate depending on the environment. We will use for this growth rate the same notation $f(E)$ as in the old model $(\ln N)^{.} = f(E)$. In our model, due to the Fisher theorem, $(\ln N)^{.} < f(E)$, i.e., preselected growth rate cannot exceed postselected, Taking into account these two properties, we can specify the form of the righthand part of the equation (3) as follows:

$$(\ln N)^{..} = \frac{\partial f}{\partial E} \dot{E} \; — \; g(E, \dot{E}) + A(E)(f(E) \; - \; (\ln N)^{.}) \qquad (4)$$

Here there are three reasons for growth rate changes:

(i)   Change in the balanced growth rate, $\frac{\partial f}{\partial E}\dot{E}$;

(ii) New disbalance in the growth rate generated by
      changing environment, $g(E, \dot{E})$. It follows from
      the Fisher theorem that $g \geq 0$, $g(E, 0) = 0$;

(iii) Adaptation process, which brings the growth rate
      towards its equilibrium value. Here it is
      assumed to be proportional to the imbalance in
      the growth rate. We call $A(E) > 0$ adaptability.

The linearization is not essential for our consideration. We use it only to clarify the meaning of the adaptability parmeter. The parameter $1/A$ can be considered then as the inertia measure. Linearization here is equivalent to the assumption that solid curves on the Fig. 1 are exponential.

Equation (4) is basically an attempt to reduce all hidden evolutionary dimensions of a population to one variable

$$x = \; f(E) \; - \; (\ln N)^{.} > 0,$$ imbalance in the growth rate. Equation (4) can be rewritten as a system of two first order equations

$$(\ell nN)^{\cdot} = f(E) - x$$

$$\dot{x} = g(E,\dot{E}) - A(E) x \qquad (5)$$

Such a reduction of a complex ecolutionary process to one extra dimension cannot be exact. Hidden dimensions should lead to a hysteresis (history dependent) character of both the imbalance generating function g and adaptability A. I hope, nevertheless, that these effects will not be very important in many real cases and most of the qualitative features of the evolutionary process from the point of view of population dynamics can be sketched by the suggested model.

The traditional approach (1) is a limiting case of the new model obtained by letting A→∞. Clearly, infinite adaptability corresponds to the case of no inertia, i.e., direct tracking of environmental variations.

I would like to mention here that the idea of using second order equations in the models of population dynamics is not new. With no reference to adaptation producing inertia as a basic mechanism it appeared independently in Clark (1971) and Ginzburg (1972) and was criticized by Innis (1972).

IV. EXAMPLES

Consider examples where we can apply the new model to the description of the adaptation processes in cases where the "exact" genetic models have been developed. My goal, here, is to compare the suggested approximate macroscopic description with the detailed description and clarify the meaning of the adaptability parameter.

DENSITY-INDEPENDENT GROWTH IN STATIONARY ENVIRONMENT

The complete genetic model was considered in detail in Ginzburg and Costantino (1979). It is based on the multiple allele one locus genetic scheme. We describe the genetic structure of the population by the vector of the gene frequencies $p = \{p_1,\ldots,p_n\}$ and use the notation $W(p)$ for the average fitness, so that $\frac{\dot{N}}{N} = W(p)$. Placed into a new environment, population will usually change its structure $p \underset{t\to\infty}{\to} p^*$ and its average fitness $W(p) \underset{t\to\infty}{\to} W^*$ under the new form of natural selection. If we assume $p^* > 0$ (polymorphism) we can obtain one interesting relationship describing the global property of the adaptation process

$$\int_0^\infty [W^* - W(p(t))]\, dt = H(p_0, p^*), \qquad (6)$$

where $H(p,p^*)$ is the entropy distance between the points p and p^* defined as follows:

$$H(p,p^*) = - \sum_{i-1}^{n} p_1^* \, \ell n \, \frac{p_1}{p_1^*} > 0 \qquad (7)$$

Let us compare this exact description with the suggested approximation. In the stationary density–dependent invironment the first two terms in the equation (4) vanish and we have

$$(\ddot{\ell n N}) = A(f - (\dot{\ell n N})), \qquad (8)$$

where A is the adaptability constant and f is the asymptotic growth rate. At the beginning of the process the growth rate ($\ell n N$ can be only less than f and it approaches f growing monotonically:

$$(\dot{\ell n N}) = f - [f-(\dot{\ell n N})_o] \, e^{-At} \underset{t\to\infty}{\to} f \qquad (9)$$

We now identify the growth rate of the population ($\dot{\ell n N}$) with the average fitness W, and the equilibrium growth rate f with the equilibrium W^*. The exact process is not necessarily exponential so that these identifications are not precisely correct. We can require, however, that the global property of the adaptation process (6), holds. We will have then:

$$\int_o^\infty [f-\dot{\ell n N}] \, dt = H \, (p_o,p^*) \qquad (10)$$

Substituting (9) to (10) we obtain the expression for the adaptability:

$$A = \frac{f - (\dot{\ell n N})_o}{H \, (p_o,p^*)} \qquad (11)$$

It has a meaning of the overall gain in the growth rate per unit of the entropy distance between initial and final genetic structures.

For the population size N(t) we obtain integrating from (9),

$$N(t) = N_o \exp[ft - \frac{f-(\dot{\ell n N})_o}{A} \exp(-At)] \underset{t\to\infty}{\sim} N_o e^{ft}. \qquad (12)$$

We see from this example that the approximate description preserves all qualitative features of the exact description but does not require exact knowledge of genetic parameters replacing it by the extra initial condition for the growth rate.

DENSITY–INDEPENDENT GROWTH IN A TIME–DEPENDENT ENVIRONMENT

In a purely time–dependent environment equation (4) becomes a first order equation with respect to the growth rate ($\dot{\ell n N}$) and can be explicitly integrated. Evolutionary inertia can certainly only lower the growth rate compared to the traditional model (1). One of the consequences is that in a periodic environment with period T, E(t+T) = E(t), the inequality

$$\frac{1}{T} \int_t^{t+T} f(E(t))dt > 0 \qquad (13)$$

is no longer a sufficient condition for survival. The new condition includes the comparison of this quantity with some kind of the integrated "genetic load":

$$\frac{1}{T} \int_{t}^{t+T} f \, dt \; > \; \frac{1}{T} \int_{o}^{T} \chi \, dt \; > \; 0 .$$
(14)

The other consequence is a significant modification in amplitude of the population size oscillations depending on the dynamics of the newly generated imbalance g and adaptability A.

The case of randomly fluctuating environment for the suggested model was considered by Braumann (1980). Introduction of "noise" for the rate of change of the growth rate (rather than for the growth rate) leads to a decreased variance and stronger autocorrelation of the process than with traditional approaches.

DENSITY-DEPENDENT GROWTH

Exact density-dependent growth model has been studied in a number of papers (Roughgarden, 1976, Ginzburg, 1977) based on the same multiple-alleles-one-locus genetic scheme. From the population dynamics point of view the most interesting effects of adaptation is the nonmonotonic character of the growth curves around an equilibrium level (carrying capacity).

Let me show how this phenomenon appears within the framework of the suggested macroscopic approach. We assume that the population size itself is the only environmental parameter influencing the population growth so that the equation (4) will take the form:

$$(\ln N)^{\cdot\cdot} \; = \frac{\partial f}{\partial N} \; \dot{N} \; - \; g(N, \dot{N}) \; + \; A(N)(f(N) - (\ln N)^{\cdot})$$
(15)

Adaptability in this case may in general depend on the population size, A=A(N). Note that the traditional logistic-like model is a special case of (15) obtained by $A \to \infty$, $(\ln \dot{N} = f(N)$. To illustrate the effect let us linearize this equation around an equilibrium N* which is the root of the equation f(N)=0. Since g(N,N) is always nonpositive, it will have a local extremum at the equilibrium point and, therefore, a zero term for the first approximation. Introducing $y = \ln(N/N^*)$ we have

$$\ddot{y} \; + \; (k + A^*) \, \dot{y} \; + \; A^* k y \; = \; 0,$$
(16)

where:

$$k = \frac{\partial f}{\partial \ln N} \bigg|_{N=N^*} \; > \; 0 \qquad \text{measures the strength of density-dependence around the equilibrium point;}$$

$$A* = A(N*)$$
is the adaptability measured at the equilibrium point.

Solution of this equation is the sum of two exponentials:

$$y(t)=(1- \frac{k}{A*})^{-1}(y_o+ \frac{1}{A*}\dot{y}_o)e^{-kt}+(\frac{k}{A*}y_o+ \frac{1}{A*}\dot{y}_o)e^{-A*t} \qquad (17)$$

It demonstrates both effects noticed on the complete genetic model: the overshooting of the equilibrium level and the temporary decrease in size due to adaptation, followed by an increase and asymptotic equilibrium at N=N* (Ginzburg, 1977).

Once again we see that the macroscopic description using one additional parameter, adaptability, captures the main qualitative characteristics of the process.

By analogy, one can go on and rewrite the prey-predator, competition and other ecosystem models including adaptability as an additional parameter, and using second order equations for each population instead of first order. This requires quite a change in intuition since growth rates are now just "initial conditions" and interactions describe environmental changes rather than environments. A general guess about the properties of such double-dimensional models is that they will show destabilization of otherwise stable equilibria leading to oscillations (or more general bounded behavior) and, possibly, extinction. It is not my goal, here, to go on so far since it may only obscure the point I am trying to make.

V. DISCUSSION

Philosophers of the last century have been involved in one discussion (among others) which is relevant to the subject of this lecture. The problem was the meaning of the second Newton's law in the form "Mass times acceleration equals force". One group considered this statement as an experimental fact, where acceleration and forces are measured independently and mass is a proportionality constant. The others insisted that the law is just a definition of the concept of force. Great people like Laplace, Poincare, Mach, were involved in the discussion which, from the modern utilitarian point of view, is irrelevant. To be consistent, though, people from the first school suggested that the first Newton's law be dropped from the list of axioms of theoretical mechanics, as a consequence of the second law (when force is zero). The second, definitional point of view seems to be winning at the present time. That is why the first law is still in the books on theoretical mechanics (see the beautiful discussion of this topic in Feyman et al., (1963)).

Following this analogy with theoretical mechanics I can qualify the major point of this lecture as a suggestion of a new definition of the "environmental force" concept as a quantity proportional to the acceleration of the population

TABLE 1. PRINCIPLES OF THE DESCRIPTION OF POPULATION DYNAMICS

	TRADITIONAL APPROACH	SUGGESTED APPROACH
DYNAMIC STATE OF A POPULATION	$N(t)$ POPULATION SIZE	$\{N(t), \dot{N}(t)=(\ell nN)^{\cdot}\}$ POPULATION SIZE GROWTH RATE
MALTHUS LAW	$\dot{N}/N = r$ WITH INITIAL CONDITION: $N\big|_{t=0}=N_0$	$(\ell nN)^{\cdot\cdot} = 0$ WITH INITIAL CONDITIONS: $N\big|_{t=0}=N_0$ $(\ell nN)^{\cdot}\big|_{t=0} = r$
GENERAL GROWTH EQUATION FOR VARYING ENVIRONMENT $E = E(t)$	$\dot{N}/N = f(E)$ WITH INITIAL CONDITION: $N\big|_{t=0}=N_0$	$(\ell nN)^{\cdot\cdot} = \tilde{F}(E, \dot{E}, (\ell nN)^{\cdot})$ WITH INITIAL CONDITIONS: $N\big|_{t=0}=N_0$ $(\ell nN)^{\cdot}\big|_{t=0} = (\ell nN)^{\cdot}_0$

growth, ($\overset{..}{\ell nN}$) (Table 1). This certainly narrows the field. Questions about the growth rate are relegated to the "initial conditions". Instead, I concentrate on the changes in the growth rate reflecting environmental variation. The analogy with mechanics extends only as far as the definition of force is concerned. Of course, in the context of population biology we expect the laws determining actual forces to bear no resemblance to physical laws.

Last century philosophers agreed then, and everybody agrees now, that the most important practical question is what stands on the righthand side of this definition, how does force actually depend on the positions and velocities of this and other bodies? Gravitations law is an example of an answer to this question.

The future success of the suggested approach depends on whether or not we will be able to answer important questions: "What actually stands in the righthand side of the equation? How do the above mentioned three components of acceleration depend on the state of a population and states of other populations when they interact?

These questions can be answered only through extensive empirical experience.

REFERENCES

Braumann, C. A. 1980. Population adaptation to a noisy environment: stochastic enalogs of some deterministic models. Proceedings of the International Statistical Ecology Program, Vol. 13 (in press).

Clark, G. P. 1971. The second derivative and population modeling. Ecology, 52:606-613.

D'Ancona, U. 1954. The struggle for existence. E. G. Bull., Leiden.

Feyman, R. P., Leighton, R. B., and Sands, M. 1963. The Feyman Lectures on Physics, Vol. 1, Addison-Wesley.

Fisher, R. A. 1930. The genetic theory of natural selection. Clarendon Press, Oxford.

Ginzburg, L. R. 1972. The analogies of the "free motion" and "force" concepts in population theory. In Coll. "Studies in Theoretical Genetics" (V. A. Ratner, ed.) Novosibirsk (in Russian).

Ginzburg, L. R. 1977. The equilibrium and stability for n alleles under the density-dependent selection. J. Theor. Biol. 68:545-550.

Ginzburg, L. R., and Costantino, R. F. 1979. On the rate of genetic adaptation under the natural selection. J. Theor. Biol. 77:307-316.

Ginzburg, L. R., and Braumann, C. A. 1980. Multilocus population and genetics: relative importance of selection and recombination. Theor. Pop. Biol. (in press).

Hutchinson, G. E. 1975. Variation on a theme by Robert MacArthur. In Coll. "Ecology and Evolution of Communities", pp. 492-521, Harvard University Press.

Innis, G. 1972. The second derivative and population modeling: another view. Ecology, 53:720-723.

Mach, E. 1893. Die Mechanik in ihrer Entwicklung historischkritisch, dergestellt. Brockhaus, Leipzig.

Polyshuk, E. M. 1977. Vito Volterra, Nauka, Moscow (in Russian).

Roughgarden, J. 1976. Resource Partitioning among competing species - a coevolutionary approach. Theor. Pop. Biol. 9:388-424.

Roughgarden, J. 1979. Theory of Population Genetics and Evolutionary Ecology: an introduction. MacMillan Publishing Company.

Slatkin, M., and Maynard-Smith, J. 1979. Models of coevolution. The Quarterly Review of Biology, 54:233-263.

Slobodkin, L. B., and Rappaport, A. 1974. An optimal strategy of evolution. The Quarterly Review of Biology. 49:181-200.

Volterra, V. 1931. Lecons sur la theorie mathematique de la lutte pour la vie. Gauthier-Villars, Paris.

Wigner, E. 1970. Simmetrics and Reflections. Indiana University Press, Bloomington, London.

TOPIC II

Problems in Population Biology and Related Disciplines

AREAS OF OVERLAP OF POPULATION GENETICS WITH

RELATED DISCIPLINES

L. Cavalli-Sforza

Department of Genetics

Stanford University School of Medicine

Stanford, California 94305/USA

I have chosen to concentrate on interdisciplinary aspects by considering areas of overlap of population genetics and some other fields of study with which it has recently established more or less close links. I am using the expression "population genetics" as synonymous with "mathematical theory of evolution," but I am also keeping in mind a wider definition that includes empirical observations which go under the same name. These observations have greatly contributed to the development of the subject, both by confirming the expectations of the mathematical approach and by providing a constant source of inspiration for new theoretical developments.

I will briefly discuss 1) the area of common interest to population genetics and molecular genetics, usually called "molecular evolution;" 2) the evolutionary aspects of ethology, which have recently become more widely known with the controversies associated with sociobiology; 3) new developments in the study of cultural transmission and evolution; 4) the interactions between epidemiology of infectious diseases and population genetics; and 5) ecology, another area in which important contacts have been developing. The areas of overlap which I have mentioned are indicated graphically in Figure 1. Within the limitations of a 2-dimensional representation, the figure also attempts to show areas of intersection between the disciplines, which themselves interact with population genetics. My review will mostly emphasize areas on which I have been directly involved.

The word "molecular evolution" and some of its first applications, like the reconstruction of phylogenetic trees of living species, and the concept of the "molecular evolutionary clock," take their origin from evolutionary interpretations of the amino acid sequences of hemoglobin and other proteins (see, e.g., Zuckerkandl and Pauling, 1965). Kimura (1968) introduced the hypothesis that many amino acid substitutions may be selectively neutral. A summary of the early history and the most recent conclusions are given in Kimura (1979a).

The hypothesis of the neutrality of substitutions involved in molecular evolution has raised a scientific controversy of great proportions between its proponents and supporters, the "neutralists" and "selectionists" (see, e.g., Bodmer and Cavalli-Sforza, 1971). Natural selection is the foundation of modern biology. It could be renounced (even though in limited circumstances) only with great caution. One source of confusion, however, is that neutralists confine their attention to "accepted" amino acid or nucleotide substitutions. These are mutations that have been successful in at least some species.. They are only a small fraction of all mutations that occur,

because clearly deleterious mutations are automatically excluded by choosing only
accepted substitutions. Thus, of three gross categories of mutants, deleterious,
neutral and advantageous, it is only the last two that are being effectively considered.
It seems likely that in most cases of substitution, the deviation from neutrality in
either direction is small.

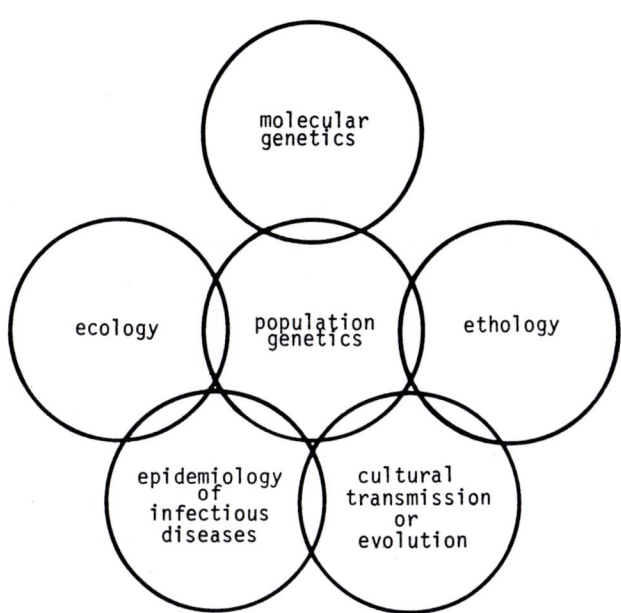

Figure 1.

Most recently, however, the hypothesis was advanced that most "neutral" alleles
are actually slightly deleterious. Coefficients of selection are assumed to be mostly
or universally negative with a specified distribution (Kimura, 1979b). A major difficulty that threatens a complete settlement of the issue is our inability under most
circumstances to measure small selection coefficients (Bodmer and Cavalli-Sforza, 1971).
Recent findings from a variety of molecular analyses (see Kimura, 1979a), however,
are in agreement with the idea that the proportion of mutations that are nearly neutral
(among the accepted ones) is not negligible. But other evidence points out that the
proportion of mutants that respond to selection is far from negligible.

Rather than looking at accepted substitution after fixation, it may pay to look at
fixations while they are happening in order to improve our chances of understanding
the mechanism of substitution. In other words, we can evaluate the importance of
selection and drift at the level of existing polymorphisms, while evolutionary substitutions are in the making. In spite of much work done on a great number of other organisms, I believe Man is still the one on which more knowledge of polymorphisms has

accumulated. Indirect approaches have been tried, based on the observed number and degree of existing polymorphisms, to be compared with those expected on the basis of known rate of evolutionary substitutions. This approach, however, is weakened by the number of assumptions which are necessary. In spite of the limitations to experimentation in Man, we have some knowledge on the selective mechanisms of some of these, due ordinarily to medical interest in them. A direct answer is thus made possible based on knowledge of selection on existing polymorphisms. One is tempted to reach the preliminary conclusion that genes showing the greatest ethnic variation (see Cavalli-Sforza, 1966; Piazza, et al. 1980) are subject to a great deal of disruptive selection, being strongly favored only in certain environments and perhaps at a disadvantage in others. Among examples of this class are Duffy, Gm and phosphatase. Genes that show medium or low ethnic variation are sometimes subject to some kind of selective balance, such as G6PD, sickle cell anemia and thalassemia, and perhaps ABO.

In practice we have evidence of some non-negligible amount of selection going on for perhaps one-third to one-half of genes studied. Absence of information for the rest does not, however, exclude selection. Much of the selection going on is tied to parasites, e.g. malaria, which also change over time, making selective advantages and disadvantages soon obsolete. The possibility, already raised by Haldane, may have to be seriously remembered that in this game selection coefficients are unlikely to remain constant over the whole process of substitution. In this case initial increases would often be selective, and final changes and fixations neutral, because in the meanwhile selective conditions have changed.

Moving over to the second area of contact, that with animal behavior and its evolutionary interpretation, I will mention E. O. Wilson's definition of the central theoretical problem in sociobiology, "How can altruism, which under certain conditons becomes increasingly prevalent and eventually appears in exaggerated forms, possibly evolve by natural selection? The answer is kinship" (Wilson, 1975, pg. 3). The question of evolution of altruism had been asked and qualitatively answered by Haldane (1932). Hamilton (1964) quantified it in his well known rule that for altruism not to be lost under natural selection, the ratio between the gain in fitness to the recipient of altruism, and the loss in fitness to the altruist, must be greater than one-half the coefficient of relationship between the altruist and the recipient. This rule was derived on the basis of optimization concepts, but was not explained in terms of population genetics. The main problem came from complexity in the definition of "inclusive fitness" that did not make it easily usable in practice. A consequence was that the rule could not be used for problems other than those of the initial advance of a rare gene, and not for the usual range of hypotheses asked in population genetics, which includes testing also for the existence and stability of internal equilibria. Perhaps the greatest limitation was that due to the lack of an explanation in terms of genetics; in the mind of most investigators, the conclusion seemed to have been reached that altruism could only develop by some kind of group selection, or at least of den-

sity dependent selection, not by strict Darwinian selection. But the introduction of
an operationally functional definition of fitness (which turns out to be gene-frequency
dependent), has helped one to prove that altruism can increase in frequency and even
fix, and can have stable or unstable polymorphisms, without need of postulating group
slection. These results are, in fact, valid under ordinary Darwinian selection (Cavalli-Sforza and Feldman, 1978a, to which I refer the reader for more detailed references). It has also been shown, by an exact treatment, that the rules by Hamilton
are only approximately correct for a diploid organism.

The same treatment can be extended to a variety of other social behaviors; in
fact, another consideration of importance is that kinship is by no means the only (and,
for vertebrates, perhaps, not even the central) mechanism by which altruism and other
social behaviors can evolve. In the same paper cited above, we have shown a model of
"good" and "bad" guys with specified interactions in fitnesses that can also be treated
by the same technique as kinship. The good (or the bad types) can fix or have polymorphic equilibria, stable or unstable. Here it is not kinship, but the mode of
social interaction between individuals of the same or different phenotypes that determines the pattern of social behavior. Apparently unnoticed by most, Hamilton had
already generated a similar model in one of his papers. The model of "hawks and doves"
by J. Maynard Smith (this symposium) also belongs to this category.

The next area of overlap, with cultural evolution, involves relationships of multiple nature. At the level of conceptualization, one can view the study of cultural
evolution as that of a "cultural organism" (for instance, a language; a set of social
customs; a technological object like a car, an airplane, etc.). Such organisms have
been "created" by other living organisms like ourselves; in fact, Man is notoriously
the animal which has developed culture way above every other animal. These "cultural
organisms" reproduce and evolve in our hands and brains, being completely dependent on
us for survival and transmission. The degree of dependence on Man of a cultural organism like a car or an airplane is not, however, entirely different from that of living
organisms like Man on carbon, hydrogen, oxygen, etc., on other living organisms, or
on a reasonable temperature and other environmental parameters.

Cars or airplanes are usually made of parts manufactured separately and eventually
assembled. The reproduction of living cells and organisms is ordinarily somewhat different, but that of bacteriophages can be described in terms similar to those above.
During reproduction of cultural organisms, modifications are possible. Some of them
are transmissible, as happens also for biological mutations. Some are voluntary attempts at introducing purposeful change (innovations), while others are random (like
biological mutations). All new, transmissible types are subject to the chance of
fixation, elimination, or of generating stable polymorphisms. The kinematics of
these phenomena is dictated by forces akin to mutation, natural selection, migration,
drift, etc., in ways similar, but obviously not identical, to those familiar for
biological evolution, as discussed at some length in a new book by Cavalli-Sforza
and Feldman (1981).

In addition to similarity, differences are also important. Natural selection can act at two levels. The cultural organism always depends on a living organism; it may well affect its Darwinian fitness, as passengers of a plane are well aware of. When an airplane crashes, the Darwinian fitness of passengers is at stake. But so is the Darwinian fitness of the airplane, since the crash may reflect badly on the acceptability of that type of plane by future passengers and airlines. A measurement of acceptability of the type of airplane would have a definition not very dissimilar from Darwinian fitness, and could constitute the Darwinian fitness of the plane type (usually taken as relative to other plane types). Such fitness is determined by choices and decisions made by the living organism, Man in this case; we call this process of choice "cultural selection" to distinguish it from natural selection, which we reserve for the living organism (where it was first introduced). Thus, natural and cultural selection are both of importance for cultural organisms. Also, migration and drift can be differentiated similarly into biological and cultural components.

Other gross differences between biology and culture are to be found in the mechanism of transmission. Transmission in biology is ordinarily close to perfect; with very few exceptions individuals generated are practically identical to those acting as models (apart from the complications of recombination). Therefore, a gene frequency tends to remain unaltered with the passage of generations, transmission being perfectly "neutral" (unless there is meiotic drive). Perfect balance in transmission is instead rarely true of a cultural trait, which is more similar to an infectious disease. Moreover, it is often transmitted also to unrelated people (and not just from parent to children, as is true of biology). In fact, there exists a multitude of mechanisms of cultural transmission, and they can be distinguished in a variety of ways: by the relationship between the teacher (or the "model" which is imitated) and the person being taught; by the age difference between them (sometimes there is a generation or more, sometimes less); by the ratio of the number of teachers or transmitters to the number of recipients, etc. The last criterion helps us differentiate among a many-to-one transmission, as in traits for which the whole social group exercises pressures on each individual; a one-to-one transmission, as in parent-child; and a one-to-many transmission, as in the school situation. Age differences, and especially the ratio of transmitters to recipients, are important in affecting strongly both the rate of change over time, the chance of polymorphisms, and the variation between non-communicating societies.

Some surveys (Cavalli-Sforza, et al., 1981; Chen et al., 1981) on college students have been used to test the models of cultural transmission developed, and for obtaining approximate estimates of parameters indicating transmission rates of parent-child, and between age peers for a set of cultural traits belonging to religion, politics, beliefs, sports, entertainment, and habits. The relative importance of parent-child transmission is highest for religion, and decreases in the six groups of traits studied in the order given. The study of age peer transmission (sibs, friends) showed it is especially important in entertainment, but not negligible for other groups of traits.

In other ways, population genetics interacts with the study of cultural transmission. Special attention has been given to cases in which there is inheritance of the capacity to learn, both in the case in which this capacity behaves as a continuous trait, influenced by one gene (Cavalli-Sforza and Feldman, 1973), or several (Cavalli-Sforza and Feldman, 1978b), or as a discontinuous trait (Feldman and Cavalli-Sforza, 1976; Uyenoyama et al., 1979). But the interaction can also be of another kind. Cultural evolution may affect biological evolution, and vice-versa. Among examples of the first direction, one usually cites the evolution towards adult lactose digestion in Caucasians and N. Africas (see Simoons, 1978), believed by many to be a consequence of the diffusion of milk consumption by adults in these areas. There are, of course, also many instances of evolution toward drug and pesticide resistance in various organisms. Most interesting would be cases of selection for specific behaviors in Man due to cultural evolution: there are several good candidates. It is practically certain, for instance, that developments in tool making abilities, and even more in speech abilities, must have been accompanied by strong natural selection and be responsible for some of the major changes we associate with hominization. Even today, or until a short while ago, genetic defects affecting the capacity to speak, hear, read or write reduced fitness very severely. Another physical trait whose evolution may have been helped by cultural innovations is the loss of hair. D. Morris (1967) lists several ways in which the "naked ape" may have first appeared, none of which is strictly cultural in origin. I would like to suggest, instead, that loss of hair is another example of cultural adaptation that may have had a selective effect on our genetic constitution. It seems a trivial consideration that Man must have started to use animal furs for protection against the cold. But why start this custom if protection by natural fur was sufficient? It is not inconceivable that the first individuals to carry animal furs may have been "naked" mutants, confronted with cold winters. But if these individuals lived where cold winters alternate with hot summers, they may have turned their "nakedness" into a selective advantage over the furry types, as they were in the situation of being protected from the heat biologically, and from the cold culturally. True of false, this suggestion can be useful for emphasizing the fact that the real selective advantage of cultural adaptation is that of extending the range of acceptable environments, and therefore the plasticity of the individual. Examples of the effects of cultural or biological evolution need not include only effects indicated by changes in natural selection. Many population explosions have been determined by technological changes. One example which is likely to have been of the greatest importance was the transition from food collection to food production, that is, from hunting and gathering economies to agriculture. A. Piazza discussed this cultural/biological change at the present meeting.

The area of interest of epidemiology of infectious diseases may seem to be wholly unrelated to population genetics. But the spread of infectious diseases is very similar to that of ideas, rumors, and, in general, cultural transmission. In most cases, of course, one can thus extend to disease the considerations we have just made for cultural traits. One expects diseases to be potentially dangerous and thus have negative effects on the fitness of an individual, while many cultural traits are likely to affect Darwinian fitness positively, or perhaps remain selectively neutral. There are, of course, exceptions, but in general the sign of selection coefficients is likely to be a major difference between an infectious disease and a cultural trait. Otherwise, there is no major (theoretical) difference. Thus, genetic variation in susceptibility to infectious disease can be treated by the same models used for genetic variation in capacity to learn, or, in general, to adopt a cultural trait (see, e.g. Cavalli-Sforza and Feldman, 1978b). There are many examples known of genetic variation in resistance to infectious disease. There are also examples of transmission of infectious disease by contagion from parent to offspring. Therefore, complex cases of transmission from parent to child, in which both genic and extragenic transmission operate side by side, can be expected not only for cultural traits, but also for infectious diseases. In species in which experimental inoculation is possible, the identification of the two mechanisms is relatively easy. Otherwise it may be difficult, and erroneous conclusions are on record in Man.

The last of the interactions of interest I have mentioned is that with ecology. Some of the papers to which we are going to listen at this symposium, by Jayakar and Matessi, offer new contributions on this topic; other important aspects have also been recently summarized systematically by Roughgarden (1979).

In conclusion, there are many ramifications of the mathematical theory of evolution. Some are generated by the evolutionary treatment of certain special biological topics which happen to be more amenable to quantification. Others arise as a conceptual extension of the theoretical treatment of evolution and other kinds of organisms. The same or similar postulates of the mathematical theory of biological evolution can be extended to other fields. But even minor differences in some of these postulates may have important effects in the final expectations.

Summary

The area of interest of population genetics overlaps with those of disciplines that range from molecular genetics to ecology, epidemiology, cultural anthropology and ethology. Developments in the areas of overlap vary considerably in extension, and will be briefly reviewed. These developments testify to the usefulness of the mathematical theory of evolution in a number of biological disciplines in which a quantitative approach is possible and rewarding.

References

Bodmer, WF, Cavalli-Sforza, LL (1971). Variation in fitness and molecular evolution. Proc. VI Berkeley Symp. on Mathematics, Statistics and Probability, Vol. 5. Univ. of California Press, Berkeley, pp. 155-175.

Cavalli-Sforza, LL (1966). Population structure and human evolution. Proc. Roy. Soc. Lond. 164:362-379.

Cavalli-Sforza, LL, Feldman, MW, (1973). Cultural versus biological inheritance: phenotypic transmission from parent to children. Am. J. Hum. Genet. 25:618-637.

Cavalli-Sforza, LL, Feldman, MW (1978a). Darwinian selection and altruism. Theor. Popul. Biol. 14:268-280.

Cavalli-Sforza, LL, Feldman, MW (1978b). The evolution of continuous variation III. Joint transmission of genotype, phenotype and environment. Genetics 90:391-425.

Cavalli-Sforza, LL, Feldman, MW, Chen, KH, Dornbusch, SM (1981). Theory and observation in cultural transmission. (manuscript in preparation).

Cavalli-Sforza, LL, Feldman, MW (1981). Cultural Transmission and Evolution: A Quantitative Approach. (to be published by Princeton Univ. Press).

Chen, KH, Feldman, MW, Cavalli-Sforza, LL (1981). A survey of cultural transmission on Taiwan students. (manuscript in preparation).

Feldman, MW, Cavalli-Sforza, LL (1976). Cultural and biological processes, selection for a trait under complex transmission. Theor. Popul. Biol. 9:238-259.

Haldane, JBS (1932). The Causes of Evolution. Harper, New York.

Hamilton, WD (1964). The genetical theory of social behavior. J. Theor. Biol. 7:1.

Kimura, M (1968). Evolutionary rate at the molecular level. Nature 217:624-626.

Kimura, M (1979). The neutral theory of molecular evolution. Sci. Amer. 241(5):98-126.

Kimura, M (1979). Model of effectively neutral mutations in which selective constraint is incorporated. Proc. Nat. Acad. Sci. USA 76:3440-3444.

Morris, D (1967). The Naked Ape. Jonathan Cape, London.

Piazza, A, Menozzi, P, Cavalli-Sforza, LL (1980). Synthetic gene frequency maps of man and selective effects of climate. (to be submitted to Proc. Nat. Acad. Sci. USA)

Roughgarden, J (1979). Theory of Population Genetics and Evolutionary Ecology: An Introduction. Macmillan, New York.

Simoons, F (1978). The geographic hypothesis and lactose malabsorption. Digestive Diseases 23:963-980.

Uyenoyama, M, Feldman, MW, Cavalli-Sforza, LL (1979). Evolutionary effects of contagious and familial transmission. Proc. Nat. Acad. Sci. USA 76:420-424.

Wilson, EO (1975). Sociobiology. Belknap Press of Harvard Univ. Press, Cambridge.

Zuckerkandl, E, Pauling, L (1965). Molecular disease, evolution and genic heterogeneity. Horizons in Biochemistry. Eds: M Kasha, B Pullman. Chicago Academic Press, Chicago.

COMPLETENESS AND CRAFT STANDARDS IN ECOLOGICAL THEORY

L.B. Slobodkin
Ecology and Evolution Department
State University of New York at Stony Brook
Stony Brook, New York 11794

I. Introduction

Clearly, good science permits us to "understand nature," i.e. to explain or predict or both. Exactly what is meant by this is unclear and varies between intellectual traditions. Since the publication of the seminal works by Volterra, theoretical ecology has continued to involve an interplay between natural history, applied mathematics, and genetics. While the curious tensions between these three traditions may not have been critical during the early pioneering stages of ecological development, they now require examination.

After discussing the relation between the intellectual craft standards in contributory disciplines of theoretical ecology, advocating the viewpoint that ecology generates its own standards, I will present two examples in which I will focus on the peculiar epistemetric properties of ecology. One of these will deal with ecosystem description and analysis and the other with the transmission of the insight of naturalists in a sufficiently formal way so as to be amenable to inclusion in theoretical models.

I will conclude that useful ecological theory does, in fact, exist and has its own logical structure, which differs in significant ways from the logical structure used in most of physical science.

II. The Conversation Between Naturalists and Theoreticians

While naturalists tend to be fascinated by detailed, particular facts and by the complexities of nature, model builders tend to try to look past the particularities to a more general format. These differences complicate communication and affect the way questions about nature are answered and formulated.

Given the limitations of talent and academic curricula, very few thoroughly learn both mathematics and natural history. Many of the most significant publications in ecological theory represent a collaborative effort, as for example that between Volterra and D'Ancona. This kind of collaboration is not simple. One of the complicating factors relates to the use of state descriptions and this will be a primary concern here, although this is not the only area of difficulty (Slobodkin 1965, 1975, and Slobodkin and Wu, 1975).

In the most general sense, to predict the behavior of an inanimate system by use of a theoretical model involves three essential steps. The system of interest must itself be defined and bounded. An initial state of the system must be defined by an appropriate set of measurements and a model used to develop predictions. This set of procedures and quality standards is usually ingrained in a theoretician during his adolescence.

Other things being equal, to a mathematician a model which generates a rich class of accurate predictions from a relatively small set of initial measurements is preferable on both aesthetic and pragmatic grounds to one which requires extensive measurement for meager conclusions. In the less applied areas of mathematics the aesthetic criteria become increasingly important. If a modification of the problem by a simplification of the system definition, or a counter-to-fact assumption, can materially enhance the attainable theoretical richness, then the modification is considered valuable and advisable. In pure mathematics the aesthetic standard is paramount.

In collaboration between a theoretician and a naturalist, there is usually no serious problem in defining the system of interest. The necessary state description, however, usually presents a problem. This arises because it is extremely difficult to discover intimate facts about nature, so that biologists feel that a fruitful lifetime of research can often be represented by a half dozen facts about a few species, often with no assurance that they apply to other species or that they are relevant to any particular question that might be asked.

When it becomes necessary for scientific, or practical, reasons to answer some specific question about either a population or ecosystem it may be the case that a naturalist has the answer readily available. Usually, however this is not the case, since the possible number of kinds of questions is so great. Explicit studies may be undertaken to seek an answer but such studies often involve long-term observations in the field or laboratory. With historically increasing frequency, the urgency and complexity of questions addressed to ecology are such as to prohibit the necessary expenditure of time and money. For many questions, even if time and resources were available, the operationality of the process of direct investigation is open to question.

Given actual constraints, often attempts at solution involve constructing a model, which is then manipulated to provide an appropriate

answer. This requires that a state descriptor be made explicit. What
ought to be in the state descriptor is set by the question being asked
and the model to be used. When the naturalist is asked to provide the
needed state information and his collection of facts does not include
what is required by the theoretician, an impasse arises which permits
several alternative procedures. One is to abandon the concept of a
model or formal theory and to rely on the insight of the naturalist to
answer the question at issue. A second possibility is to attempt to
develop a theory from the available information, even if this departs
from familiar mathematical forms. In theoretical ecology both of these
approaches are relatively rare. The first suffers from being untestable,
and smacks of relying on a "guru" rather than "science". The second is
likely to violate the craft standards of the model builder, or at least
make the process more difficult for him. I will return to discuss both
of these in later sections.

Here I briefly consider a third and very common alternative. Namely, when a mathematically trained theoretician, with a model to hand,
asks a natural historian for the information needed to construct a state
vector and is told the appropriate information is not available, the
apparent lack of information may be taken as a license to simplify the
problem so that it will fit into the available framework. The properties
of this theoretical framework are often dictated by mathematical convenience and craft standards.

Occasionally the actual information from nature is too rich for
the kind of state descriptor that the model builder wants to use. Once
again the craft standards of the mathematician usually prevail. For
example, age structure differences, non-linearities, and biological
peculiarities are often deliberately ignored in order to develop a
mathematically tractable format (i.a. May 1976, May et al. 1979).

Occasionally the biological inquiry suggests either a new use for
an interesting mathematical technique or, after slight simplification,
produces a problem of mathematical beauty.

Some of the published material in mathematical ecology, like formal
population genetics, is best considered a sub-area of applied mathematics
with its own internal standards of quality, internally generated questions and answers. They need not be expected to provide explicit answers
to biologically generated questions, but this leaves the problem of how
models are to be constructed to answer ecological questions that are of
biological or practical, but not mathematical, interest.

Obviously there is neither need for, nor value in a model of nature which precisely simulates the natural world. Borges (1975) has discussed the making of a map as large and detailed as the province it represents. However, while map makers select the kind of information they retain, the criteria of retention are mainly the needs of the map user rather than those of the cartographer. In the following sections I will consider how ecology can respond to the pragmatic needs of its users. The users are of two general classes; those concerned with ecological management and those concerned with the testing of theoretical conclusions. I am attempting to examine "user-oriented" ecological theory.

III. Complete Description in Natural History

A general assumption in the above discussion was that the information acquired by naturalists can be effectively transmitted to persons who have not shared the experience of naturalists. Running counter to this assumption, however, is what might be called the naturalists' mystique; namely, that the only way to learn what the naturalists have learned after 20 years is to follow their footsteps for 20 years. When one eminent naturalist was asked how he recognized a good muskrat habitat, he seriously said "I can think like a muskrat," I did not doubt him, but the answer was not helpful. There exists a very real problem of making sure that the assertions of naturalists are publicly verifiable. Unless it is possible for the naturalist to permit someone else to share his insights by some process other than that of becoming his disciple, the scientific value of these insights remains questionable.

The information of natural history is in fact often presented in lengthy descriptions of particular organisms, expeditions, collections, etc. It is a more than trivial task to search the scientific literature for information about particular organisms. Given the fact that there are of the order of 2 million species, the search might even seem to be an endless and impossible task. However, I believe, for two reasons based on the properties of organisms, that in fact natural history need not be a mass of indigestable details. The obvious reason is that, by and large, the classical system of biological classification works reasonably well, so that, while certain details of muskrat biology may be the esoteric knowledge of only an experienced muskrat expert, many of the properties associated with rodents, mammals, chordates and eucaryotes in general are well known. I will not belabor this point further.

The second, more speculative, point I will illustrate with an example from my own work (Slobodkin, 1980). My students and I have been concerned with hydra as experimental animals for many years. Part of the motivation for studying these animals has been that there is already an enormous history of previous study going back to the early 18th century. Not only have hydra been carefully studied in the past but by all reasonable criteria they seem somewhat simpler than most Metazoans. It would therefore seem that we might actually get to the point in the study of hydra in which we might assert that in fact we "know" the natural history of these animals.

This point seems to elude us however since new and surprising facts continue to emerge. Within the past two years we have been able to document predatory interactions between particular hydra species and escape behavior in which one species crawls away from another. Neither of these phenomena, at least to the best of my knowledge, has been found before. Nevertheless, we can claim to understand the natural history of hydra in a more complete way than that of most groups of organisms. It is therefore of interest to ask whether we can meaningfully and usefully organize this information so that it can be easily transmitted.

Hydra share with other animals reproductive activities, feeding, physiological responses to their environment, wound healing and so forth. What questions can we answer about hydra which we cannot answer about say the Pogonophora which have essentially not been studied at all? Can we demonstrate that in fact we understand the well-studied hydra in some deeper sense than we understand the biology or organisms that have not been studied from the standpoint of natural history? Obviously if no such demonstration can be made then we must question the value of studying natural history.

It is possible to construct ecological theories for which detailed natural history is irrelevant, on the basis of optimization assumptions (see for example Maynard Smith in this volume and the references therein). Prediction of specific isolated traits (i.e. particular organs, habits, or anatomical features) in particular organisms is not generally a convincing test of optimization theory since it is generally agreed that the meaning of any trait only becomes clear if the trait is seen in context. Without contextual understanding it is impossible to be confident that a particular trait relates to the theory itself rather than to something quite extraneous. This has recently become most apparent in the polemical literature related to Wilsonian-sociobiology.

control mechanism. That is, if there is strong dominance by the hypo-
stome, budding is restricted and the food that would have supported the
budding process can only be used for growth.

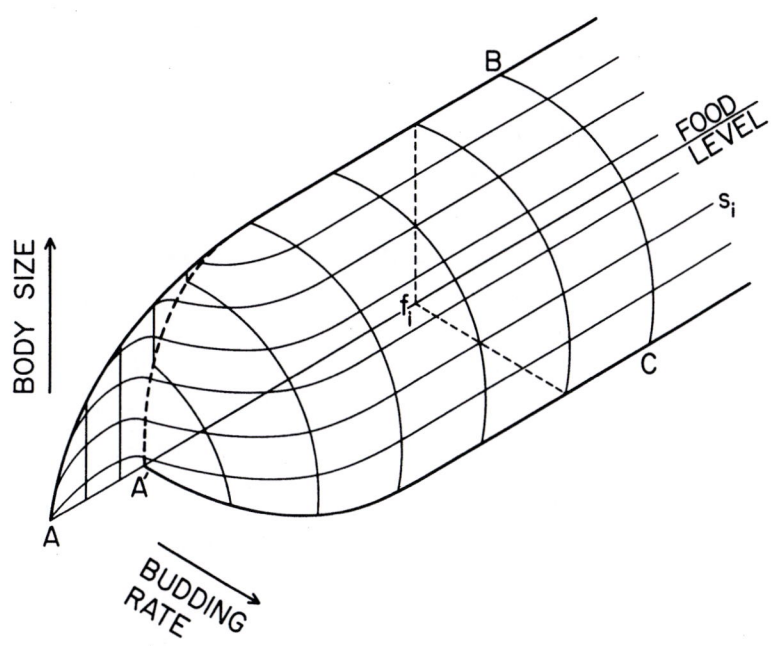

Fig. 1. The three axes are <u>food level</u> and the <u>body size</u> and <u>budding
rate</u> attained by individual animals all at constant temperature and
kept at constant food until an approximate steady state in their budding rate has been reached. The surface flattens against the food
level-body size plane at low food levels, since hydra can be maintained
at food levels which permit survival but not budding. At food levels
below A hydra die. As food level increases, the smaller species of
hydra begin to bud before the larger ones. At sufficiently high food
levels the growth and reproductive rates reach an asymptote. The
meridianal lines (As_i, etc.) represent what I believe to be the trace
of particular genotypes on this surface.

Does the fact that a male baboon walks ahead of his troop mean that he
is "leading" or that he is "scouting" or that he is "protecting" or
that "he wants to be alone"? A full context for the activity is required before the forward position of the male can be used to test any
theory.

The question that concerns me here is whether an appreciation of
the full context of behavior can be transmitted from persons who have
studied the organism to persons who have not studied the organism. We
cannot expect to be able to present the full context for properties of
mammals or of poorly studied organisms if we cannot do so for hydra or
other simple well-studied organisms.

The problem is not trivial. Simply a list of facts denies any
meaning to the idea of context. "Context" implies some kind of organization in which the nature of the organization itself is significant.
As a heuristic device I attempted to diagram as much information as
possible about hydra. To do this I examined triplets of measurements
which might generate a three-dimensional field on which other information could be plotted. After trying a large number of possible presen-
tations, the only choice of axes that seemed suitable for this purpose
was that shown in Fig. 1.

Most properties of organisms and environments do not lend themselves to linear ordering so that arbitrarily chosen triplets of
properties of either hydra or their environment did not generate
c o h e r e n t surfaces of any recognizable kind. Even if I restrict my
choices to orderable axes, say temperature, size, and food supply as
one possible triplet, they did not generate coherent closed surfaces.

In Figs. 1 and 2 I summarize almost two decades of study in my
laboratory of various aspects of the biology of hydra and also of the
work of many other investigators (cf. references in Slobodkin, 1980)
in as complete and explicit a way as I can. I start with several facts,
valid for some hydra, although they have not been demonstrated for all
species. I believe that they will hold on the basis of what we know
about how related animals tend to resemble each other and they permit
me to rationalize my choice of axes for Fig. 1.

(1) Hydra have an asymptotically increasing relation between food
supply and both growth rate and budding rate at any particular temperature, kind of food, and water chemistry.

(2) Between species, there is an inverse relation between growth
rate, and budding rate. This is intimately related to the apical

Increasing temperature lowers body size and increases budding rate
for several species. It may, therefore, rotate or pull the surface of
Fig. 1 towards the small-body-size-rapid-budding edge. Alternations in
water chemistry may also distort the surface in a reasonably simple
manner.

In Fig. 2 I have tentatively mapped closed regions on the surface
shown in Fig. 1 which describe the responses of hydra.

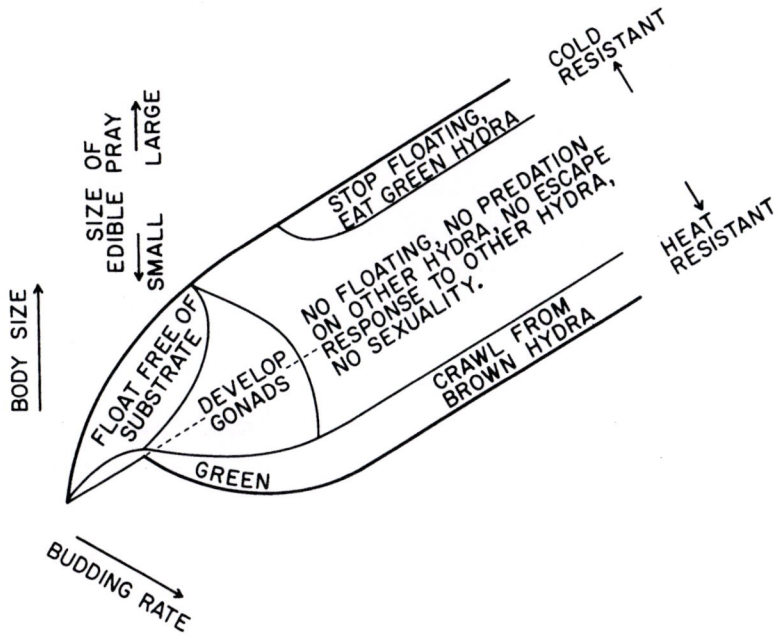

Fig. 2. Some examples of properties of hydra that seem to map onto the
adaptive response surface shown in Fig. 1.

The surface drawn in Figs. 1 and 2 is an Adaptive Response Surface
which arises purely from observation of hydra. It is not a consequence
of any more general theory. That is, no optimization theory or theory
of population genetics or niche theory or adaptive landscape theory
predicts how to draw the surface, although there is reason to suspect
that a surface of this type is possible in general (see below). It is

possible to rationalize the particular responses, but the rationaliza·
tions are independent of the description. That is, tne transmission of
information about hydra is free of optimality assumption or models, but
can be used to organize and present the kind of information required to
construct theoretical models.

We have just provided the information to permit the reader to think
like a hydra to some extent. Obviously hydra are not as clever as
muskrat. But perhaps available information about muskrats can be
presented in an equally public way.

Since the immediate concern is purely descriptive there is no
guarantee that the same set of axes would be equally useful in dealing
with some other set of organisms than hydra, although on the other hand
they might be useful. The question is an empirical one.

IV.   Ecological Descriptions as Objects of Theoretical Analysis

I believe that I demonstrated in Section III that there may exist
ways of describing ecological systems which are derived from basically
biological considerations. The adaptive response surface is rich in
information and admits of the addition of further information. It also
permits this information to be communicated in an explicit way.

I will now relate the concept of Adaptive Response Surface (ARS),
introduced as a technique for communicating ecological information, to
some other approaches to ecological and evolutionary theory.

If ARS such as Fig. 1 are real they relate to and support the
contentions of King and Wilson (1975) about evolutionary mechanisms.
These authors suggest that quantitatively small DNA differences between
species can result in major morphological differences, if the DNA
differences act to control developmental properties and thereby the
mode of expression of other genes.

I am suggesting that many of the apparent differences between
hydra species are related to the single mechanism of strength of hypostomal dominance, so that in these organisms, between species differences can be largely attributed to genetic control of a regulatory
process. In the case of the hydra the relevant developmental control
can be explicitly identified.

For any group of organisms there will exist an Adaptive Response
Surface if there are a relatively small number of major genetic controls of a few developmental and physiological properties which will

in turn determine other properties, in the context of the organisms'
environment. Wherever it is the case that quantitative differences in
regulatory processes affect a group of related species an ARS may be
expected. This is obviously speculative but is amenable to investigation.

In hydra the genotypic control of hypostomal dominance seems to
regulate the interdependence between size and budding rate which in
turn determines how suitable various environmental circumstances are
for different kinds of hydra.

Only for purposes of discussion, I momentarily abandon the requirement of strict operationality and will speak in terms of generalized
abstract properties of organisms and environments in order to discuss
the relation between the concept of the empirical description as summarized in the Adaptive Response Surface and three central theoretical
concepts of ecology and evolution. The Hutchinsonian Niche, Sewall
Wright Adaptive Landscape and Fisher's Fundamental Theorem of Natural
Selection.

Consider an Instantaneous Environmental Space each point of which
is defined by a set of all measurements that might be relevant to any
hydra--light intensity, temperature, probability of encountering various
types of prey or dangers and water chemistry are among the appropriate
measures. Actual points in the natural environment relate to this space
by a many-one mapping. Even if this explicit description and mapping
were possible, they would be of very limited use, since the adaptive
value of various properties of hydra depend on the temporal and spatial
distributions of environmental properties--not on instantaneous values.
The space of all possible distributions and co-occurrences of all possible instantaneous values--call it the Environmental Distribution Space
has an absurdly large number of dimensions. The subset of that space
in which any hydra population can maintain itself is the Fundamental
Niche of Hydra (Hutchinson 1957).

The situation is somewhat eased by considering that we are more
concerned with nature than with abstract spaces, so we need not consider any portion of the abstract space for which there are no environmental mapping points. This does not diminish the dimensionality but
does discard much of the volume (Cf. Hutchinson 1968).

Now consider the relation between the set of all possible hydra
genotypes and each point in the Environmental Distribution Space. Any
single point can be though of as a potential set of circumstances which
could be either found in nature or set up in the laboratory and in

which in principle, all possible multiples of hydra genotypes could be experimentally tested. If these genotypes represent different species, no assertions could be made about relative fitness, since fitness in normal population genetic usage is not defined between species but only between genotypes within species (Lewontin, 1974). This restriction again sweeps away many of the possible multiples of genotypes but still leaves an impossibly large number to be ranked for relative fitness, assuming the techniques to measure such fitness were available (Slobodkin and Rapoport, 1974).

Hydra are divisible into groups of genotypes. Consider one such group, say Hydra oligactis, and then consider the i-th genotype from that group and consider that this particular genotype is tested for relative fitness against all other H. oligactis genotypes over the points in the Environmental Distributions Space, permitting an assignment of relative fitness for genotype i at each such point j. The environmental points could then be considered as a multidimensional map upon which the specific relative fitness values of genotype i can be plotted as elevations. This will produce a kind of landscape which will state which environments are best (i.e. show highest fitness) for genotype i.

Since I am focussing on the relative fitness of a particular genotype in different environments, this is not the same as the concept of "Adaptive Landscape" developed by Wright (1932). If the environment is kept constant, separate landscapes can be constructed for each alternative genotype of H. oligactis. The Adaptive Landscape of Sewall Wright relates to the distribution of genotypes within a polymorphic population in a particular environment. The elevation, in that case, refers to particular genetic combinations which will have locally higher fitnesses than others. The Sewall Wright landscape demonstrates that even knowing the complete characteristics of the environment does not uniquely predict the course of evolution in a genetically polymorphic population. For present discussion I assume that the genotypes showing peaks on the Sewall Wright landscape in a particular environment will be on the average phenotypically more similar to each other than they would be to those in a different environment. (Note: If I should use Maynard Smith's version of the concept of Adaptive Landscape in which the environments of Ostrich, Kangaroo and Antelope are considered identical (sic) then the above argument is not of value.)

The relative rate of gene frequency change in the absence of mutation and migration at each environmental point will depend on the

variance of between genotype fitnesses at that point. This plausible
sounding hypothesis is suggested by, but not demonstrable from, Fisher's
Fundamental Theorem (1930) since Fisher's study makes simplifying
assumptions about recombination which make it impossible to rigorously
apply in the present discussion. Nevertheless one might expect gene
frequencies to alter so as to sort out genotypes between environments,
leaving each genotype predominantly at the region of its adaptive peak.
Locally less fit genotypes at each location would be expected to become
rare, eventually minimizing fitness variance and rates of gene frequency
change at all points.

I make the plausible assumptions that more similar phenotypes can
deal effectively with more similar environmental problems and that
similar genotypes produce similar phenotypes in similar environments.
I assume also that hydra actually conform to the surfaces of Figs. 1
and 2 and that there also exists a descriptor of the environmental requirements of hydra that has the property of a surface.

On these assumptions Fig. 1 is isomorphically one to one mappable
onto a surface defined by a set of environmental measures, in the sense
that nearest points on the one surface will correspond to nearest points
on the other. It should therefore be possible to predict from environmental measurements the phenotypic properties of an optimally fit hydra
for that environment. Conversely, we also should be able to predict
from the properties of the hydra a class of optimal environments.

In each portion of this discussion I have tried to keep statements
about genotype, phenotype and environment distinct, connecting them by
explicit relationships. I feel that some of the confusion in ecological theory has been caused by failure to maintain this distinction.

Figs. 1 and 2 relate to measurements of individual organisms, not
populations, despite the fundamental concern of ecology with populations.
Budding rate is not equivalent to any of the functions of rate of increase normally used in population dynamics since these consider death
as a component of increase. Death is considered here to be the resultant of a series of environmental accidents to which the individual
animals may be more or less susceptible depending on their position on
Fig. 1. Death is considered as a largely environmental event--perhaps
predation, being washed away, starving, etc. An attempt to incorporate
death as a part of the ARS is therefore difficult since death involves
both environmental and phenotypic properties in the same measure.

Fig. 1 does however provide insight into population processes.
While the exact death rate will depend on miscellaneous environmental

events not explicitly listed, it is to be expected that at least some of these events are more likely to affect starved rather than well fed hydra. Any population of hydra in the region of the line BC (Fig. 1), can be expected to shift its relation to its own food supply toward point A if sources of mortality are sufficiently ineffective. As it does so, budding rate will decrease, as will food consuming capacity, and the size range of acceptable food items. The system may stabilize at almost any point if appropriate sources of mortality are present.

Which hydra species are expected to be present in any location will depend on the size of food particles available and the sources of mortality. Water flow patterns will also be important--considering, for example, that a reasonably swift laminar flow will act as a selective mechanism for removing large floating animals. Temperature increase may shift competitive outcomes as a function of its effect on both hydra and their potential prey.

In short, after verification of Figs. 1 and 2, the properties of hydra required to construct population growth models of a very realistic kind can be read off these figures and can be readily combined with actual circumstances of interest. Figs. 1 and 2 do not constitute a model of hydra population growth but are a meta-model (in the sense of Slobodkin 1958).

In general, an Adaptive Response Surface is a multi-dimensional surface to which the individual organisms of some group are confined evolutionarily and ontogenetically. It permits mapping of closed regions which define the occurrence and context of specific properties or activities of the organisms.

There are two kinds of theoretical problems in evaluating whether or not a particular data presentation is an ARS or not, statistical or biological.

The statistical problems are concerned with measuring the probability that a particular cloud of data points actually represents a particular multi-dimensional surface drawn through the cloud. I will not deal with that problem here.

Biologically, I believe that an Adaptive Response Surface must have the following characteristics:

It must be complete for a taxon, in the sense that any attempt to construct an ARS for the class Aves, for example, must define the phenotype of all possible birds. It should not have either holes or islands in it. In terms of Fig. 1 this means I could not claim to have

constructed an ARS for hydra if I had to refer explicitly to species'
names in constructing the surface.

It is quite likely that any attempt to construct such a surface
for birds as a whole would require so many dimensions as to be effectively meaningless, although it might be done for the smaller subgroups--
say penguins, flamingos, or warblers.

The dimensions of an Adaptive Response Surface are empirically
determined. In the case of Fig. 1, since hypostomal dominance can in
effect be measured by the body-size budding-rate ratio, the genetic
property "degree of hypostomal dominance" need not appear as an explicit
axis. Food level is environmental, and the size and budding rate are
phenotypic. Extra genetic dimensions would have possibly freed me from
the necessity to discuss greenness and floating explicitly in Fig. 2
and permitted me to read these properties directly from the axes, but
at the cost of clarity.

Not every set of possible axes is appropriate for the construction
of an ARS nor will every arrangement of appropriate axes produce a com-
prehensible surface.

It seems apparent that the organisms which can be included on the
same surface are ecologically related. However, they do not necessarily
constitute a guild, since guilds are defined in terms of role and role
is determined in part by environmental properties not used in defining
the surface. Nor do they necessarily compete with each other. For
example, there may be very little food overlap between large and small
hydra. Hydra do, in fact, both form a guild and compete under certain
circumstances but this is an empirical matter, not predictable a priori
from the idea of the ARS. It may be the case that all organisms that
share a surface can, under some circumstances, constitute a guild or
compete. It is certainly the case that members of the guild and sets
of competitors need not be on the same surface.

There is, however, a definite formally necessary relation between
organisms that share a surface. Namely, they share a set of restrictions on their evolution and ontogeny such that they are relatively free
to move on the surface but not orthogonal to it. It is this type of
restriction that Bateson (1963) referred to as the economics of somatic
evolution and similar concepts are central to optimization and evolutionary theory (Lewontin, 1978; Stearns, 1977).

In this section I have attempted to relate the concept of Adaptive
Response Surface, developed for hydra in section III, to other

theoretical modes of description of the ecology of specific organisms.

V. The Problem of Describing Ecosystems

Ecosystems are even more difficult to describe completely than are their component populations. Nevertheless specific questions about ecosystems must necessarily be asked and answered.

The sense of what it means to understand an ecosystem and how this understanding can aid in answering specific questions will be considered in this section which is a summary of arguments presented by Botkin et al, 1979; Maguire et al, 1980; and Slobodkin et al, 1980.

Given a particular ecosystem, assuming we know its boundaries, we might want to know how it will be altered under some particular environmental perturbation, which might mean anything from changing hunting or fishing regulations to building a military base or garbage dump; or we might want to know how its properties conform to some scientific prediction--a theory of species packing, an energy flow diagram or a gene distribution pattern. Obviously the most useful kind of observation of that ecosystem, and the ways in which these observations would be used, may be expected to vary with the question being asked.

For many questions, a model of the system may prove more satisfactory in providing answers than direct observations confined to real time. Obviously, models are of value in deciding about the possible effects of perturbation since otherwise we would have to perform the perturbation on a comparable system.

Is there a uniquely best kind of ecosystem model? Since we cannot generally anticipate the questions to be asked, might it be possible to build a complete model which will be equally useful for dealing with all questions in advance of specification of any question?

In general a complete model is not technically feasible since each, of up to several thousand, species in the ecosystem may interact directly or indirectly with any of the others in many measureably different ways. Also the inanimate storage pools will interact with each other and with the organisms present. The number of kinds of interactions which may themselves be of interest makes it effectively impossible to construct a realistic or complete model which will be any simpler to understand than the ecosystem itself. Because of this difficulty a series of indices of ecosystem condition have been defined which have permitted the construction of more tractable models. Among these indices are caloric content, species diversity, information content (curiously defined), biogeochemical fluxes and evolutionary optimality criteria (e.g. Pielou, 1969; Innes, 1975; Margelef, 1975). A common feature of these indices is that the necessary number of observations required to describe the system for purposes of the model or theory is materially reduced below what would be required in constructing any complete model. This is of importance since the actual measuring of ecosystems usually involves perturbation.

Many indices are relatively low in information content, in the sense that even if we knew the index there remains a great deal we do not know. For example knowing the species diversity, carbon flow and biomass together will not tell us if we are in a forest, swamp, coral reef or high grass prairie.

The use of an index involves a choice of procedures and assumption as to the relative theoretical importance of the index chosen as compared with others that might have been chosen. Therefore, since at present there exists no theory that is sufficiently powerful to use any particular index to generate answers to all possible questions, the relative importance of the different indices is contingent on the importance to be attached to the different questions that might be asked about the system. We have already seen that there is no particular restriction on these so that there is no generally optimal index, or even set of indices, for ecosystem description.

If we are asked to make assertions about some particular system it would seem to be advantageous to be able to use our expertise with other ecosystems in this new context. This can be done to the degree that we can make assertions about how various indices may be expected to behave, or to the degree that the material studied in this ecosystem can be determined to have properties identifical with those of previously studied systems. Unfortunately only weak generalizations about the behavior of ecosystems indices have been developed so far and it is very difficult to establish identity between most components of ecosystems (with exceptions to be indicated below). The herbivores in one ecosystem are often quite different from the herbivores in another. Maynard Smith (1978) could assume an identity between kangaroos and antelopes for the purposes of his theoretical inquiries, but this identity is not as useful for purposes of management or perturbation analysis.

So far I have recited a series of difficulties, complications and negative assertions. I will now suggest that there exists a uniquely useful descriptor for any ecosystem which is rich in information, which permits bringing to bear on the ecosystem literally centuries of past research; which is formal in the sense of being statable as a simple list; which is theoretically neutral in the sense of not imposing constraints on the types of questions that might be asked of the ecosystem; and is useful both in the sense of being of some help with regard to any question that might be asked of the ecosystem and of permitting certain types of questions that could not otherwise be asked.

After that imposing introduction I request that the reader seriously consider what will seem at first reading to be an anticlimactic platitude.

I suggest that this paragon of apparent operational and theoretical virtues is a partial list of the species observed in the area under question. I will now defend this apparently atavistic assertion.

A species name, despite being subject to change as taxonomic revisions occur, is enormously rich in information. It provides access, through the scientific literature, to the work of naturalists studying organisms of that kind and similar kinds over the past three centuries. It also provides information about all the properties these organisms share with the broader taxonomic groups to which the particular species belongs. This pool of information also includes statements about necessary environmental conditions and biological prerequisites of the organisms. In fact there is no cheaper or more effective way of gaining flexible, useful information about an ecosystem than making a list of the species that can relatively easily be found there.

Consider what is learned from the first species named on the list. We know roughly its temperature and food requirements, and we know whether or not it is terrestrial or marine or aquatic. We can therefore eliminate, as possible complicators of our consideration of this ecosystem, more than 1 million species as having requirements incompatible with the known property of the organism we have found. In all cases, finding that first organism need have essentially no impact on the ecosystem itself.

Finding a second species will reduce the class of possible species yet to be found to the logical product of the species that might coexist with both it and the first species, adding more to our list of impossible new finds. Further extension of the species list will provide more information but probably at a diminishing rate. The fiftieth species found adds less new information about the characteristics of that ecosystem than the second or tenth.

At this point the 2 million possible kinds of inhabitants that might have been present have been divided into four portions. The largest portion consists of organisms one can be sure are absent. There will be several thousand species that may or may not be expected to be found on further investigation. There is also a class of organisms that have not yet been found but we believe must be present, since there presence is a prerequisite for the occurrence of some organism we have actually seen. Finally, there is a small list of actually observed species.

We also will have, from the data associated with past investigations of the observed species, and those whose presence may be inferred, a reasonably good idea of the physical and chemical properties of the ecosystem--probably a much better idea than we would have had if we spent a corresponding amount of time and effort on chemical, geological, and meteorological analyses.

A species list is therefore seen as a cheap, rapid, information-laden approach to defining an ecosystem.

This procedure works for two basic reasons. First, each species is related to the world in a slightly different way, but all share the property of continuity. Each species can be thought of an an environmental sensor, whose persistance in a particular place is a reliable indication of the condition and immediate past history of that place. To acquire knowledge of each species' properties would be prohibitively time-consuming, expensive and possibly environmentally perturbing, but we have free quick access to information gained by past studies.

So far I claim a species list to be a uniquely valuable definition of any ecosystem for any purpose. The more complete the list the better, but even an incomplete list is very good.

The information implicit in the species list is generally not derived from the ecosystem under investigation but rather uses previous studies made in other locations. This not only saves time and money but also avoids, to some extent, the problem of excessive perturbation of an ecosystem during an investigation.

I do not require the assumption that the role of all species are invariant between ecosystems. Certain plants vary in their growth habits in known ways and diets of predators are notoriously different from place to place. The expectation that a species may change from place to place can be taken into account in any particular study.

There is an assumption that species have been more or less correctly designated. The effect of an error in species identification will depend strongly on the problems being studied. If, for example, one is concerned with the role of fungi as decomposers, the differences in toxicity between various Amanita mushrooms is probably not critical. Species definition of the Amanitas would require greater care if the problem at hand was the establishment of a mushroom restaurant.

A species list is theoretically neutral in the sense that it is implicitly a rich collection of information, some of which is almost certainly relevant to any ecological problems but none of which in any way constrains the class of questions that might be asked.

From the information implicit in the species list one may be able to provide explicit answers to specific questions of managerial importance. At the least, this information will define what must be studied to answer a specific question and will avoid fruitless repetition of effort.

An observed species list partially defines an ecosystem. The failure of complete definition may be of several kinds. If two ecosystems have identical observed species list they may differ in the set of unknown species. If two ecosystems have species lists which overlap but are not identical they may actually share identical complete lists since the nonoverlapping species in each case may be among the not-yet-observed-species in the other. Nevertheless a broadly overlapping species list strongly indicates some kind of similarity between ecosystems. Ecosystems which broadly share a species list are referred to by Botkin et al. (1979) as being in the same "ecosystem cluster".

While finding the first few species of the species list is nondestructive, being sure one has the complete list involves serious perturbation, so that a guaranteed complete species list is not actually accessible for any but the simplest of ecosystems. Identity of "species cluster" is the best one can do.

For essentially all interesting questions, subsequent investigation beyond the definition of the species list will be needed. No model can be properly formulated in the absence of a question but natural history of the animals found in the ecosystem is likely to be of some value for almost any question.

Ecosystems with identical species lists may differ in their responses. A forest may have one specimen of wild cherry and a

thousand maples and will be expected to differ in many respects from
one with a thousand wild cherry trees and only one maple.

Ancillary information, selected for a particular purpose and
specifically collected from the ecosystem at issue to provide information not implicitly available in the species list, may be termed the
"state variable vector" for that ecosystem and for a specific problem.
This is never a complete state vector, since different measurements
would have been made were the question different.

The mathematicians' standard of elegance returns, since, given the
information in the species list, shorter state variable vectors which
can still permit the analysis to solve a particular question are preferable. That is, a minimum of new information gathering is advisable both
from the standpoint of ecosystem perturbation and expense and from the
standpoint of mathematical elegance, providing the resultant analysis
actually can solve problems.

I have described a process of ecosystem investigation which consists of combining the information of natural history (embodied in the
species list) with measurements made on site (the state variable
vector) to produce an ecosystem descriptor tailored to the requirements
of a particular theoretical or practical problem. This procedure
circumvents the necessity for constraining ecosystem theory within the
craft standards of mathematicians rather than those of biologists and
abandons the unrealistic search for complete ecosystem models.

It also relegates simplified indices of the state of ecosystems to
the status of objects for study, rather than substitutes for natural
history information. For example, it may meaningfully be asked how
diversity indices vary with species and with the state of ecosystems
but it need not be assumed that a diversity index must be relevant to
a conservation problem.

It might be noted that the species lists themselves can also serve
as objects of study. Freckman et al. (1980) have used them to analyze
a problem in species packing theory. Botkin, et al. (Ms.) investigate the abstract geometry of the hypercube generated by the class of
all species lists. I will now discuss some aspects of species lists in
that context.

The species list derived from direct field observation is the
cheapest and most effective starting point for studying any ecosystem.
It will be termed the "observed species list" and each such list will
be considered as a vector of ones representing the presence of observed

species i, j, k, etc.; a_i, a_j, a_k, etc. List B will have entries b_i, b_j, b_k, etc. Confining our attention to the naive list, it is possible to measure the square of an Euclidean distance between two such lists as $D^2(A,B)$. For this purpose the logical sum (A∨B) of two lists is considered as the list of species found in either A or B. Then n (A∨B) is the number of species in (A∨B).

The square distance between the two observed lists is the number of disagreements between the two lists.

An absolute distance of say 5 is more significant if the species lists A and B are short than if they are longer. Relative distance between two naive lists A and B can be determined as a fraction of the maximum possible distance that might have occurred between the two lists. This maximum distance is equal to $(A∨B)^{\frac{1}{2}}$. If, for example, in two such lists there are a total of 12 species the maximum possible distance (i.e., no corresponding species in the two lists) is $12^{\frac{1}{2}}$.

If there are 5 species in list A and 10 in list B, but three species are common to both lists then

$$D^2(A,B) = 7(1-0)^2 + 3(1-1)^2 + 2(0-1)^2 = 9$$

$$D = 3$$

Relative distance is $\dfrac{D(A,B)}{D_{max}(A,B)} = \sqrt{\dfrac{9}{12}} = .87$

On the observed list appear only species actually seen, not those inferred. If I were to assign a 0 to all species not seen, then my naive list would have c.10^6 entries--the overwhelming preponderance of which are 0's (but obviously none of which are 0's for all possible lists).

The distance, and relative distance, between any two lists is not changed by considering the global species list, but we are permitted to pose certain questions about the distribution of actual lists on the hypercube generated by the global list. The number of vertices of the global hypercube is enormous, of the order of 2^{10^6}. The number of species found in any area small enough to admit of ecologically significant short term interaction, (i.e., any ecosystem which is likely to pose any managerial or theoretical problem) is of the order of 10^3 or 10^4. We can ask how are the relatively tiny number of observed species lists distributed over the immense number of vertices of the global hypercube?

This question is more tractable if we consider the distribution of distances between lists. If there were no ecological connection between species, the distribution of the distances between species lists would be unimodal and the probability of finding any particular species on any particular list would be proportional to its abundance in individuals. However, it is almost certain from what is known of the interdependence of organisms, that the distribution of distances between observed species list is actually bimodal. Either a relatively large number of species will be shared between lists or very few species will be shared. The peak in the region of maximum distances will be in the distance range 10^1 - 10^2. (Since D_{max} is the square root of (A∨B) and maximal species lists are of length of order 10^3 - 10^4.)

The location of the short distance peak, and the degree to which the distance distributions are altered by using relative rather than absolute distance, are open questions but the above discussion is sufficient to indicate that there exist theoretical questions generated from a consideration simply of the naive species lists themselves.

The primary value of the observed species list is to act as a guide to the ecological literature. Among the information to be gained from this literature is an inferred species list consisting of the directly observed species plus species whose presence or absence can be inferred with some certainty from information about those which have actually been found.

Also, there are species whose probable presence or absence can be inferred but whose precise identity is not clear. That is, plants may be inferred from the presence of animals, but only if the animals are specific monophages will a precise species of plant be inferrable. There will also be a residuum of species whose presence or absence is not clear.

What does the transition from observed to inferred species lists do to the distances between pairs of species of naive lists and to the distribution of between-list distances? In inferred species lists we expect more entries than in observed lists, but the magnitude of 10^3 to 10^4 for maximal length of observed lists was taken from exhaustive samples (Elton, 1966). We therefore do not expect much basic difference in the distance distribution when we replace observed by inferred species lists.

A, B, C, etc. will designate inferred species lists. The distance between A and B is designated D(A,B) and each species in the list A, whether definitely known to be present or inferred to be present can be designated by a_i, a_j, a_k, etc. Two lists that share an enormous number of absences are relative very close to each other, but now we are considering them from the standpoint of the large hypercube and are permitted to use what we know of ecology. It seems likely that those 0's which are generated in common by two species lists and by several different species on each list represents species which are normally found in a different category of ecosystems from the two lists examined. This is suggested by the obvious fact that almost any organism on almost any naive species list of terrestrial ecosystems, will generate 0's for essentially the complete set of marine species. Lists containing marine organisms are representatives of those ecosystems which are maximally distant from the terrestrial ecosystems.

We can represent parts of the process of using the scientific literature to transform the observed into the inferred species list by considering that each species on the observed list will be represented in the inferred list by itself plus a number of other species. How many others, and which others, and whether these will be inferred presences or inferred absences, will vary with what is known about each species on the observed list and with its ecological characteristics. Some tell us almost nothing; either because almost nothing is known about them or because they are ecologically uninformative. E. coli, for example, is perhaps the best understood organisms in the world from the standpoint of genetics, cellular biology and biochemistry but unfortunately it is almost ubiquitous.

We know that species i on the observed list is represented by some number of species on the inferred list but we cannot write a general functional relation describing the transition from observed to inferred species lists because the information provided by each species is structured in significant ways. Each species found, in fact (given the information pool), generates a kind of information vector of its own with up to 10^6 entries, each of which is a 1 for known present or 0 for known absence.

E. coli generates a great number of uncertain entries and can therefore not be used as an indicator of much of anything.

We can consider the vectors $x(a_i)$ generated by the information about i in the observed species list, A. The number of species in the inferred list $\underset{\sim}{A}$ is given by

$$(x(a_i)) \vee (x(a_j)) \vee \ldots)).$$

A will consist of both 0's and 1's, unlike observed incomplete species
lists considered separately, which consist of 1's and for which the
absence of the species can only be inferred from comparison with some
other list.

Define $X(A)$ as the set of vectors $x(a_i)$, $x(a_j)$, etc. derived from
the scientific literature about species a_i, a_j, etc. The entries in
$x(a_i)$ will be $x_{i,k}$, $x_{i,e}$, etc. where $x_{i,k}$, for example, can take the
value of 1 or 0 depending on the necessary presence or absence of
species k given the presence of species i. We expect that for all i
and j, if we consider only those k, l, m, etc. for which both species
i and j provide definite information, the Euclidian distance between
$x(a_i)$ and $x(a_j)$ is expected to be zero, if i and j both occur in the
same observed list A. That is we do not expect one actually observed
species to infer the presence of some other species whose absence is
inferred by some other observed species. If this seems to be occurring, either the ecosystem is unstable, or the scientific literature is
wrong, or the samples straddled two different ecosystems. Therefore
if we compare the $x(a_i)$, $x(a_j)$, etc. we find that they may differ in
which species are listed but no $x(a_i)$ can have a definite 0 at the place
where $x(a_j)$ has a definite 1, for all i and j.

The level of cohesion or integrity of an ecosystem may be represented by considering the structure of $X(A)$. Consider that there are
various possible ways in which $X(A)$ can be examined. For example, if
it is found that the particular species in A all generate the same list
of definite presences and absences, and all the species actually present
in the list A are predicted as present in each $x(a_i)$ in X, then I would
believe the system under examination to be more tightly integrated than
one in which most of the species generate a long list of possible species
but very few necessary species.

Focussing on individual species, those that generate a very short
list of species with which they may or may not be associated, but a
relatively long list of necessarily co-occurring or incompatible species,
can be considered to have rather narrow ecological associations. Compare Kirtland's warblers, Bongo antelope or coral reef fishes with
species that do not clearly predict the presence of other species.

I have discussed the generation of an inferred species list from
an observed species list considering observed species one at a time.
Obviously it is possible that particular pairs, triples or larger combinations of species may have implications different from those of the
individual species considered separately. This awaits investigation.

If a set of species is ordered in terms of breadth of ecological associations, is it the case that there is a high correlation between rank in breadth of associations and frequency of co-occurrence? That is, do narrow association species tend to occur together? If species i requires the presence of species j, k, and ℓ, is it also usually the case that j, k, and ℓ require the presence of i? This is an empirical question.

VI. <u>Summary</u>

Ecological systems are so complex and fragile and the questions that may be asked about them are so diverse that it is difficult to use the normal craft standards of mathematical theory construction in an ecological context, therefore special formalisms dictated by the peculiarities of ecology may be of value. I have discussed two examples.

The first example relates to the problem of how natural history information may be formulated so as to permit relatively complete and public transmission. For hydra this may be possible by use of an Adaptive Response Surface in three dimensions on which many properties of the animals may be mapped.

I discussed the relation of Adaptive Response Surfaces to some aspects of a concept of ecological niche, adaptive landscape, and genetical natural selection. I also considered the problem of determining adaptive response surfaces for organisms other than hydra.

The second relates to the problem of ecosystem description. The simple species list seems to be the best possible descriptor for any ecosystem since it is concise, information rich and theoretically neutral. Species lists can also be considered as objects of theoretical interest in their own right.

Throughout these discussions I have attempted to incorporate the full richness of ecological information available, rather than attempting to simplify the argument for theoretical convenience. I cannot guarantee that this procedure is optimal but it seems that it may be of some interest.

At best, the attempt to avoid simplifying ecology for mathematical convenience might result in new and interesting approaches to mathematics as well as to predictive power in ecology. At the very worst however the tension between the elegant theory construction that is possible in a simplified mathematical context and the rich, but mathematically crude, descriptions of ecology may interplay fruitfully and avoid excesses in self confidence on the part of both mathematician and naturalist. The attempt of each to understand the other and to translate their work so as to be understood by the other is itself a worthwhile intellectual endeavor.

Acknowledgements

I have benefited from the criticism of Lev Ginzburg. Some of the research from my laboratory was supported by the U.S. National Science Foundation General Ecology Program. The examination of ecosystem theory was supported by the U.S. National Aeronautic and Space Agency.

This is contribution no. 351 of the Ecology and Evolution Program of the State University of New York, Stony Brook.

References

Bateson, G. 1963. The role of somatic change in evolution. Evolution 7:529-539.

Botkin, D., S. Golubic, B. Maguire, B. Moore, H. Morowitz and L.B. Slobodkin. 1979. Closed regenerative life support systems for space travel: their development poses fundamental questions for ecological science. (COSPAR) Life Sciences and Space Research 17: 3-12.

Borges, J.L. 1975. A Universal History of Infamy. Penguin Books, London.

Elton, C. 1966. The Pattern of Animal Communities. Methuen, London.

Fisher, R.A. 1930. The Genetical Theory of Natural Selection. Oxford: Clarendon Press.

Freckman, D., L.B. Slobodkin and C. Taylor. 1980b. Pesticide use and the stability of species-rich and species-poor communities of nematodes. Proc. Int. Soil Zoology Coll. VII (In Press).

Hutchinson, G.E. 1957. Concluding remarks. Cold Spring Harbor Symp. Quant. Biol. 22:415-427,

Hutchinson, G.E. 1968. When are species necessary? Chapter 12 in Population Biology and Evolution. R.C. Lewontin, ed., Univ. of Syracuse Press, pp. 177-186.

Innes, G.S., ed. 1975. New Directions in the Analysis of Ecological Systems. Simulation Council Proceedings, Vol. 5.

King, M-C. and A.C. Wilson. 1975. Evolution at two levels in humans and chimpanzees. Science 188:107-116.

Lewontin, R.C. 1974. The Genetic Basis of Evolutionary Change. Columbia Univ. Press, N.Y.

Lewontin, R.C. 1978. Fitness, survival and optimality, in Analysis of Ecological Systems. D. Horn, R. Mitchell, G.R. Stairs, Ed. Ohio State Univ. Press, Columbus.

Maguire, B., L.B. Slobodkin, H.J. Morowitz, B. Moore, and D.B. Botkin. 1980. A new paradigm for the examination of (closed) ecosystems. Symposium on Microcosms in Ecological Research. John Giesy (ed.). Technical Information Center, U.S. Dept. of Energy (In Press).

Margalef, R. 1975. Perspectives in Ecological Theory. Univ. Chicago Press, Chicago.

May, R.M. (Ed.). 1976. Theoretical Ecology, Principles and Applications. Saunders.

May, R.M., J.R. Beddington, C.W. Clark, S.J. Holt, R.M. Laws. 1979. Management of multi-species fisheries. Science 205:267-277.

Maynard Smith, J. 1978. Optimization theory in evolution. Ann. Rev. Ecol. and Syst. 9:31-56,

Pielou, E.C. 1969. An Introduction to Mathematical Ecology. Wiley-Interscience, New York

Slobodkin, L.B. 1958. Meta-models in theoretical ecology. Ecology 39:550-557.

_____. 1965. On the present incompleteness of mathematical ecology. Am. Sci. 53:347-357.

_____. 1975. Comments from a biologist to a mathematician. pp. 318-329 in Ecosystem Analysis and Prediction. S. Levin, ed. Soc. Ind. and Appl. Math. Philadelphia.

_____. 1980. Problems of ecological description. I. The adaptive response surface of Hydra. Mem. Ist. Ital. Idrobiol. (In Press).

Slobodkin, L.B., D. Botkin, B. Maguire, B. Moore, H.J. Morowitz. 1980. On the epistemology of ecosystem analysis in Estuarine Ecosystems, V.S. Kennedy, ed. Academic Press, New York (In Press).

Slobodkin, L.B. and A. Rapoport. 1974. An optimal strategy of evolution. Quart. Rev. Bio. 49:181-200.

Slobodkin, L.B. and L. Wu. 1975. An elementary reconstruction of population dynamics: A conversation between a mathematician and a biologist. Simulation Council Proceedings 5(2):159-166,.

Stearns, S.C. 1977. The evolution of life history traits. Ann. Rev. Ecol. and Syst. 8:145-171.

Wright, S. 1932. The roles of mutation inbreeding, crossbreeding and selection in evolution. Proc. Sixth Int. Congr. Genetics 1:356-366.

A THEORETICAL APPROACH TO THE DYNAMICS
OF SINGLE POPULATIONS

C. Matessi
Laboratorio di Genetica Biochimica
ed Evoluzionistica. CNR.

Via S. Epifanio 14, Pavia, Italy.

INTRODUCTION

Although a large part of mathematical ecology, the theory of
competition in particular, rests upon models of growth of single populations, the theoretical foundations of this class of models are
rather weak. Their logical status in the whole theory tends to be that
of "primitive objects". Almost the sole constraint for them is that
they should express in a simple way the basic property of natural populations, namely self regulation through density dependent factors
(Wangersky, 1978). Thus, single population models are not themselves
the product of a logical sequence from more basic principles, rooted in
the several branches of the biology of single organisms such as physiology and ethology. The pathways which where opened in this direction at
the origin of mathematical ecology (e.g. Volterra, 1938, 1939; Kostitzin, 1940a, b) seem abandoned.

This is an unsatisfactory state of affairs. When we deal with the
population dynamics of a particular species or class of species we are
unable to tell which of the many available models is most suitable
unless we go through a complicated process of graduation based on a
collection of demographic data (e.g. Ayala et al., 1973). All we know
about the natural history of this species is almost irrelevant for the
purpose. If we eventually succeede in picking up a satisfactory model,
it is impossible for us to tell which value the parameters of the model
should take if some external condition, such as amount of food, where
to take a different value. Thus field or experimental ecology, excluding
demography, and theoretical population dynamics can be of very little
help to each other at a general level.

This weakness is felt throughout the whole fabric of theoretical
ecology. Many results in the theory of ecological strategies have
rather poor foundations from a logical point of view, although they
might be biologically quite sound. In principle we should say that a
certain strategy is optimal for a certain species if and only if phenotypes using that strategy would outcompete all others. But we cannot
prove this unless we can say how any particular strategy will affect
the dynamics of the population. Thus for example we need a way to tell
that, since with a certain body size so many calories of food can be
gathered at the cost of so many metabolic calories, then a population
of individuals with that particular body size will grow according to
an equation of a particular form with parameters of a particular value.
We cannot, in principle, simply assume that the fitness of these individuals will be proportional to the net caloric input (Schoener, 1969;
Lynch, 1977). As another example consider the theory of limiting similarity and, in general, niche theory. On the one hand, it took such an
impetus only since when MacArthur and Levins put forward a model in
which the parameters of a logistic competition model are analysed in
terms of niche structure, and therefore logically derived this model
from assumptions of lower level (MacArthur and Levins, 1967). On the
other hand this same theory has been criticised because its validity
seems to depend so much from the logistic model itself (Abrams, 1975).
But then, either we develop theories of limiting similarity for a lot
of basic models or we try to show that a basic logistic model is quite
good for species of a certain class, or other assertions of this kind.

Recent developments respond to this kind of problems. For example
Ayala et al. (1973) tested an array of models with Drosophila populations and held the opinion that a certain model which performed well
could be of broad validity. They also attempted a rough classification
of animals with respect to the value that a certain parameter of their
population growth curve (the point of inflection) should have (see
also Wangersky, 1978 and May et al., 1979). But, apparently, data
gathered by Schoener (1973) seem to disprove these generalisations.
Schoener on the other hand (1973, 1976) developped a theory which produced a family of single and multipopulation models based on quite

explicit principles and whose parameters are operationally well defined
and could therefore be measured a priori (Schoener, 1974). A similar
philosophy underlies the theoretical and experimental work of deJong
(1976 a, b) on competition for food in Drosophila. In this study I will
follow this path and develop a model of population growth starting from
detailed assumptions at quite a low level. I will translate these in to
a micromodel for the interaction of various components of the process
which leads to population growth and will use this to finally derive
a macromodel for the dynamics of the population.

1. THE WAY OF LIFE OF AN IDEALISED POPULATION

I am concerned with organisms depending on a basic resource, such
as food, which is consummable but capable of renewing itself. I assume
that the population dynamics of these organisms is entirely ruled by
competition for this sole resource. Population growth then is viewed
as the end product of a process in which energy and materials are
collected and put to use to affect survival and fertility of individuals
in the population. An idealised version of this process is made out of
three basic ingredients:

(i) the kinetics of the resource, that is the manners in which it is
      produced and destroyed;

(ii) the foraging for the resource and its metabolism;

(iii) the demography of the consumer population, that is the manners
      in which the metabolised resource affects death and fertility
      rates in the population.

If specific formal assumptions are made about these three components
and their connections, a law of growth of the population can be
derived.

Time scales and spatial framework

From this picture it follows immediately that, since amount of
resource and number of consumers affect each other, the dynamics
involves in principle at least two state variables. Thus a law of

growth involving only population size can only be derived under special
conditions which must be clarified and will not be satisfied by all
kinds of consumer species. These two state variables in general can be
separated if two distinct time scales are involved so that components
(i) and (ii) above have a much shorter characteristic time scale than
component (iii), that is births and deaths occur at a much slower pace
than appearance and disappearance of resource items. Partially to
account for this property, I assume that the consumer species has
discrete generations whereas the kinetics of the resource occurs in
continuous time.

A concrete picture will show how separation of the state variables is accomplished. I imagine that the resource is available to the
whole population, at any given generation, in a definite portion of
space, a patch. Within a patch the resource has a kinetics which
enshures that a constant equilibrium abundance is rapidly attained if
the patch is left unexploited. At inception of a generation, reproductive consumers invade a patch and lay eggs there. The newborn will
consume part of the resource, while it undergoes its usual turnover, and
grow. Some deaths might occur in the meanwhile. When development is
completed to reproductive maturity, the population will leave the
patch and lay eggs either in a previously unexploited, but otherwise
identical patch or in the same patch but after a lapse of time, so that
the unexploited equilibrium abundance of resource is restored. No other
resource controls this last part of the process. The essential point is
that at the beginning of each generation the same amount of resource is
available, although, obviously, resource availability will change in the
course of the generation.

My analysis will consider processes which develop within a generation, and these will have a continuous time scale. The input of these
processes will be a certain number of eggs and a fixed amount of resource, the output a certain number of surviving adults endowed with a
certain fertility, both being functions of the initial number of eggs.
Given these two quatities the number of eggs for the next generation can
be computed, thus obtaining a recursion equation for the consumer population size, the law of growth which was sought for. This formal pro-

cedure is akin to that used by Kostitzin (1940) for an otherwise
different problem.

Kinetics of the resource and foraging

The resource is produced outside the patch and merely shed in it
at a constant rate. This assumption facilitates somewhat the matematics
but also is in character with a strictly mechanistic approach. Resource
productivity can thus be quantified with operationally well defined parameters and demographic notions such as resource carrying capacity and
intrinsic reproduction rate are avoided. On the other hand the class
of consumer species compatible with the model is restricted. They cannot
be true predators since do not feed on reproductive units of a living
resource. Thus either they consume dead matter or prey upon surplus
segments of a living population of organisms. Maybe herbivores can
also be fit into this model. Apart from predation there also occurs
some decay at a rate which is constant per unit of resource. This might
be due to either chemical decomposition or to consumption by some
other consumer which however is not limited by this factor.

Individuals of the consumer population ignore each other. Since
they are immature, their sole activity is search for the resource, which
is assumed to be uniformly distributed within the patch. I do not consider functional response or satiation phenomena of any sort. Thus all
encountered food items are collected and the amount of food consumed
per unit time, per individual, will be proportional to the volume of
space explored per unit time, and to the concentration of the resource
in the patch.

Consumer metabolism

The collected food is converted into various bodily components of
the individual consumer. I lump all these diverse components into a
single quantity labelled as (individual) biomass. It is therefore
obvious that mortality and fertility rates will be affected by amounts
of food collected in the past only indirectly, through this single
quantity. Biomass also serves as a memory. Starvation suffered in an
early part of the generation will affect future mortality and fertility.

Individual biomass is a key variable in the process and its dynamics must therefore be described. It increases in the unit time by an amount proportional to the collected food. It also is consumed because of metabolic costs including of course foraging activity. It seems that metabolic expenditures are proportional to a power function of body size with exponent roughly around 0.7 (Schoener, 1969), but there are instances of an exponent of one (Nagy and Milton, 1979). This value is much more convenient mathematically, thus I assume that overall costs (losses of biomass per unit time) are proportional to biomass. In general one could conceive that foraging activity (volume of space explored in the unit time) of growing individuals is a function of their body size or their age. For example measured filtering rate (a component of overall foraging activity) of various individuals of a Dafnia species increased with their body size (Lynch, 1977). I did not consider this complication and assumed that foraging activity is a constant, as stated above.

Consumer death rates and fertilities

Certain assumptions relate death rates and fertilities to individual biomass. The basic idea is simple. Scarcity of food will result in exaustion of individual energy deposits and wearing away of the various structures. These effects can be measured in a simplistic model by decreases of individual biomass with respect to some standard. Since individuals are growing I assume that there is a fixed standard growth curve (i.e. an age specific standard biomass) which is a property of the species. Whenever, in the course of development, the actual biomass falls below this limit curve, there will be a positive risk of mortality proportional to the (relative) deficit. Mortality is zero for a biomass above this standard. This might seem an odd feature but without it the mathematics would become rather messy. Thus all mortality is due to competition for food. One could complicate matters by assuming that beside a lower standard there is an upper standard as well, such that mortality would be positive for biomasses either too small or too large and zero in the middle. The standard growth curve should not be arbitrary in order to be consistent with realized growth curves. Thus I assume that the standard growth curve gives the biomass an individual would have at each age if a given and costant amount of food had been available all the time. I will refer to this constant amount of food as *minimum food requirement* (MFR); it is a typical property of the species. It is conceivable that different ages have different MFR. However, a costant MFR for a growing individual means a MFR per unit biomass decreasing with age, which does'nt seem too far from reality, beside being mathematically useful.

Adulthood is reached when the actual growth curve reaches a plateau, or stationary biomass value. Fertility is treated in a similar way as mortality. It is assumed to be proportional to the excess of adult biomass above a standard value. This is assumed to coincide with the stationary (adult) value in the standard growth curve. There is no need for mortality and fertility being controlled by the same standard biomass value. One could conceive organisms which are well fit for reproduction when their fitness for survival is poor, such as humans, and on the opposite side, organisms which can survive well but not reproduce, such as Drosophilas which can pupate at very low sizes but then lay very few eggs. Some kind of generalisation of this sort could be easily introduced in the model.

2. THE MATHEMATICS OF INTRAGENERATION PROCESSES

The assumptions detailed above are easily translated into a system of ordinary differential equations with respect to time. Intrageneration events occur along a time axis, t, with origin ($t=0$) at the beginning of a generation. They are completely described by three state variables:

$y(t)$ = *amount of food at time t;*
$x(t)$ = *biomass of an individual consumer at time t;*
$n(t)$ = *number of consumers alive at time t.*

All consumers have of course the same biomass since they are born at the same instant $t=0$, environment is homogeneous and the model is deterministic. The time variable can also be thought of as the age of the consumer cohort. An addictional function of time is needed for describing the standard growth curve:

$\theta(t)=$ *standard individual biomass at time (age) t.*

The state variables shall satisfy the following system of differential equations (derivatives with respect to time are denoted by e.g. $\dot{x}$ etc.):

$$\dot{y}=\omega-\delta y-\gamma ny, \qquad (1.1)$$

$$\dot{x}=-\varepsilon x+\alpha y, \qquad (1.2)$$

$$\dot{n}=\begin{cases} -\mu n(\theta-x)/\theta & \text{if } x<\theta \\ \\ 0 & \text{if } x\geq\theta. \end{cases} \qquad (1.3)$$

The parameters appearing in the equations are thus defined:

$\omega=$ *amount of food shed into a patch per unit time,*

$\delta=$ *fraction of food autonomously decomposed per unit time,*

$\gamma=$ *individual feeding rate, i.e. fraction of patch volume searched through per unit time by an individual consumer,*

$\varepsilon=$ *total metabolic losses per unit biomass and unit time,*

$\alpha=$ $c\gamma,$

$c=$ *amount of consumer biomass obtained from a unit amount of food,*

$\mu=$ *death rate per individual per unit (relative) biomass deficit.*

The standard age specific biomass, θ, is required to satisfy the following differential equation:

$$\dot{\theta}=-\varepsilon\theta+cQ, \qquad (2)$$

where:

$Q=$ *minimum food requirement per individual, a species specific constant.*

Equation (2) gives a standard growth curve consistent with the realised growth curve as defined by Equation (1.2). The equation for the resource gives the dynamics in unxploited patches if n is set equal to 0:

$$\dot{y}=\omega-\delta y.$$

This shows immediately that the equilibrium abundance of food in unexploited patches is ω/δ. Each generation of consumers finds as much resource at birth. Equation (1.3) expresses the fact that death risks occur only if biomass is below the age specific standard. The state of the system at inception of a generation must also be specified. Thus we have the following initial conditions:

$$y(0)=\omega/\delta, \qquad (3.1)$$

$$x(0)=\theta(0)=0, \qquad\qquad\qquad\qquad (3.2)$$

$$n(0)=N_k, \quad k=1,2,\ldots \;, \; a \; generation \; index. \qquad (3.3)$$

Initial biomass is set equal to 0 for mathematical convenience and without loss of generality. Equation (3.2) also expresses the assumption that eggs are perfect whatever the health status of their parents is. With initial condition (3.2) for θ, Equation (2) can be readily solved uniquely:

$$\theta(t)=\frac{c}{\varepsilon}Q(1-e^{-\varepsilon t}). \qquad\qquad\qquad (4.1)$$

Since I assume that sexual maturity occurs when a stationary value of biomass is reached, the standard adult biomass, $\hat{\theta}$, is obtained from Equation (4.1) by letting $t\to\infty$. Thus:

$$\hat{\theta}=\frac{c}{\varepsilon}Q=\frac{\alpha Q}{\varepsilon\gamma}, \qquad\qquad\qquad\qquad (4.2)$$

from the definition of α.

In Equation (3.3) N_k is the number of eggs laid at the beginning of the $k\text{-}th$ generation. The purpose of System (1) together with (3) is to provide a mathematical relation between N_k and N_{k+1}. Fertility is assumed to be proportional to the excess of adult biomass over the adult standard $\hat{\theta}$. Notice that fertility will be zero if an adult has biomass equal to or less than $\hat{\theta}$. Thus θ does not give an optimal biomass but a lower limit for an "healthy" status. Once fertility and number of surviving adults are known, N_{k+1} can be immediately computed. Thus one needs to find the stationary state (state at $t=\infty$) of System (1) under initial conditions (3), after having proved that there exists one. System (1) is rather peculiar. The number of consumers n can only decrease or stay constant. Further, its solutions are not smooth functions of time. The second derivative of n will be discontinuous in general (unless $x(t)$ is tangent to $\theta(t)$ at intersection points). This will also affect higer derivatives of x and y. This mathematical peculiarity makes the system biologically meaningful . Its stationary state depends on the initial conditions and hence on N_k which makes the computation of a recursion formula for the population size possible. Most frequently instead, a system of differential equations has stationary states (equilibria) independent from initial conditions. The stationary value of n is the number of surviving adults, the stationary value of x, together with $\hat{\theta}$ provides individual fertility.

Hidden properties of the model are discovered by asking whether the standard growth curve can ever be realized "in nature", that is under System (1). Firstly consider that if $x(t)$ coincides with $\theta(t)$ at all t, there will be no mortality, because of (1.3), and n will stay constant. By inspection of (1.2) and (2) one concludes that $x(t) \equiv \theta(t)$ if $y(t) \equiv Q/\gamma$. But $y(t)$ is constant if $\dot{y}(t) \equiv 0$ thus one finds, from (1.1), that $x(t) \equiv \theta(t)$ if the number of consumers n satisfies $\omega - \delta Q/\gamma - nQ = 0$, i.e. if:

$$n = P = \frac{\omega}{Q} - \frac{\delta}{\gamma} . \tag{5}$$

Thus P is the size of a population of immature consumers which in the given environment can grow according to the standard growth curve and therefore reach maturity with zero mortality but also with zero fertility. It shall therefore be referred to as *limiting population size*. It will be shown later that P is also the maximum size for the adult population that the given environment will allow to emerge. Thus a consumer species can exist at all on such an environment only if $P > 0$ i.e. if $\omega/\delta > Q/\gamma$. Since Q/γ is the total amount of food that is needed in the patch in order that each individual gets its MFR in a unit time (taking into account that an individual can only explore a limited portion γ of the patch in a unit of time), this relation merely says that the patch must harbour more food than the minimum consumer requirement. The parameters P and Q clearly play a key role in the model.

The results that can be obtained analitically from System (1) under conditions (3) can now be stated. The proof is given in the appendix in four theorems and one corollary.

Result 1

Provided that P > 0, with any initial number n(0) > 0 (number of eggs) there is a positive stationary value $\hat{n} = \lim_{t \to \infty} n(t)$ which depends on n(0). A stationary value of y (food) and x (individual biomass) also exists and depends on $\hat{n}$:

$$\hat{y} = \lim_{t \to \infty} y(t) = \frac{\omega}{\delta + \gamma \hat{n}} , \tag{6.1}$$

$$\hat{x} = \lim_{t \to \infty} x(t) = \frac{\alpha}{\varepsilon} \hat{y} = \frac{\alpha}{\varepsilon} \frac{\omega}{\delta + \gamma \hat{n}} . \tag{6.2}$$

Result 2

If the initial number satisfies $n(0) \leq P$ then $n(t) \equiv \hat{n} = n(0)$. If the initial number satisfies $n(0) > P$ then $\hat{n} \leq P$.

The first result says that the problem of finding a relation linking the number of individuals in successive generations has always a solution since the number of adults and their fertility can always be uniquely determined as a function of the number of eggs. The second result says that any number of eggs up to the limiting population size will grow to maturity without mortality. Mortality will only arise if the number of eggs exceeds P and will be strong enough to keep down the number of adults to a value not exceeding P.

An explicit result with respect to fertility can be easily derived from Result 1. Since fertility is proportional to $\hat{x} - \theta$, one obtains from (6.2) and (4.2) that:

$$Fertility \; \propto \; \frac{\alpha}{\varepsilon} \, \frac{\omega}{\delta + \gamma \hat{n}} - \frac{\alpha}{\varepsilon} \, \frac{Q}{\gamma} \; .$$

After simple manipulations and use of (5) one proves the truth of the following

Result 3

Adult fertility is given by:

$$Fertility \; \propto \; \hat{\theta} \gamma \, \frac{P - \hat{n}}{\delta + \gamma \hat{n}} \; .$$

This is a consistent value for a fertility since Result 2 ensures that it will always be nonnegative, because $\hat{n} \leq P$ for all $n(0) > 0$. One also sees again that if the adult population reaches the limiting size which the environment permits to this species, there will be zero fertility.

Given Result 3, the number of eggs for the next generation can be readily computed:

$$N_{k+1} = r\hat{\theta} \, \frac{\gamma \hat{n}(P - \hat{n})}{\delta + \gamma \hat{n}} \; ,$$

where r is the number of eggs per unit biomass (excess of) per individual. This can be put in simpler form if we substitute to γ its value computed from Equation (5). Thus

$$N_{k+1} = r\hat{\theta} \, \frac{PQ\hat{n}(P - \hat{n})}{P\omega - PQ(P - \hat{n})} \; .$$

This immediately suggests a new meaningful parameter. Let:

$$H= \frac{PQ}{\omega} \ .$$ (7)

Since PQ is the food consumed from a population of limiting size in the unit time and ω is the food produced in the unit time, H measures the fraction of the food produced in the unit time that a species can consume in the same time; it is therefore a measure of the exploitation pressure that a species is able to develop in a given environment. For this reason I label it *exploitation potential*. H is a characteristic property of a given species-environment pair. It has the pleasant property of being always positive (by definition) and less than one. This should be obvious from its interpretation but can also be immediately seen from (5). If further one defines $\rho = r\hat{\theta}$, which has the same meaning as r when biomass is measured in units of adult standard biomass, the number of eggs for the next generation is given by:

$$N_{k+1}= \rho H \ \frac{\hat{n}(P-\hat{n})}{P-H(P-\hat{n})}$$ (8)

Equation (8) is an implicit recurrence equation for consumer population size since Result 1 says that $\hat{n}$ is a function of $n(0)=N_k$. Result 2 makes it explicit only for certain values of N_k. In fact $\hat{n}=n(0)=N_k$ for all $0 \leq N_k \leq P$. A partial solution to the initial problem of finding a law of growth for the consumer population is then

$$N_{k+1}= \rho H \ \frac{(P-N_k)N_k}{P-H(P-N_k)} \qquad for \ 0 \leq N_k \leq P.$$

The full solution for the case of $N_k > P$ cannot be obtained analitically. Numerical methods can help.

3. NUMERICAL ANALYSIS OF INTRAGENERATION PROCESSES

The method

        System (1) and the associated Equation (2) have together 7 parameters, which makes a parameter space of 8 dimensions including N_k, too many for computer trials. A heavy reduction is however quite easy without loss of generality. The three state variables and time are all dimensioned and since measuring units are arbitrary, (1) and (2) can be reduced to their dimensionless form. I take ω/δ, $\hat{\theta}$, P and $1/\delta$ as the measuring units for y, x and θ, n and t respectively and denote:

$$u(t)=n(t)/P ,$$

$$U_k=N_k/P , \quad k=1,2,\ldots$$

Other variables are denoted as before. System (1), Equation (2) and initial conditions (3) reduce to:

$$\dot{y}=1-y-\frac{H}{1-H} uy , \qquad\qquad (9.1)$$

$$\dot{x}=-\varepsilon x+\frac{\varepsilon}{1-H} y , \qquad\qquad (9.2)$$

$$\dot{u}=\begin{cases} -\mu u(\theta-x)/\theta & for \ x<\theta \\ \\ 0 & for \ x\geq\theta , \end{cases} \qquad (9.3)$$

$$\dot{\theta}=\varepsilon(1-\theta) , \qquad\qquad (9.4)$$

$$\theta(0)=x(0)=0 , \ y(0)=1 , \ u(0)=U_k \qquad (9.5)$$

Metabolic and death rates ε and μ can take in principle any positive value. Remembering that the decay rate of the resource is now one, the ordering $0<\mu\leq\varepsilon\leq1$ is plausible, since the rate 1 refers to a resource which is probably of simpler organisation than the consumer species and ε refers to elementary components of the consumer biomass whereas μ refers to the whole organism. The interesting values of U_k are those larger than one since for lower values the solution is already known.

Thus the parameter space which should be explored is

$$0<H<1 , \ 0<\mu\leq\varepsilon\leq1 , \ U_k>1.$$

The restriction for ε and μ is arbitrary, although plausible, and conclusions cannot be generalised to different situations. The actual numerical explorations concerned each of the 100 grid points defined by all combinations of the following parameter values:

$H:$ 0.1 , 0.3 , 0.5 , 0.7 , 0.9 ;

$\varepsilon:$ 0.1 , 0.3 , 0.5 , 0.7 , 0.9 ;

$\mu:$ 0.7ε , 0.8ε , 0.9ε , ε .

For each parameter combination about 26 initial values, $u(0)=U_k$, where considered. System (9) was run on a computer and a run was stopped when the stationary value $\hat{u}$ of $u(t)$ was found. The criterion for stopping was based on the mathematical fact that either $\lim\limits_{t\to\infty} u(t)=1$

or in a finite time $x(t)$ becomes larger tha $\theta(t)$ and $u(t)$ becomes smaller than one. As soon as this occurs $u(t)$ stays at a constant value, which therefore is $\hat{u}$. This is proved in the appendix. The first event never occured.

The results

In all numerical trials the relationship between $\hat{u}$ and the initial value $u(0)$ had the same properties which can be summarised as follows:

(i) *$\hat{u}<1$ for all $u(0)$; that is the number of surviving adults from any population initially exceeding the limiting size P is strictly less than P.*

(ii) *$\hat{u}$ is a decreasing, concave upward function of $u(0)$; that is as the initial excess over limiting population size increases, the number of survivors actually decreases at a decreasing rate.*

(iii) *$\hat{u}$ seems to be rapidly approaching a constant minimum value; that is the number of survivors tends rapidly to a value independent from the initial population size.*

The true purpose of this numerical analysis however, is not that of obtaining pictures but rather an analitical relation between the number of surviving adults and the initial number of eggs in order to make explicit the law of population growth (8). A reasonable approach is to use statistical tecniques to fit some analitical model to the set of points "observed" in the numerical trials. Linear regression is a simple and safe procedure, but then some transformation is needed to straighten out the observed curved lines. The following linear relation performed quite well:

$$\frac{1}{1-\hat{u}} = a+\frac{b}{u(0)-1} \quad , \qquad\qquad (10.1)$$

which implies:

$$\hat{u}= \frac{b+(a-1)(u(0)-1)}{b+a(u(0)-1)} \quad . \qquad\qquad (10.2)$$

The correlations between transformed variables, computed on about 26 points for each parameter combination, are very high, always exceeding 99.9%. Equation (10.2) can therefore be taken as a good approximation to the exact relation. The weakness of this numerical approach lies elsewhere. The parameters a and b in Equations (10) are devoid of any physical meaning. All that is known is their geometrical meaning and the fact that they depend on the physical parameters H, ε and μ. The asymptotic value of $\hat{u}$ is $(a-1)/a$. Thus necessarily $a>1$ and as a increases the number of survivors tends to P. The derivative of $\hat{u}$ at $u(0)=1$ is $-1/b$, thus $b>0$ and as b decreases the more rapidly $\hat{u}$ reaches its asymptote. Since both a and b depend on H, ε and μ their values cannot vary independently from each other or from the primitive parameters. From the numerical results it appears that both a and b become very large as H tends to one, and in general seem to increase with H.

4. A LAW OF GROWTH FOR A POPULATION OF CONSUMERS

Combining together the results of Sections 2 and 3, one finds that a population living under the regime described in Section 1 will grow according to the law:

$$N_{k+1} = \begin{cases} \rho H \dfrac{(P-N_k)N_k}{P-H(P-N_k)} & \text{if } N_k \leq P, \qquad (11.1) \\[4mm] \rho H \dfrac{P(N_k-P)\{Pb+(a-1)(N_k-P)\}}{\{Pb+(a-H)(N_k-P)\}\{Pb+a(N_k-P)\}} & \text{if } N_k > P, \qquad (11.2) \end{cases}$$

where:

N_k = *number of newborn at generation* $k=0,1,\ldots$,

P = *maximum adult population size* ,

H = *exploitation potential, i.e. proportion of resources produced in the unit time which is appropriated by the population in the same time under certain standard conditions* ,

ρ = *intrinsic fertility, i.e. fertility at an adult biomass twice a certain standard* ,

a,b = *functions of exploitation potential, consumer metabolic rate and consumer intrinsic death rate.*

The parameters satisfy certain constraints and properties, namely:

(i) *$0<H<1$* ,

(ii) *$a>1$ and $a\to+\infty$ as $H\to 1$* ,

(iii) $b>0$ *and* $b \to +\infty$ *as* $H \to 1$.

Piecewise defined growth laws are not new to theoretical ecology (e.g. May, 1976). This is peculiar in several respects, however. The two pieces (11.1) and (11.2) are separated from the point $N_k = P$. At this particular size the population will be extinct in the next generation. Much more important however is the fact that very different ecological events take place in the population when it undergoes one or the other dynamics. Equation (11) results from the composition of two processes: survival to adulthood and reproduction. Given N newborn, the number of survivors to adulthood is:

$$n = \begin{cases} N & \text{if } N \leq P \\ \\ P\,\dfrac{Pb+(a-1)(N-P)}{Pb+a(N-P)} & \text{if } N > P \text{ ,} \end{cases}$$

thus $n \leq P$ for all N. Given n adults, the number of newborn they will produce is:

$$N' = \rho H \frac{(P-n)n}{P-H(P-n)}$$

Thus, as long as $N \leq P$, i.e. when (11.1) holds, mortality is independent of population size, and in fact it is zero. On the other hand, fertility decreases from a maximum of $\rho\,\dfrac{H}{1-H}$, in the limit $N=0$, to a minimum of zero, when $N=P$. Opposite processes take place when $N>P$, i.e. (11.2) holds. Mortality increases from a minimum of zero, in the limit $N=P$, to a maximum of $\{1 - \dfrac{a-1}{a}\ \dfrac{P}{N}\}$, as N tends to infinity. On the other hand, fertility increases from a minimum of zero, for $N=P$, to a maximum of $\rho\,\dfrac{H}{a-H}$, as N tends to infinity. A substantial increase of fertility occurs only when N is in the neighborhood of P.

Thus when Equation (11.1) holds the population is regulated by density dependent fertility while mortality is constant and minimal. When Equation (11.2) holds the population is regulated by density dependent mortality, which mostly takes place in the early part of the life cicle. Fertility instead is either constant or even increasing with density. It is then very important to establish whether a population will be necessarily governed by both kinds of laws, alternating each other in time, or whether there can exist populations which always grow according to only one of the two laws. It turns out that the crucial parameter in this respect is the intrinsic fertility ρ.

An exaustive description of the population dynamics implied by Equations (11) can be obtained in the usual way by finding out equilibria and their stability properties. A special attention must also be given to the conditions under which population size stays in the region $0<N<P$ or wanders beyond P. A straightforward analysis produces the following results:

(i) $0<\rho\leq\rho_0=\dfrac{1-H}{H}$.

There exists only one equilibrium, $\hat{N}_0=0$. It is stable. The population goes extinct.

(ii) $\rho_0<\rho<\rho_1=\dfrac{3-2H+\sqrt{9-8H}}{2H}$.

There exist only two equilibria: $\hat{N}_0$ and $\hat{N}_1=P-\dfrac{P}{H(1+\rho)}$. $\hat{N}_1$ is positive and always less than P. It is also stable whereas $\hat{N}_0$ is unstable. N_k converges to $\hat{N}_1$.

(iii) $\rho_1\leq\rho<\rho_3$.

Only the two equilibria $\hat{N}_0$ and $\hat{N}_1$ exist, but none is stable. N_k fluctuates permanently. The existence of a boundary ρ_3 can be proved but ρ_3 can only be determined implicitly as:

$$\rho_3=l(\hat{u})=\frac{\{b+(a-H)(\hat{u}-1)\}\{b+a(\hat{u}-1)\}\hat{u}}{H\{b+(a-1)(\hat{u}-1)\}(\hat{u}-1)}$$

where $\hat{u}$ is the unique solution for $u>1$ of $l'(u)=0$

(iv) $\rho>\rho_3$.

Two new equilibria come to existence, $\hat{N}_2=Pu_2$ and $\hat{N}_3=Pu_3$, along with $\hat{N}_0$ and $\hat{N}_1$. Both are larger than P. They can only be defined implicitly since u_2 and u_3 are the unique solutions, for $u>1$ and $\rho>\rho_3$, of $\rho=l(u)$. Of the four equilibria the smallest three, $\hat{N}_0$, $\hat{N}_1$ and $\hat{N}_2$, say, are unstable. Stability of $\hat{N}_3$ is difficult to ascertain in general. However it is quite easy to prove that if $a>1+\sqrt{1-H}$ $\hat{N}_3$ is stable whenever it exists, independently of the value of ρ. Notice that this lower bound to a is quite small, never exceeding 2. I never found such low values for a in the numerical explorations, thus it is quite possible that this condition is always satisfied. In any case it must hold most of the times. In the border case $\rho=\rho_3$, the two equilibria $\hat{N}_2$ and $\hat{N}_3$ merge into a single equilibrium.

(v) If $\rho\leq\rho_2 = \frac{(1+\sqrt{1-H})^2}{H}$, the population size will either be always smaller than P or become so in just one generation. If instead $\rho>\rho_2$ there are values of $N_k<P$ such that $N_{k+1}>P$. It can be proved that $\rho_1<\rho_2<\rho_3$. It follows from (iii) that when $\rho_1\leq\rho<\rho_2$ the population fluctuates permanently but is always less than P and thus remains constantly governed by Equation (11.1). When instead $\rho_2\leq\rho<\rho_3$ the population size fluctuates permanently and is sometimes less than P, sometimes larger, thus alternating the regime of Equation (11.1) with that of Equation (11.2). Furthermore it follows from (iv) that when $\rho>\rho_3$, provided that $a>1+\sqrt{1-H}$, the population size will become quite soon larger than $\hat{N}_2>P$ and from this point on will remain in this region, converging to $\hat{N}_3$. Thus, under these conditions, the population is always governed by Equation (11.2) with the possible exception of a transient phase in which it is under Equation (11.1).

Thus, summarising these findings, populations with small intrinsic fertility have a dynamics as described by Equation (11.1). Populations with large intrinsic fertility have in general a dynamics as described by Equation (11.2). Both these kinds of populations will converge smoothly to an equilibrium size. In particular populations of the second kind will behave so however large their intrinsic fertility is. Populations with intermediate intrinsic fertilities will have a permanently fluctuating size and their dynamics can be either always of type (11.1) or alternatively of types (11.1) and (11.2).

5. DISCUSSION

Model (11), the endproduct of this study, is a consequence of a number of hypotheses about the life history of an idealized consumer. The most important among these is the idea that food availability affects mortality and fertility by moving individual biomasses below or

above a certain age specific standard. Thus, acting as a memory of
recent shortages or excesses of food, biomass distributes in a non linear way their effects upon mortality and fertility. For example, if a
severe shortage of food causes intense mortality, survivors will
benefit a rapid gain in biomass and therefore an increased fertility.
All peculiarities of model (11) derive essentially from the presence of
this basic mechanism.

Most population dynamics models in discrete time become unstable,
engendering more or less irregular oscillations, when certain parameters, usually a measure of intrinsic growth rate, become large (May and
Oster, 1976). Instability occurs in model (11) also, when the intrinsic
fertility ρ is sufficiently high. This is transitory, however, since for
still larger ρ in most cases a stable behaviour appears again. The
reason is that as ρ increases the whole biology of density regulation
also changes. At high intrinsic fertilities control is taken over by
premature mortality and ensuing early losses are compensated by a later
improvement of actual fertility of survivors. In a sense, this theory
suggests the hypothesis that the conceptual operation of changing the
value of a parameter keeping the shape of a model constant, may not
be biologically legitimate, since different ranges of certain parameters are associated with different kinds of demographic processes.

These properties imply the possibility of a sharp, qualitative
test for the theory. If a substantial number of real consumer species
had a population dynamics in agreement with the theory, one should
expect a correlation between intrinsic fertility and certain other features of the life history. According to the theory, in fact, consumer
species should cluster around either of two basic types. The first type
is characterised by:
*1a) high intrinsic fertilities; 1b) density dependent mortality among
juveniles; 1c) fertilities which are either density independent or
even increasing with density.*
The second type should have opposite properties, namely:
*2a) low intrinsic fertilities; 2b) low, density independent mortality;
2c) density dependent fertilities.*
The theory at least indicates the possibility that a single basic ecological plan may encompass a broad spectrum of life history strategies,

such as that delimited by the two estreme types above, and that the whole ensemble may be spanned by changing a single parameter such as intrinsic fertility above.

Finally it is worthwhile to emphasize that two novel parameters, by which most of the consumer-resource interaction is described, have been derived in this study, namely the *limiting population size P*, which delimits the number of individuals that a given available production can sustain, and the *exploitation potential H*, which measures the ability of a species to exploit the available production.

APPENDIX

The proof of Results 1 and 2 of Section 2 is given here in four Theorems and one Corollary. These concern some properties of the solutions $(x(t), y(t), n(t))$ of the following system of differential Equations $(\dot{x} \equiv dx/dt \ etc.)$

$$\dot{x} = -\varepsilon x + \alpha y \ ,$$
$$\dot{y} = \omega - \delta y + \gamma n y \ ,$$

$$\dot{n} = \begin{cases} 0 & for \ x \geq \theta, \\ \\ -\mu n \{1 - \frac{x}{\theta}\} & for \ x < \theta, \end{cases}$$

$$\dot{\theta} = -\varepsilon \theta + \alpha Q \ , \qquad where \ Q = \frac{\omega}{\delta + \gamma P} \ , \ and \ P > 0 \ ;$$

$$x(0) = \theta(0); \ y(0) = \omega/\delta; \ n(0) > 0;$$
$$\varepsilon, \alpha, \omega, \delta, \gamma, \mu > 0.$$

Theorem 1.

Part 1.

If for some $t_0 > 0$, $n(t_0) \leq P$ and $x(t_0) < \theta(t_0)$, there exists a finite $t' > t_0$ such that:

(i) $x(t) < \theta(t)$ for all $t_0 \leq t < t'$ and $x(t') = \theta(t')$

(ii) $n(t') < n(t_0)$

Part 2.

If for some $t_0 \geq 0$, $n(t_0) \leq P$ and $x(t_0) \geq \theta(t_0)$ then:

(i) $x(t) \geq \theta(t)$ for all $t \geq t_0$

(ii) $n(t) = n(t_0)$ for all $t \geq t_0$

If $n(t_0) < P$, inequality in (i) is a strict one.

Proof of Part 1.

Since $\dot{n}(t) \leq 0$ for all $t \geq 0$, then $n(t) \leq n(t_0)$ for all $t \geq t_0$. Therefore $\dot{y} \geq \omega - \delta y - \gamma n(t_0) y$ for all $t \geq t_0$. Let $\tilde{y}$ be defined by:

$$\dot{\tilde{y}} = \omega - \delta \tilde{y} - \gamma n(0) \tilde{y}, \quad \tilde{y}(t_0) = y(t_0).$$

Thus $y(t) \geq \tilde{y}(t)$ for all $t \geq t_0$ and therefore $\dot{x} \geq -\varepsilon x + \alpha \tilde{y}$ for all $t \geq t_0$. Let $\tilde{x}$ be defined by:

$$\dot{\tilde{x}} = -\varepsilon \tilde{x} + \alpha \tilde{y}, \quad \tilde{x}(t_0) = x(t_0).$$

Thus $x(t) \geq \tilde{x}(t)$ for all $t \geq t_0$. It is quite easy to verify that $\tilde{x}(t) \to \frac{\alpha}{\varepsilon} \frac{\omega}{\delta + \gamma n(t_0)}$ as $t \to \infty$. Thus, if $n(t_0) < P$, $\tilde{x}(\infty) > \frac{\alpha}{\varepsilon} \frac{\omega}{\delta + \gamma P} = \theta(\infty)$.

Let instead be $n(t_0) = P$. Since $x(t_0) < \theta(t_0)$ and $x(t)$ is continuous, there certainly exists a $\tau > 0$ such that $x(t) < \theta(t)$ for all $t_0 \leq t \leq t_0 + \tau$. But then $\dot{n}(t) < 0$ for all $t_0 \leq t \leq t_0 + \tau$ and thus $n(t_0 + \tau) < P$. Thus the previous argument can be repeated if $\tilde{y}$ and $\tilde{x}$ are defined with respect to $t_0 + \tau$ rather than t_0. Hence $x(t) \geq \tilde{x}(t)$ for all t sufficiently larger than t_0 and $\tilde{x}(\infty) > \theta(\infty)$. Thus there certainly exists a finite $t' > t_0$ such that $x(t') = \theta(t')$ and $x(t) < \theta(t)$ for all $t_0 \leq t < t'$. It follows that $\dot{n}(t) < 0$ for all $t_0 \leq t < t'$ and thus that $n(t') < n(t_0)$.

Proof or Part 2.

Either for all $0 \leq t \leq t_0$, $x(t) \geq \theta(t)$ or, for some positive $t' < t_0$, $x(t') < \theta(t')$. In the first case, $x(0) = \theta(0)$ and $\dot{x}(0) = \alpha \omega / \delta > \alpha Q = \dot{\theta}(0)$. In the second case there exists a t'' such that $t' < t'' \leq t_0$, $x(t'') = \theta(t'')$ and $x(t) \geq \theta(t)$ for all $t'' \leq t \leq t_0$, so that $\dot{x}(t'') \geq \dot{\theta}(t'')$. In any case then, there exists a t_1 such that $0 \leq t_1 \leq t_0$ and:

(i) $x(t_1) = \theta(t_1)$ and $\dot{x}(t_1) \geq \dot{\theta}(t_1)$

(ii) $x(t) \geq \theta(t)$ for all $t_1 \leq t \leq t_0$

From (i) it follows that $\alpha y(t_1) \geq \alpha Q$. From (ii) it follows that $\dot{n}(t) = 0$ for all $t_1 \leq t \leq t_0$ and therefore $n(t) = n(t_0) \leq P$ for all $t_1 \leq t \leq t_0$. From this and from the fact that $n(t) \leq n(t_0)$ for all $t > t_0$ since $\dot{n}(t) \leq 0$ for all $t \geq 0$, it follows that $\dot{y} \geq \omega - \delta y - \gamma n(t_0)y$ for all $t \geq t_1$. Let now $\tilde{y}$ be defined by

$$\dot{\tilde{y}} = \omega - \delta \tilde{y} - \gamma n(t_0)\tilde{y}, \quad \tilde{y}(t_1) = Q \leq y(t_1).$$

Thus, $y(t) \geq \tilde{y}(t)$ for all $t \geq t_1$. But,

$$\tilde{y}(t) = Q + \left\{ \frac{\omega}{\delta + \gamma n(t_0)} - Q \right\} \{1 - exp(-(\delta + \gamma n(t_0))(t - t_1))\},$$

and therefore $\tilde{y}(t) \geq Q$ for all $t \geq t_1$, since $\omega/(\delta + \gamma n(t_0)) \geq Q$. Hence, $y(t) \geq Q$ and if $n(t_0) < P$, $y(t) > Q$, for all $t \geq t_1$. It follows that $\dot{x} \geq -\epsilon x + \alpha Q$, for all $t \geq t_1$, with strict inequality if $n(t_0) < P$.

But θ satisfies

$$\dot{\theta} = -\epsilon\theta + \alpha Q, \quad \theta(t_1) = x(t_1),$$

so that $x(t) \geq \theta(t)$ for all $t \geq t_1$, with strict inequality if $n(t_0) < P$. From this it follows that $n(t) = n(t_1) = n(t_0)$ for all $t \geq t_1 \leq t_0$.

Theorem 2.

For each $n(0) > 0$, $n(t)$ converges to some positive limit $\hat{n}$ as t tends to ∞.

Proof.

Since $\dot{n} \geq -\mu n$ for all $t \geq 0$, $n(t) \geq n(0)e^{-\mu t} > 0$ for all $t \geq 0$ and $n(0) > 0$. On the other hand, n is non increasing for all positive t. Thus n must have a non negative limit for $t \to \infty$. If $n(t) \to 0$ as $t \to \infty$, there certainly exists a t_0 such that $n(t_0) < P$. It follows from Theorem 1 that there exists a finite $t_1 \geq t_0$ such that $n(t_1) \leq n(t_0)$ and $n(t) = n(t_1)$ for all $t \geq t_1$. But $n(t) > 0$ for all $t \geq 0$ so that $n(t_1) > 0$. Therefore $n(t) = n(t_1) > 0$ for all $t \geq t_1$, which contraddicts the hypothesis that $n(t) \to 0$.

Theorem 3.

For each $n(0) > 0$, $y(t)$ and $x(t)$ converge to a limit as t tends to ∞.

Proof.

For Theorem 2, $n(t)$ tends to a positive limit $\hat{n}$ for $n(0) > 0$.

Now

$$y(t) = \frac{\omega}{\delta} \exp\left(-\int_0^t p(u)\,du\right) + \omega \exp\left(-\int_0^t p(u)\,du\right) \int_0^t \exp\left(\int_0^u p(s)\,ds\right) du,$$

where $p(u) = \delta + \gamma n(u) \geq \delta + \gamma \hat{n} = p(\infty) > 0$. Thus, $\int_0^t p(u)\,du \to \infty$ as $t \to \infty$, and therefore

$$\lim_{t \to \infty} y(t) = \omega \lim_{t \to \infty} \frac{\int_0^t \exp\left(\int_0^u p(s)\,ds\right) du}{\exp\left(\int_0^t p(u)\,du\right)} = \omega \lim_{t \to \infty} \frac{\frac{d}{dt}\left\{\int_0^t \exp\left(\int_0^u p(s)\,ds\right) du\right\}}{\frac{d}{dt}\left\{\exp\left(\int_0^t p(u)\,du\right)\right\}} =$$

$$= \omega \lim_{t \to \infty} \frac{\exp\left(\int_0^t p(u)\,du\right)}{p(t)\exp\left(\int_0^t p(u)\,du\right)} = \frac{\omega}{p(\infty)} = \frac{\omega}{\delta + \gamma \hat{n}} > 0.$$

Furthermore,

$$x(t) = \alpha e^{-\varepsilon t} \int_0^t y(u) e^{\varepsilon u}\,du$$

and $\int_0^t y(u) e^{\varepsilon u}\,du \to \infty$ as $t \to \infty$. Therefore

$$\lim_{t \to \infty} x(t) = \alpha \lim_{t \to \infty} \frac{\int_0^t y(u) e^{\varepsilon u}\,du}{e^{\varepsilon t}} = \alpha \lim_{t \to \infty} \frac{\frac{d}{dt}\left\{\int_0^t y(u) e^{\varepsilon u}\,du\right\}}{\frac{d}{dt} e^{\varepsilon t}} =$$

$$= \alpha \lim_{t \to \infty} \frac{y(t) e^{\varepsilon t}}{\varepsilon e^{\varepsilon t}} = \frac{\alpha}{\varepsilon} y(\infty) = \frac{\alpha}{\varepsilon} \frac{\omega}{\delta + \gamma \hat{n}}.$$

Corollary.

If $n(0) \leq P$, $n(t) = n(0)$ for all $t \geq 0$, and $y(t)$ tends to $\dfrac{\omega}{\delta + \gamma n(0)}$ and $x(t)$ tends to $\dfrac{\alpha}{\varepsilon} \dfrac{\omega}{\delta + \gamma n(0)}$.

Proof.

The fact that $n(t) = n(0)$ for all $t \geq 0$ follows immediately from Part 2 of Theorem 1, with $t_0 = 0$, since $x(0) = \theta(0)$. Convergence of y and x then follows from Theorem 3.

Theorem 4.

When $n(0) > P$, $\lim\limits_{t \to \infty} n(t) \leq P$.

Proof.

Let suppose that $\lim\limits_{t \to \infty} n(t) = P + \upsilon > P$. Then, from Theorem 3

$$\lim_{t \to \infty} \frac{\theta - x}{\theta} = \frac{\varepsilon}{\alpha} \frac{\delta + \gamma P}{\omega} \left\{ \frac{\alpha}{\varepsilon} \frac{\omega}{\delta + \gamma P} - \frac{\alpha}{\varepsilon} \frac{\omega}{\delta + \gamma (P + \upsilon)} \right\} = \frac{\gamma \upsilon}{\delta + \gamma (P + \upsilon)} > 0.$$

Thus $\lim\limits_{t\to\infty} \dot{n}(t) < 0$, which is in contraddiction with the existence of $\lim\limits_{t\to\infty} n(t)$.

SUMMARY

A model for the population dynamics of an idealized consumer species with discrete generations is derived from a set of assumptions with respect to: (i) the kinetics of a food source; (ii) the ways in which food is acquired by a number of individual consumers; (iii) the ways through which acquired food affects survival and fertility in the population. In particular the assumption is made that mortality and fertility depend directly from body size relative to a certain age specific standard. These assumptions are translated into a system of ordinary differential equations for: the amount of food; the individual body size; the number of individuals. The solution of this system provides the number of surviving adults and their body size as a function of the number of eggs at inception of the current generation. With these two quantities the number of eggs for the next generation can be computed and the required recurrence equation is thus obtained. The resulting model has some peculiar properties. The form of the dynamic equation at low population numbers is different from that at high population numbers, and the two forms correspond to quite different life history features. Depending on levels of intrinsic fertility a population can have one of the two pure forms or a mixture of both. Thus with the same basic ecological plan a whole array of life history strategies can be spanned by changing a single parameter, namely the intrinsic fertility.

ACKNOWLEDGEMENTS

Dr. M. Bugatti, while working at its thesis, did most of the computer programming needed for Sec. 3. Dr. F. Scudo very carefully read an early draft of this study and helped with many criticisms.

REFERENCES

Abrams, P. 1975. Limiting similarity and the form the competition
coefficients. Theor. Pop. Biol. $\underline{8}$: 356-375.

Ayala, F.J., Gilpin, E. and Ehrenfeld, J.G. 1973. Competition between
species: Theoretical models and experimental tests. Theor. Pop.
Biol. $\underline{4}$: 331-356.

de Jong, G. 1976 . Natural selection and viability as consequences
of competition for food. Ph. D. Thesis. University of Utrecht.

de Jong, G. 1976 . A model of competition for food. I. Frequency
dependent viabilities. Amer. Natur. $\underline{110}$: 1013-1027.

Kostitzin, V.A. 1940 . Sur la loi logistique et ses generalisations.
Acta Biotheoretica. $\underline{5}$: 155-159.

Kostitzin, V.A. 1940 . Sur la ségrégation physiologique et la variation des espèces. Acta Biotheoretica. $\underline{5}$: 160-168.

Lynch, M. 1977. Fitness and optimal body size in zooplankton populations. Ecology $\underline{58}$: 763-774.

Mac Arthur, R. and Levins, R 1967. The limiting similarity, convergence and divergence of coexisting species. Amer. Natur. $\underline{101}$: 377-385

May, R.M. 1976. Models for single populations. In "Theoretical Ecology", R.M. May (ed), Blackwell Sc. Pub., Oxford, pp. 4-25.

May, R.M. and Oster, G.F. 1976. Bifurcations and dynamic complexity
in simple ecological models. Amer. Natur. $\underline{110}$: 573-599.

May, R.M., Beddington, J.R., Clark, C.W., Holt, S.J., Laws, R.M.
1979. Management of multispecies fisheries. Science. $\underline{205}$: 267-277.

Nagy, K.A. and Milton, K. 1979. Energy metabolism and food consumption by wild howler monkeys. Ecology. $\underline{60}$: 475-480.

Schoener, T.W. 1973. Population growth regulated by intra-specific
competition for energy and time: Some simple representations.
Theor. Pop. Biol. $\underline{4}$: 56-84.

Schoener, T.W. 1974. Competition and the form of habitat shift.
Theor. Pop. Biol. $\underline{6}$: 265-307.

Schoener, T.W. 1976. Alternatives to Lotka-Volterra competition:
Models of intermediate complexity. Theor. Pop. Biol. $\underline{10}$: 309-333.

Volterra, V. 1938. Population growth, equilibria and extinction under

specified breeding conditions: A develpment and extension of the
theory of the logistic curve. Human Biology. <u>10</u>: 1-11.1938

Volterra, V. 1939. Calculus of variations and the logistic curve.
Human Biology. <u>11</u>: 173-178.

Wangersky, P.J. 1978. Lotka-Volterra population models. Ann. Rev.
Ecol. Syst. <u>9</u>: 189-218.

STOCHASTIC EQUATIONS IN NEUROBIOLOGY

AND POPULATION BIOLOGY

L.M. Ricciardi

Istituto di Scienze dell'Informazione
dell'Università,Salerno, Italy

1. Introduction and Background

Rather than spending time to describe at length specific models of biophysical interest I thought it would be more profitable to discuss certain aspects of
mathematical modeling whose interest surely extends far beyond the simple examples
I shall bring up from the fields of neurobiology and population biology. I shall
thus talk about stochastic equations and their use for model building. For the sake
of brevity I shall limit myself to considering only first order equations. On the
other hand, little of the present considerations can be extended to the multidimensional case.

I should like to mention that many people, including myself, have so far made
use of stochastic equations to model biological and physical phenomena. Despite the
fact that everybody seems to imply that everything is "well known" about interpretation and use of stochastic differential equations, the number of papers dealing
with this subject has been steadily increasing during the last decade, particularly
in the biological literature. As far as I am concerned, the more I think about it
the more I find gaps and unsatisfactory results, when non linear differential equations are employed. Hence, I came to the conclusion that it is advisable to work with
simpler models and to prove directly all the results of interest. By proving "direc
tly" I mean that I first confine myself to considering discrete stochastic equations. The meaning and the range of validity of the following continuous approximations become than clearer.

To introduce the necessary terminology and notation, let me refer to a one-
dimensional state-and-time-continuous stochastic process $X(t)$, with $t \in [0, \infty)$ and
let $f_n[X(t_1); X(t_2); \ldots; X(t_n)]$ be the joint n-th order probability density function (p.d.f.) of $X(t_n)$ for all arbitrarily considered n-tuples of instants

$t_1, t_2, \ldots, t_n$. Such function is known if $X(t)$ is completely specified. Conversely, if one knows the n-th order p.d.f. f_n, for all n and all instants t_i, then $X(t)$ is specified since, for instance, any statistical average of $X(t)$ can be calculated. The process can thus be characterized by an infinite sequence of p.d.f.'s of increasing order $f_1\left[X(t_1)\right]$, $f_2\left[X(t_1); X(t_2)\right]$,..., $f_n\left[X(t_1); X(t_2); \ldots; X(t_n)\right]$,...with

$$\int f_n\left[X(t_1); X(t_2); \ldots; X(t_n)\right] dX(t_j) = f_{n-1}\left[X(t_1); \ldots;\right.$$

$$\left. X(t_{j-1}); X(t_{j+1}); \ldots; X(t_n)\right]$$

for all $1 \leqslant j \leqslant n$, the integral on the l.h.s. being extended over the entire domain of the r.v. $X(t_j)$. Hence, in general we are confronted with the quite impossible task of determining the functions $f_n\left[X(t_1); X(t_2); \ldots; X(t_n)\right]$ for <u>all</u> n and t_i. However, the situation improves a great deal when Markov processes are considered. Indeed, for all n and $t_1 < t_2 < \ldots < t_n$ one then has:

$$f\left[X(t_n) \mid X(t_{n-1}); X(t_{n-2}); \ldots; X(t_1)\right] = f\left[X(t_n) \mid X(t_{n-1})\right] \qquad (1.1)$$

where the conditional p.d.f. on the l.h.s. is as

$$f\left[X(t_n) \mid X(t_{n-1}); X(t_{n-2}); \ldots; X(t_1)\right] =$$

$$\frac{f_n\left[X(t_1); X(t_2); \ldots; X(t_n)\right]}{f_{n-1}\left[X(t_1); X(t_2); \ldots; X(t_{n-1})\right]} . \qquad (1.2)$$

The function on the r.h.s. of (1.1) is called, for evident reasons, the transition p.d.f. of $X(t)$. In general, this will be a function of the four variables $x_n = X(t_n)$, $x_{n-1} = X(t_{n-1})$, t_n and t_{n-1}. From (1.1) and (1.2) it follows that a Markov process is completely specified by the univariate p.d.f. $f_1\left[X(t)\right]$ <u>and</u> the transition p.d.f. $f\left[X(t) \mid Y(\tau)\right]$ since for all n and for all $t_1 < t_2 < \ldots < t_n$ one has:

$$f_n\left[X(t_1); X(t_2); \ldots; X(t_n)\right] = f\left[X(t_n) \mid X(t_{n-1})\right] f\left[X(t_{n-1}) \mid \right.$$

$$\left. X(t_{n-2})\right] \ldots f\left[X(t_2) \mid X(t_1)\right] f_1\left[X(t_1)\right]. \qquad (2.3)$$

These considerations disclose the importance of the transition p.d.f. as a tool to obtain the description of a Markov process. In order to show how this function may be determined, let me denote by $t_o < \tau < t$ three otherways arbitrary instants and set $x_o = X(t_o)$, $y = X(\tau)$, $x=X(t)$. It is then easy to prove that the following Smolukowski equation holds:

$$f(x,t \mid x_o,t_o) = \int dy \; f(y,\tau \mid x_o,t_o) \; f(x,t \mid y,\tau), \qquad (1.4)$$

This is to be viewed as a compatibility condition on f rather than an equation in the unknown f. Equivalent, but more expressive, forms of Eq. (2.4) can be obtained by some straightforward manipulations. Indeed, the following differential expansions hold (cf., for instance, Ricciardi,1967):

$$\frac{\partial f}{\partial t} = \sum_{n=1}^{\infty} \frac{(-1)^n}{n!} \frac{\partial^n}{\partial x^n} \left[A_n(x,t) \; f \right]$$

$$(1.5)$$

$$\frac{\partial f}{\partial t_o} + \sum_{n=1}^{\infty} \frac{A_n(x_o,t_o)}{n!} \frac{\partial^n f}{\partial x_o^n} = 0$$

where

$$A_n(z,u) = \lim_{\Delta t \to 0} \frac{1}{\Delta t} \int (v-u)^n \; f(v,t+\Delta t \mid u,t) \; dv \quad (n=1,2,..) \quad (1.6)$$

is the infinitesimal moment of order n. If $X(t)$ is temporally homogeneous, i.e. $f(x,t \mid y,\tau) = f(x,t-\tau \mid y,0) \equiv f(x,t-\tau \mid y)$ Eqs. (1.5) read:

$$\frac{\partial f}{\partial t} = \sum_{n=1}^{\infty} \frac{(-1)^n}{n!} \frac{\partial^n}{\partial x^n} \left[A_n(x) \; f \right]$$

$$(1.7)$$

$$\frac{\partial f}{\partial t} = \sum_{n=1}^{\infty} \frac{A_n(x_o)}{n!} \frac{\partial^n f}{\partial x_o^n} .$$

From now on we shall always refer to temporally homogeneous processes.

The presence of arbitrarily high order derivatives does not allow one to "solve" Eqs. (1.7) to determine the transition p.d.f. Hence, the question when Eqs. (1.7) are actually partial differential equations of the customary type and what is the order of the equations when this is the case. A theorem, first proved by Pawula (1967), provides an answer to this question which seems to be in conflict with one's intuition: If for all n the infinitesimal moments $A_n (x,t)$ exist, the vanishing of any even order infinitesimal moment implies $A_n (x,t) = 0$ for $n > 2$. This implies that whenever Eqs. (1.5) or (1.7) exhibit a finite number of derivatives, they are second order equations at most. Since the first order equation cases describe deterministic systems, the only non-trivial case for which partial differential equations regulate the dynamics of the process is that of diffusion processes. Apart from a number of problems arising for singular equations (cf.Feller 1951,1952, 1954), diffusion processes thus appear as those Markov processes whose transition p.d.f. can be obtained as the solution of either equation

$$\frac{\partial f}{\partial t} = -\frac{\partial}{\partial x}\left[A_1(x) \ f\right] + \frac{1}{2}\frac{\partial^2}{\partial x^2}\left[A_2 (x) \ f\right]$$

(1.8)

$$\frac{\partial f}{\partial t} = A_1(x_o) \frac{\partial f}{\partial x_o} + \frac{A_2(x_o)}{2}\frac{\partial^2 f}{\partial x_o^2}$$

that satisfies the initial condition

$$\lim_{t \to 0} f (x,t \mid x_o) = \delta (x-x_o).$$

(1.9)

The question remains how does one determine the first and second order moments ("drift" and "infinitesimal variance",respectively). Indeed, Eqs. (1.8) have been derived aiming at the determination of the unknown transition p.d.f. On the other hand, to write Eqs. (1.8) drift and infinitesimal variance are to be calculated first which, due to definitions (1.6), seems to require in turn the knowledge of the transition p.d.f. This apparent tautology is eliminated if one remarks that in definitions (1.6) the transition p.d.f. over an infinitesimal time interval is involved. As we shall see by means of the example brought up in Section 2, this function may at times be calculated by first principles, which permits one to write down Eqs. (1.8) and thus determine f (x,t $\mid$ x_o) by making use of condition (1.9). In other instances, the coefficients of Eqs. (1.8) are evaluated by writing differential or difference stochastic equations. This will be discussed in Section 3 where some considerations of interest to problems of model building in population biology will be presented.

2. A Stochastic Model for Neuronal Activity

Assuming that the reader is familiar with the general terminology (cf., for instance, Ricciardi and Sacerdote 1979 and references quoted therein), I shall consider a neuron possessing p+q dendrites on which excitatory and inhibitory post-synaptic potentials of magnitudes $e_k > 0$ (k=1,2,...p) and $i_\ell < 0$ (=1,2,...,q), respectively, are generated by Poisson distributed excitatory and inhibitory synaptic stimuli characterized by rates α_k (k=1,2,...,p) and β_ℓ (ℓ = 1,2,...,q), respectively. If x is the membrane potential at a certain time, the arrival at that time of an excitatory input along the k-th excitatory pathway determines the instantaneous transition $x \rightarrow x + e_k$ (k=1,2,...,p) whereas the instantaneous transition $x \rightarrow x+i_\ell$ (ℓ=1,2,. ...,q) depicts the effect of an input signal carried by the ℓ-th inhibitory synapsis. The neuron's membrane potential X(t) thus undergoes a random walk in continuous time. Since X(t) is Markov and temporally homogeneous, Eq. (1.4) yields:

$$f (x,t+\Delta t \mid x_o) = \int_{-\infty}^{\infty} dz \; f (x,\Delta t \mid z) \; f (z,t \mid x_o) \tag{2.1}$$

where x_o = X(0). Denoting by θ the membrane's time constant and taking as zero the resting potential, the above assumptions imply:

$$f(x, \Delta t \mid z) = \left\{1-\Delta t \left[\sum_{k=1}^{p} \alpha_k + \sum_{k=1}^{q} \beta_k\right]\right\} \delta \left[x-(z-z \frac{\Delta t}{\theta})\right] \tag{2.2}$$

$$+ \Delta t \sum_{k=1}^{p} \alpha_k \; \delta \left[x-(z-z \frac{\Delta t}{\theta} + e_k)\right] + \Delta t \sum_{k=1}^{q} \beta_k \; \delta \left[x-(z-z \frac{\Delta t}{\theta} + i_k)\right].$$

We now make use of (2.2), carry out the integrations on the r.f.s. of (2.1) and use the approximation $(1-\Delta t/\theta)^{-1} \approx 1+\Delta t/\theta$ to find:

$$\frac{\partial f}{\partial t} = \frac{\partial}{\partial x} (\theta^{-1} x f) + \sum_{k=1}^{p} \alpha_k \left[f (x-e_k,t \mid x_o) - f(x,t \mid x_o)\right] \tag{2.3}$$

$$+ \sum_{k=1}^{q} \beta_k \left[f (x-i_k,t \mid x_o) - f(x,t \mid x_o)\right]$$

or:

$$\frac{\partial f}{\partial t} = \sum_{n=1}^{\infty} \frac{(-1)^n}{n!} \frac{\partial^n}{\partial x^n} \left(A_n \ f \right), \tag{2.4}$$

where we have set:

$$A_1 = \frac{-x}{\theta} + \eta_1$$

$$A_r = \eta_r \tag{2.5}$$

$$\eta_n = \sum_{k=1}^{p} \alpha_k \ e_k^n + \sum_{k=1}^{q} \beta_k i_k^n \qquad (n=1,2,\ldots)$$

Eq. (2.4) is the differential expansion of the Smolukowski equation for the instance considered here. In order to shade some light on the input-output behavior of the considered neuron, it is convenient to resort to a diffusion "approximation" and set:

$$\eta_r = 0 \qquad (r = 3,4,\ldots)$$

$$|\eta_1| < \infty \qquad , \ 0 < \eta_2 < \infty . \tag{2.6}$$

However, it is to be remarked that (2.6) can also be obtained via a suitable limit process involving the magnitudes of the PSP's and the rates of arrival of the synaptic inputs (Ricciardi,1977). Due to (2.6), from (2.4) we obtain the partial differential equation:

$$\frac{\partial f}{\partial t} = -\frac{\partial}{\partial x} \left[\left(-\frac{x}{\theta} + \eta \right) f \right] + \frac{\sigma^2}{2} \frac{\partial^2 f}{\partial x^2} , \tag{2.7}$$

where we have set $\eta_1 = \eta$ and $\eta_2 = \sigma^2$. Hence, the neuron's membrane potential X(t) is a normal process with

$$E\left[X(t) \right] = \eta\theta - (\eta\theta - x_o) \ \exp\left(-\frac{t}{\theta} \right)$$

$$Var\left[X(t) \right] = \frac{\theta\sigma^2}{2} \left[1 - \exp\left(-\frac{2t}{\theta} \right) \right]. \tag{2.8}$$

Eq.(2.7) regulates the time course of the "unrestricted" process X(t). To determine the neuron's firing distribution one has to solve a first passage time problem. In other words, denoting by S the neuron's threshold, let T be the time when first the membrane potential attains the value S starting from $X(0)=x_o$:

$$T = T(S,x_o) = \inf\left\{ t: X(t) > S \mid X(0)=x_o \right\},$$

and let $g(s,t \ x_o)$ be its p.d.f.:

$$g(s,t \mid x_o) = \frac{\partial}{\partial t} \Pr\left\{ T \leqslant t \right\}.$$

As shown elsewhere (Ricciardi,1977), if X(t) is described by Eq. (2.7) a closed form solution to the first passage time problem exists only if the threshold has the form:

$$S(t) = A\, e^{-t/\theta} + B\, e^{t/\theta} \tag{2.9}$$

with A and B arbitrary constants. However, this cannot be taken as a neuronal threshold. The neuron's firing problem has thus to be studied by some approximate procedure. Without entering here into any details, I should like to mention that two alternative approaches are possible. The first consists of solving numerically the Volterra equation

$$f\left[S(t),t \mid x_o\right] = \int_0^t d\tau\; g\left[S(\tau),\tau \mid x_o\right]\, f\left[S(t),t-\tau \mid S(\tau)\right]$$

in the unknown function g. Although this is not a simple job due to the singular nature of the kernel in the neighborhood of the origin, some suitable algorithms have been developed and implemented (Anderssen et al., 1973; Favella et al., in preparation). The second approach, useful when the threshold is taken as a constant (small net excitation) aims at the calculation of the moments of the firing time T. This can be done since the moments generating function can be explicitly determined (cf.Ricciardi and Sacerdote,1979). Although the final results are too cumbersome to be reproduced here, I would like to mention that a rather detailed study on the input-output behavior of the considered model neuron has been successfully performed (Ricciardi and Sacerdote,1979).

3.   Population Growth and Stochastic Equations

In Section 2, by making use of a neurobiological terminology an example has been given in which the coefficients appearing in the differential expansion of the Smolukowski equation could be determined via the specification of the transition p.d.f. for an infinitesimal time interval. In this Section I shall instead construct diffusion process- and thus write down drift and infinitesimal variance- by a different procedure based on stochastic differential and difference equations. However, a few remarks should first be made to recall known results of the theory of random processes. The reader will find a comprehensive discussion of this subject in Stratonovich (1963,1968), Wong (1974) and Arnold (1974) and in the references quoted therein.

Let ∂ be a dynamical system and let its state $x(t)$ be described by the Stratonovich's stochastic differential equation

$$\frac{dx}{dt} = f(x) + g(x) \quad N(t),$$ (3.1)

where $N(t)$ is a stationary delta-correlated normal process (white noise) with zero mean and intensity σ^2:

$$E\left[N(t)\right] = 0$$
$$E\left[N(t) \ N(t')\right] = \sigma^2 \ \delta(t-t')$$ (3.2)

and where $f(x)$ and $g(x)$ are given deterministic functions. By using a suitable calculus named after Stratonovich one can then show that $x(t)$ is a time homogeneous diffusion process whose drift and infinitesimal variance are given by:

$$A_1(x) = f(x) + \frac{1}{4} \ \frac{dA_2(x)}{dx}$$
$$A_2(x) = \sigma^2 \ g^2(x),$$ (3.3)

respectively.

Another frequently used method for including a random "force" in the state evolution equation of the considered system ∂ consists of writing the so called Ito's equation

$$dy = f(y) \ dt + g(y) \ dW(t)$$ (3.4)

where W(t) is the zero-mean Wiener process whose covariance $E\left[W(t_1)\ W(t_2)\right]$ is given by σ^2 min (t_1, t_2). Since N(t) cannot be identified with the derivative of W(t), Eqs. (3.1) and (3.4) are not equivalent. As shown in the quoted references, by using the so called Ito's calculus one can see that Eq.(3.4) implies that the state of $\mathcal{X}$ is modelled by the diffusion process y(t) whose drift and infinitesimal varian ce are

$$B_1(y) = f(y) \neq A_1(y)$$

$$B_2(y) = \sigma^2\ g^2(y) = A_2(y),$$

(3.5)

respectively. Unless g=const, functions A_1 and B_1 differ in a substantial manner. The effect of such diversity was dramatically pointed out by Feldman and Roughgarden (1975) with reference to a population growth process in random environment. Indeed, taking $f(z) = Kz - z^2$ and g(z)=z, Eqs. (3.1) and (3.4) model a logistic growth process in the presence of a randomly varying carrying capacity K(t) such that $E\left[K(t)\right]$=K. However, if Eq. (3.1) is used, the population size is modelled by the diffusion pro cess X(t) specified by:

$$A_1(x) = x\ (K + \frac{\sigma^2}{2})\ -x^2$$

$$A_2(x) = \sigma^2\ x^2.$$

Instead, if Eq. (3.4) is considered, the resulting diffusion process Y(t) is such that:

$$B_1(y) = y(K-y)$$

$$B_2(y) = \sigma^2\ y^2.$$

It can then be seen (May,1973) that for the latter the steady-state distribution

$$F(y) = \lim_{t \to \infty}\ f(y,t\mid x_o)$$

exists if $K > \sigma^2/2$. Hence, if $K > \sigma^2/2$ (small environmental fluctuations) the ultimate extinction probability is null. As for the former, the steady-state distribution exists irrespectively of the values of K and σ^2 so that ultimate extinc-tion can never occur (cf.also Ricciardi,1977; Nobile and Ricciardi,1979).

This example clearly shows that Eqs.(3.1) and (3.4) are models of <u>different</u> dynamical systems. However, a glance at (3.3) and (3.5) leads us to the conclusion that the pair of equations

$$\frac{dx}{dt} = f(x) + g(x) \ N(t) \tag{3.6}$$

$$dx = \left[f(x) + \frac{\sigma^2}{2} \ g(x) \ g'(x) \right] dt + g(x) \ dW(t)$$

are equivalent for modeling purposes. The same is true for the equations

$$dy = f(y) \ dt + g(y) \ dW(t)$$

$$\frac{dy}{dt} = \left[f(y) - \frac{\sigma^2}{2} \ g(y) \ g'(y) \right] + g(y) \ N(t). \tag{3.7}$$

However, Eqs.(3.6) lead to the moments (3.3) whereas from (3.7) moments (3.5) follow.

The question remains of what stochastic equations are to be used to account for random perturbations acting on a dynamical system whose deterministic behavior is expressed by first order differential equations. To answer this question let us assume that $\mathcal{O}\!\!\backslash$ is a population growing in a finite carrying capacity environment and let $x_{n\tau}$ be the number of individuals counted by an observer at the instants $t=n\tau$ ($\tau > 0$; n=0,1,2,...). In the absence of any other information, one may mo-del this growth process by the difference equations:

$$\Delta x_{n\tau} = A \tau \ f(x_{n\tau}) \qquad (n=0,1,...) \tag{3.8}$$

or by the differential equation:

$$\frac{dx}{dt} = B \ f(x), \tag{3.9}$$

A and B being parameters (relating to the Wrightian fertility and to the Malthusian parameter) to be experimentally determined. Since (3.8) and (3.9) are taken to describe the very same population, we set $x(n\tau) = x_{n\tau}$, $\forall n$.

This procedure amounts to imposing that the solution to Eq.(3.9) at the discrete times $t=n\tau$ yields the values determined by the discrete model (3.8). What we wish to obtain is a relationship between the parameters A and B securing that the identity between the considered values actually holds. By integrating Eq.(3.9) over a ti me interval of duration we obtain:

$$B = \frac{1}{\tau} \int_{x_{n\tau}}^{x_{(n+1)\tau}} dz \left[f(z) \right]^{-1}$$

or, on account of (3.8):

$$B = \frac{A\, f(x_{n\tau})}{\Delta x_{n\tau}} \int_{x_{n\tau}}^{x_{(n+1)\tau}} dz \left[f(z) \right]^{-1} \qquad (3.10)$$

where $\Delta x_{n\tau}$ is given by the r.h.s. of (3.8). A Taylor series expansion of the r.h.s. of (3.10) then easily yields:

$$B = A - \frac{1}{2}\, f'(x_{n\tau})\, A^2 \tau + o\,(1). \qquad (3.11)$$

This relation shows that, except for the Malthusian growth process, B is density-dependent.

Let us now suppose that the considered process is intrinsically discontinuous and modify (3.8) by the "random environment" assumption $A\tau \rightarrow A'_{n\tau}$. Here $A'_{n\tau}$ (n=0,1,...) is a sequence of independent identically distributed random variables with (Capocelli and Ricciardi, 1978 and 1979):

$$Pr\left\{ A'_{n\tau} = \sigma\sqrt{\tau} \right\} = \frac{1}{2} + \frac{A\sqrt{\tau}}{2\sigma}$$

$$Pr\left\{ A'_{n\tau} = -\sigma\sqrt{\tau} \right\} = \frac{1}{2} - \frac{A\sqrt{\tau}}{2\sigma} \qquad (3.12)$$

and $\sigma > 0$ is an arbitrary parameter. From (3.12) one easily finds:

$$E\left[A'_{n\tau} \right] = A\tau$$

$$E\left[(A'_{n\tau})^2\right] = \sigma^2\tau$$

$$(3.13)$$

$$E\left[(A'_{n\tau})^{2+p}\right] = o(\tau) \qquad p=1,2,\ldots$$

Note that by the outlined procedure the deterministic growth process $x_{n\tau}$ described by Eqs. (3.8) has been substituted by the stochastic process $X_{n\tau}$ modeled by the equations:

$$\Delta X_{n\tau} = A'_{n\tau} \ f(X_{n\tau}) \qquad (n=0,1,\ldots).$$

$$(3.14)$$

Furthermore, from (3.13) it follows

$$\lim_{\tau \to 0} \tau^{-1}\left\{E\left[\Delta X_{n\tau} \mid X_{n\tau} = x\right]\right\} = A \ f(x)$$

$$(3.15)$$

$$\lim_{\tau \to 0} \tau^{-1}\left\{E\left[(\Delta X_{n\tau})^2 \ X_n \mid = x\right]\right\} = \sigma^2 \ f^2(x)$$

$$\lim_{\tau \to 0} \tau^{-1}\left\{E\left[(\Delta X_{n\tau})^{2+p} \mid X_{n\tau}=x\right]\right\} = 0 \qquad (p=1,2,\ldots).$$

Comparing (3.15) with definitions (1.6), we conclude that in the limit as $\tau \to 0$ (and consequently $n \to \infty$) the <u>Markov</u> process $X_{n\tau}$ converges to the diffusion process $X(t)$ whose drift and infinitesimal variance are given by

$$A_1(x) = A \ f(x)$$

$$A_2(x) = \sigma^2 \ f^2(x).$$

Recalling (3.5) and (3.7) we thus see that $X(t)$ is modeled by either equation

$$dX(t) = A \ f(x) \ dt + f(x) \ dW(t)$$

$$\frac{dX(t)}{dt} = \left[A - \frac{\sigma^2}{2} \ f(x) \ f'(x)\right] \ N(t).$$

Hence, the conclusion that Ito's equation (and the corresponding calculus) is the

natural tool for modeling the continuous approximation to an intrinsically discontinuous growth process in random environment.

Let us now assume that the considered process is intrinsically continuous
and let us take Eq. (3.9) as the deterministic model of it. The following system of
difference equations then follows:

$$B\tau = \int_{x_{n\tau}}^{x_{(n+1)\tau}} dz \left[f(z)\right]^{-1} \qquad (n=0,1,\ldots)$$

and the random environment assumption yields:

$$B'_{n\tau} = \int_{Y_{n\tau}}^{Y_{(n+1)\tau}} dz \left[f(z)\right]^{-1}, \qquad (n=0,1,\ldots)$$

with

$$Pr\left\{B'_{n\tau} = \sigma\sqrt{\tau}\right\} = \frac{1}{2} + \frac{B\sqrt{\tau}}{2\sigma}$$

$$P\left\{B'_{n\tau} = -\sigma\sqrt{\tau}\right\} = \frac{1}{2} - \frac{B\sqrt{\tau}}{2\sigma}.$$

It is now easy to see that the following equations hold:

$$\lim_{\tau \to 0} \tau^{-1}\left\{E\left[\Delta Y_{n\tau}\mid Y_{n\tau} = y\right]\right\} = f(y)\left[B + \frac{\sigma^2}{2} f'(y)\right]$$

$$\lim_{\tau \to 0} \tau^{-1}\left\{E\left[(\Delta Y_{n\tau})^2 \mid Y_{n\tau} = y\right]\right\} = \sigma^2 f^2(y)$$

and that all higher order infinitesimal moments vanish. This implies that $Y_{n\tau}$
now converges to the diffusion process $Y(t)$ defined by either equation

$$\frac{dY(t)}{dt} = \left[B + N(t)\right] f(Y)$$

$$dY(t) = \left[B + \frac{\sigma^2}{2} f'(Y)\right] f(Y) \, dt + f(Y) \, dW(t).$$

Therefore, the conclusion follows that an intrinsically continuous growth process

in random environment should be modeled by Stratonovich's equation (and corresponding calculus).

What if one ignores whether the system is intrinsically continuous or intrinsically discontinuous? The foregoing considerations clearly indicate that
either equation

$$dX(t) = A \ f(X) \ dt + f(X) \ dW(t)$$

$$\frac{dY(t)}{dt} = \left[B + N(t) \right] f(Y)$$

may be used, provided A and B are not taken as indefendent but as related to one
another as specified by (3.11).

As a concrete straightforward axample of the foregoing considerations, let
us consider a logistic growth process and set:

$$f(z) = z(1-K^{-1} z), \quad B=m, \quad A=w.$$

Eqs.(3.8) and (3.10) then read:

$$\Delta x_{n\tau} = w\tau \ x_{n\tau} \ (1-K^{-1}x_{n\tau})$$

$$m = \frac{w \ x_{n\tau}}{\Delta x_{n\tau}} (1-K^{-1}x_{n\tau}) \int_{x_{n\tau}}^{x_{(n+1)\tau}} dz \left[z(1-K^{-1}z) \right]^{-1}.$$

After some straightforward calculations one then finds:

$$w = \frac{1- e^{-m\tau}}{(1-e^{-m\tau}) \ K^{-1}x_{n\tau} + e^{-m\tau}} \ .$$

Let us now make a random environment assumption and change $w\tau$ into $W_{n\tau}$ and $m\tau$
into $M_{n\tau}$, where $W_{n\tau}$ and $M_{n\tau}$ are i.i.d. random variables with $E\left[W_{n\tau} \right] = w\tau$ and
$E\left[M_{n\tau} \right] = m\tau$. From (3.11) it then follows:

$$E\left[M_{n\tau}\right] = w\tau - \frac{\sigma^2}{2}(1-2\ K^{-1}x)\tau + 0(\tau)$$

if $W_{n\tau}$ is looked upon as independent. If, instead, $M_{n\tau}$ is viewed as independent, one finds:

$$E\left[W_{n\tau}\right] = m\tau + \frac{\sigma^2}{2}(1-2\ K^{-1}x)\tau + 0(\tau).$$

The relations existing between Malthusian parameter and Wrightian fertility thus easily follows:

$$m = \lim_{\tau \to 0} \tau^{-1} E\left[M_{n\tau}\right] = w - \frac{\sigma^2}{2}(1-2\ K^{-1}x)$$

and

$$w = \lim_{\tau \to 0} \tau^{-1} E\left[W_{n\tau}\right] = m + \frac{\sigma^2}{2}(1-2\ K^{-1}x).$$

References

Anderssen,K.S., De Hoog,F.R. and Weiss,R.(1973). On the numerical solution of Brownian motion processes, J.Appl.Prob.10, 409-418.

Arnold,L.(1974). Stochastic Differential Equations. Wiley,N.Y.

Capocelli,R.M. and Ricciardi, L.M.(1978). On the role of noise in systems dynamics. Proc.Int.Cong.Cybern.Soc.Tokyo, 1058-1064.

Capocelli,R.M. and Ricciardi,L.M.(1979). A cybernetic approach to population dynamics modeling.J.Cybernetics 9, 297-312.

Feldman,M.W. and Roughgarden,J.(1975). A population's stationary distribution and chance of extinction with remarks on the theory of species packing. Theor. Pop.Biol. 7, 197-207.

Feller,W.(1951). Two singular diffusion processes. Ann.Math. 54, 173-182.

Feller,W.(1952). Parabolic differential equations and semigroups of transformations. Ann.Math. 55, 468-518.

Feller,W.(1954). Diffusion processes in one dimension. Trans.Amer.Math.Soc. 77,1-31.

May,R.M.(1973). Stability and complexity in model ecosystems.Princeton Univ.Press, Princeton,N.J.

Nobile,A.G. and Ricciardi,L.M.(1979). Growth and extinction in random environment. Proc.INFO II,Patras,Greece.

Pawula,R.F.(1967). Generalizations and extensions of the Fokker-Planck-Kolmogorov equations. JEEE Trans.Information Theory, 13, 33-41.

Ricciardi,L.M.(1977). Diffusion processes and related topics in Biology. Springer, Heidelberg.

Stratonovich,R.L.(1963). Topics in the theory of random noise,   I. Gordon & Breach, N.Y.

Stratonovich,R.L.(1968). Conditional Markov processes and their applications to the theory of optimal control.Elsevier,N.Y.

Wong,E.(1971).Stochastic processes in information and dynamical systems. Mc Graw-Hill, N.Y.

MODELS FOR VECTOR-BORNE PARASITIC DISEASES

K. Dietz
Tübingen University

INTRODUCTION

There are several reasons for concentrating on the class of vector-borne diseases from a modelling point of view:

1) They still figure among the health problems of highest priority in most countries outside Europe, North America and Australia;

2) They require specialized measures for prevention which are mostly directed against the vector populations with an aim to reduce contact between humans or contacts between the reservoir population(s) and humans;

3) The factors which regulate their transmission are usually known qualitatively so that dynamic modelling has a sound basis to start from;

4) Many quantitative problems have to be solved before alternative methods for prevention and control (already existing or to be developed) can be evaluated in a rational way.

The transmission of vector-borne parasites can be regarded like a dynamic system which describes the interactions of at least three classes of populations: parasite, human and vector. The rate of contacts between humans achieved by the vector population(s), determine the degree of stability of the parasite population(s). Some parasite populations show a remarkable capacity for self regulation. Wide environmental variations have sometimes very small effects on the prevalence of the parasite populations. If one would like to plan interventions in such complicated feed-back systems one needs a thorough understanding of its behaviour over the full range of contact rates, i.e. vectorial capacities. But this basic epidemiological knowledge is missing for most parasitic diseases. Many epidemiological investigations have of course been carried out, but usually in such a way that it is impossible to study the interaction of the vector population(s) and the parasite population(s). Sampling of vectors and parasites was not standardized and seldom carried out at the same time in the same place. If one would like to improve the epidemiological understanding of parasitic diseases it is necessary to set up appropriate field studies which can provide the necessary data to answer for instance the following questions:

What is the critical vectorial capacity below which transmission cannot maintain itself?

How long does it take to eliminate the parasite reservoir after interruption of transmission?

By how much does one have to reduce the vectorial capacity in order to reduce the incidence or the prevalence to a specified level?

None of these questions can be answered satisfactorily at present for any parasitic disease.

Control measures have been and are being carried out (sometimes successfully) without this basic epidemiological understanding. The improvement of this understanding does not automatically help to improve the control methods, but some pay-off will be the explanation provided for control failures and the prevention of wastage of resources in useless control activities. If one would like to apply the modelling approach for the selection of alternative control strategies to be implemented, one has to be aware of two crucial points:

1. The effects of the alternative control measures cannot be predicted accurately since they will depend on a number of unpredictable and uncontrollable factors like weather and human cooperation. One can however make relative predictions, like "other things being equal, method A is more effective than method B".

2. In order to compare alternative methods of control one needs essentially a one-dimensional objective function which can be evaluated for the various methods. Or one has to be satisfied in listing the effects of the alternative measures for the various age groups, (morbidity, disability, blindness, etc.) and leave it to the public health decision maker to make his choice. This is only feasible for a small number of alternative choices.

Dynamic transmission models may improve the estimate of the effects of alternative measures on various outcome variables. Whether this improvement is significant depends on the objective functions of public health decision makers. Since this is usually not explicit, it is difficult to judge how much precision is needed in predicting the effects of alternative interventions.

In the following we discuss some specific problems of modelling activities which have been carried out in relation to malaria, schistosomiasis and onchocerciasis.

PREVALENCE AND DENSITY

Most epidemiological models are based on a classification of the human population into a few states: susceptible, infective, immune etc. This is justified as long as there is a simple relationship between an infection and the chance of getting the resulting disease. For parasitic diseases the intensity of an infection, i.e. the number of parasites in the host, is a key variable in determining the risk of developing disease symptoms. There may be villages where everybody above a certain age is infected, but the prevalence of the disease may vary considerably due to different parasite loads.

The first malaria model by Ross (1911) only considered prevalence of the infection $y(t)$:

$$\frac{dy}{dt} = \beta y(1-y) - \gamma y. \tag{1}$$

Here β denotes the contact rate and γ the recovery rate from an infection. Recovered individuals are susceptible again. Eq. (1) has the following equilibria

$$y_1 = 0;$$
$$y_2 = 1 - \gamma/\beta.$$

The second is stable for $\beta/\gamma > 1$, i.e. when the number of secondary cases of one infective during his infectious period is greater than one.

If we assume that the contact rate has an exponential distribution in the population, then the number of parasites per individual has a geometric distribution. We denote the average of this distribution by m. Then we have

$$m = y/(1-y),$$

and

$$y = m/(1+m).$$

Hence eq. (1) yields the following equation for the average parasite load:

$$\frac{dm}{dt} = \beta m - \gamma m (1+m).$$

This implies that the death rate per parasite increases linearly with the parasite density in the host. The equilibrium parasite load for $\beta > \gamma$ is

$$m^* = \beta/\gamma - 1.$$

This model is applicable for diseases where the inoculation rate is proportional to the average parasite load and where immunity increases the death rate of the parasites. If one assumes however, that there is no density dependent death rate of the parasite and that the inoculation rate is proportional to the prevalence of the infection, then we have the following equation:

$$\frac{dm}{dt} = \beta m/(1+m) - \gamma m.$$

Here we have the same equilibria as before, but the prevalence is now described by the equation

$$\frac{dy}{dt} = \beta y (1-y)^2 - \gamma y (1-y).$$

For the evaluation of eradication projects we are particularly interested in the rate of decline of the prevalence for $\beta = 0$. The two models yield the following expressions

$$y(t) = y_o e^{-\gamma t}$$

and

$$y(t) = [1 + (1/y_o - 1) e^{\gamma t}]^{-1}.$$

The second model yields a recovery rate which decreases for increasing y. This phenomenon has been discussed for the first time by Macdonald (1950). For a description of Macdonald's approach see Fine (1975). Macdonald considers a stable situation with a constant inoculation rate λ and derives an equation for the age-prevalence curve. If one follows his assumption, the number of infections in an individual of age a is given by the equation

$$\frac{dm}{da} = \lambda - \gamma m$$

with solution $m(a) = (\lambda/\gamma)(1-e^{-\gamma t})$. If exposure is uniform and inoculations follow a Poisson process, then the number of infections has a Poisson distribution with mean $m(a)$. Hence the age-specific prevalence is

$$y(a) = 1-e^{-m(a)}.$$

From this one can derive the average length of an infectious period for a tending to infinity:

$$T = (e^{\lambda/\gamma}-1)/\lambda.$$

Dietz et al. (1974) took the inverse of this value as an approximation to the variable recovery rate which a model for the parasite density would yield. If one compares the age-specific prevalence for the approximation

$$y(a) = (1-e^{-\lambda/\gamma})\left[1-\exp\left(\frac{-\lambda a}{e^{\lambda/\gamma}-1}\right)\right]$$

with

$$y(a) = 1-\exp[-(\lambda/\gamma)(1-e^{-\gamma a})],$$

one finds that the difference is negligible in the parameter range of interest. E.g. for $\lambda = \gamma = 1$ per year the maximum difference is about 0.016 at age 2. The approximation underestimates the rate of approach to equilibrium.

If one studies the dependence of

$$m^* = \max(0, \beta/\gamma - 1)$$

and

$$y^* = \max(0, 1-\gamma/\beta)$$

as a function of the contact rate, one finds that the density is much more sensitive to changes and uncertainties of β. Let C_{m^*}, C_{y^*} and C_β denote the coefficients of variation respectively. Then for $\beta/\gamma > 1$ we have

$$C_{m*} = C_{\beta*}$$

and

$$C_{y*} = (\beta/\gamma-1)^{-1} C_{\beta*}.$$

For $\beta/\gamma = 1$, the partial derivatives of m* and y* with respect to β do not exist. For $\beta/\gamma < 1$, $C_{m*} = C_{y*} \neq 0$.
These relationships can be interpreted in terms of description and control. Changes in the contact rate produce similar changes in the parasite density independent of the contact rate as long as $\beta/\gamma > 1$. Changes in prevalence however are inversely proportional to $(\beta/\gamma-1)$ for given changes in the contact rate. This has important practical implications: If the contact rate is far above its critical level γ^{-1}, large reductions will show no appreciable effects in prevalence. In such a situation it is however possible to estimate β with relatively small error because there are many vectors to be sampled. Thus it is possible to give a good description of the prevalence and of the effort required to reduce the contact rate to the desired level, but which may turn out to be difficult to achieve. On the other hand, for contact rates little above the critical level, small changes result in large changes of the prevalence. From the point of view of control this is desirable but this also implies that both the contact rate and the prevalence can no longer be described satisfactorily. The vector densities may be at their limit of detectability and the prevalence is likely to show large fluctuations around a low average.

A MODEL FOR MALARIA PARASITE DENSITY

In view of the limitations of prevalence models I proposed a model for the parasite densities whose mathematical properties have been investigated by Elderkin et al.(1977).
Numerical studies show satisfactory agreement with data.
Let y(t,a) denote the average trophozoite density of an individual of age a at time t, and let r(t,a) be the rate at which trophozoites are eliminated from an individual with age a at time t. If h(t) is the time-dependent inoculation rate, then we have

$$\frac{\partial y}{\partial t} + \frac{\partial y}{\partial a} = h(t)-r(t,a)y(t,a).$$

Here it is assumed that the inoculation rate is not age-dependent. Multiplication of the trophozoites within the host is not taken into account explicitly, since it is not the objective of the model to describe transient fluctuations of the parasite density. We aim at a description of the average density on the scale of the life length of an individual. It is assumed that the presence of trophozoites increases the death rate, which can be interpreted as the level of immunity. Loss of immunity is also possible according to the rate β, but only to a minimum level of the trophozoite death rate r_o:

$$\frac{\partial r}{\partial t} + \frac{\partial r}{\partial a} = \alpha y - \beta (r - r_o).$$

The trophozoites produce gametocytes according to a rate which decreases exponentially with increasing death rate r. This assumption has the desired consequence that individuals with a high level of immunity are less infective. Gametocytes die at a rate δ:

$$\frac{\partial g}{\partial t} + \frac{\partial g}{\partial a} = \gamma y e^{-rT} - \delta g.$$

The boundary conditions are

$$y(t,0) = 0,$$
$$r(t,0) = r_o,$$
$$g(t,0) = 0,$$

i.e. individuals at birth are free of trophozoites and gametocytes and have the basic immunity level r_o.

We are particularly interested in equilibrium solutions, hence we neglect derivatives with respect to t:

$$\frac{dy}{da} = \lambda - ry$$

$$\frac{dr}{da} = \alpha y - \beta (r - r_o)$$

$$\frac{dg}{da} = \gamma y e^{-rT} - \delta g.$$

The equilibrium inoculation rate λ is proportional to the average gametocyte density, averaged over all ages. Let G denote the equilibrium age distribution of the population and let V be the contact rate between individuals through the vector population. Then

$$\lambda = V \int_0^\infty g(a)\,dG(a).$$

If the death rate of individuals is a constant, say μ, then

$$\lambda = V\mu \int_0^\infty e^{-\mu a} g(a)\,da.$$

Elderkin et al.(1977) solved the problem of specifying the critical level for the contact rate V_0 above which nontrivial endemic levels exist:

$$V_0 = \gamma^{-1}(\delta+\mu)(r_0+\mu)e^{r_0 T}.$$

It would be interesting to explore the average trophozoite density

$$\int_0^\infty y(a)\,dG(a)$$

and the average gametocyte density

$$\int_0^\infty g(a)\,dG(a)$$

as a function of the contact rate V. There is numerical evidence that the latter is not increasing monotonically.

NONHOMOGENEOUS CONTACT RATES

We shall illustrate with a model by Barbour (1978) for schistosomiasis that nonhomogeneous contact rates between individuals may increase the expected number of offspring of one parasite.

Commonly the implicit assumption is made that exposure rates and contamination rates are proportional to each other with the same factor for the total population. E.g. Barbour uses the following equations:

$$\dot{X}_i = \alpha \sum_{j=1}^{L} \lambda_{ij} Y_j / A_j - \gamma X_i,$$

$$i = 1, \ldots, M \tag{2}$$

$$\dot{Y}_j = \beta \sum_{i=1}^{M} X_i \lambda_{ij} (1 - Y_j / \rho_j A_j) - \delta Y_j,$$

$$j = 1, \ldots, L$$

with the notation:

X_i number of female schistosomes within person i

M   number of people living in the area

Y_j number of infected snails in pond j

L   number of ponds

α average exposure rate per person

β average contamination rate per person

λ_{ij} amount of time per day spent by person i in pond j

A_j accessible water area in pond j

ρ_j snail density in pond j

γ death rate of female schistosomes in the human host population

δ death rate of infected snails.

A more realistic model would replace the matrix $\{\lambda_{ij}\}$ by two matrices $\{\epsilon_{ij}\}$ and $\{\kappa_{ij}\}$ where

ϵ_{ij} is the amount of time per day during which person i is exposed in pond j

and

κ_{ij} is the rate at which person i contributes to the contamination of pond j.

In order to simplify the subsequent argument we restrict ourselves to one pond (L=1). Then (2) reads as follows

$$\dot{X}_i = \alpha \varepsilon_i Y/A - \gamma X_i; \quad i=1,\ldots,M;$$

$$\dot{Y} = \beta \sum_{i=1}^{M} X_i \kappa_i (1-Y/\rho A) - \delta Y.$$

We use the same normalisation as Barbour:

$$\sum_{i=1}^{M} \varepsilon_i = \sum_{i=1}^{M} \kappa_i = M.$$

The net reproductive value of one parasite is then given by

$$\mu = \frac{\alpha \beta}{\gamma \delta A} \sum_{i=1}^{M} \varepsilon_i \kappa_i$$

$$= \frac{\alpha \beta M}{\gamma \delta A} (1+SD(\varepsilon)SD(\kappa)r_{\varepsilon,\kappa}),$$

(3)

where SD means standard deviation and $r_{\varepsilon,\kappa}$ is the correlation coefficient. If $r_{\varepsilon,\kappa} = 1$, as Barbour assumes, then

$$\mu = \frac{\alpha \beta M}{\gamma \delta A} (1+Var(\lambda)).$$

This expression is minimal for homogeneous contact rates ($Var(\lambda)=0$). According to (3) this minimal value can be reached in any one of three ways: (1) homogeneous exposure, (2) homogeneous contamination, (3) zero-correlation of exposure and contamination. For negative correlation the threshold parameter is even less than this value, but this is unlikely in reality. The estimation of μ for a particular transmission unit is an important objective of quantitative epidemiological studies, since it allows to determine the amount of control required to reduce μ below its critical value of one.
According to (4) it is necessary to estimate the standard deviations of the exposure and the contamination rates and their correlation. If one only estimates the exposure rates and assumes that they are equal to the contamination rates, then one obtains an upper bound for the

threshold parameter. For certain applications this may be appropriate.
If one would like to relate the contact rates to parasitological observations then it is important to use the total population as a sampling
frame. Sampling at contact sites only leads to biased estimates.
If one applies the same approach to a vector-borne disease which is
transmitted by bites of the intermediate host, then the distinction between contamination and exposure is superfluous. Here the variance of
the exposure rate to bites enters the formula for the not reproductive
rate. If this variance is large it is likely to be more economical to
concentrate control measures to those individuals which contribute most
to the transmission.

A MODEL FOR ONCHOCERCIASIS

The present model is based on a working paper of the Expert Committee on Epidemiology of Onchocerciasis (Dietz, 1975). It provides a tool
to study theoretically the interrelationships of the following factors,
namely:

1. non-homogeneous exposure of the human population to *Simulium* bites

2. maturation period of the parasite in man

3. chance of a female worm to be fertilized

4. density-dependent production of microfilariae

5. density-dependent development of infective stage larvae in the vector

6. differential dispersal of nulliparous and parous flies

Only the assumptions and the corresponding equations are described
below. Qualitative and quantitative predictions of the model will be
published elsewhere.

Every individual is characterized by two parameters: age and distance from the breeding site. The human population is assumed to be in equilibrium with age distribution L(a). As a simple indicator of the exposure to *Simulium* bites we take the average distance of an individual to
the breeding site. It is assumed that the fly population originates from
one breeding site and that the human population is evenly distributed
around it. As unit of measurement of the distance we take the maximum
flight range of the vector during one feeding cycle. We assume that the
vector returns to the breeding site after each blood-meal and then chooses
again a host located within a circle of radius one around the breeding
site. For simplicity, we assume that all flight directions are equally

likely, so that we can restrict ourselves to the specification of the distance y of an individual from the centrally located breeding site.

Exposure to *Simulium* bites is independent of age and sex of the human host. Let $\lambda(y,t)$ denote the rate at which infective larvae of either sex are injected into an individual at time t at distance y from the breeding site. The sex ratio of infective stage larvae is 1:1. Both male and female parasites need to undergo a maturation period of length T_1 which they survive with a probability q. We assume that all females are fertilized, if at least one male is present in the host. The number of males is assumed to have a negative binomial distribution. Both male and female mature parasites die at a constant rate σ. The number of microfilariae produced per fertilized female decreases with the total number of fertilized females present in the host. There is a maximum number C of microfilariae which may be contained in one unit volume of skin.

Let $\mu(t)$ denote the emergence rate of vector females per human individual within the unit circle around the breeding site. Let p be the survival probability for one feeding cycle. There is no differential mortality. Blood-meals are taken at regular intervals of length F. At each meal, vector females make a random choice of the host. The probability that the host belongs to the human population is denoted by b. The vector chooses a host at distance y according to the density function b_0 if it is the first blood-meal and according to b_1 for all subsequent blood-meals. The mean distance for the density b_1 is assumed to be smaller than the mean distance for b_0.

The microfilariae have to undergo a maturation period in the vector before they can be infective. Let T_2 denote the number of feeding cycles required for maturation. Infective stage larvae leave the vector at the blood-meal coinciding with the completion of the maturation time.

We assume that the probability of a microfilaria to be transmitted by a vector is a decreasing exponential function of the microfilaria density of the host. Thus, the transmission rate is density dependent.

Let u(y,a,t) denote the number of mature female parasites in an individual at distance y of age a at time t. According to our assumption about the chances of fertilization, the expected number of fertilized females v(y,a,t) in an individual at distance y of age a at time t is given by

$$v(y,a,t) = u(y,a,t)\left[1 - \left(\frac{\gamma}{\gamma+u(y,a,t)}\right)^{\gamma}\right].$$

Let m(y,a,t) denote the microfilaria density in an individual at distance y of age a at time t. Then our assumptions imply

$$m(y,a,t) = C\{1-\exp[-Dv(y,a,t)/C]\},$$

where D is the microfilaria density per fertilized female for small numbers of parasites. Let A be the maximum proportion of microfilariae transmitted and let B be the rate of decline of this proportion, as the number of microfilariae increases. Then the inoculation rate $\lambda(y,t)$ is given by the following formula:

$$\lambda(y,t) = \frac{b_1(y)}{2y}\,\bar\lambda(t)$$

with

$$\bar\lambda(t) = \mu(t-T_2)\ b^2\ p^{T_2+2}\int_0^\infty\int_0^1 \bar b(y)f(m(y,a,t-T_2))\,dy\,dL(a).$$

Here

$$\bar b(y) = \frac{1}{p}\,b_o(y) + \frac{1}{1-p}\,b_1(y)$$

and

$$f(m(y,a,t)) = Am(y,a,t)\exp[-Bm(y,a,t)].$$

The dynamic equation for u(y,a,t) is then given by

$$\frac{\partial u}{\partial a} + \frac{\partial u}{\partial t} = \frac{q}{2}\,\lambda(y,t-T_1)-\sigma u(y,a,t),$$

with suitable boundary and initial conditions.

In order to investigate equilibrium solutions for constant emergence rate μ one may proceed as follows:

For given $\bar\lambda$, one calculates $\lambda(y)$, then successively u(y,a), v(y,a) and finally the required emergence rate μ which is required to yield a given inoculation rate. By repeating this process for a sufficiently wide range of $\bar\lambda$ values, one can determine critical emergence rates below which transmission cannot maintain itself.

The equilibrium solutions can be fitted to the cross-sectional studies of several villages with varying transmission levels. The dynamic version of the model allows then to make projections in time about the effect of interventions.

REFERENCES

BARBOUR, A.D.(1978). Macdonald's model and the transmission of bilharzia. *Trans. Roy. Soc. Trop. Med. Hyg.*, **72**, 6-15.

DIETZ, K.(1975). Epidemiological models. Working Paper of the Expert Committee on Epidemiology of Onchocerciasis, ONCHO/WP/75.31, 1-3.

DIETZ, K. et al.(1974). A malaria model tested in the African savannah. *Bull. Wld Hlth Org.*, **50**, 347-57.

ELDERKIN, R.H. et al.(1977). On the steady state of an age dependent model for malaria. In *Nonlinear systems and applications. An International Conference.* V. Lakshmikantham, ed., Academic Press, New York, 491-512.

FINE, P.E.M.(1975). Superinfection - A problem in formulating a problem. *Trop. Dis. Bull.*, **72**, 475-488.

MACDONALD, G.(1950). The analysis of infection rates in diseases in which superinfection occurs. *Trop. Dis. Bull.*, 47, 907-15.

ROSS, R.(1911). *The prevention of malaria.* 2nd edition. John Murray, London.

THE DYNAMICS AND CONTROL OF

DIRECT LIFE CYCLE HELMINTH PARASITES

Roy M. Anderson

Zoology Dept., Imperial College,

London University, Prince Consort Rd.,

London SW7

Introduction

It is not widely appreciated that directly transmitted tapeworm and roundworm (nematode) parasites are some of the most prevalent of all human infections within many tropical, subtropical and temperate regions of the world. The roundworm *Ascaris lumbricoides*, for example, which is found in both tropical and temperate climates where there is adequate moisture and low standards of hygiene and sanitation, is one of, if not the most common of all human infections (Muller, 1975; Peters, 1978). Furthermore, the five most prevalent helminth parasites of man are all nematode species which are transmitted directly between hosts (Table 1). In 1975, W.H.O. statistics record that more than a third of the world's population was infected with one or more of these species (Peters, 1978) (Table 1).

In communities where such infections are endemic, the prevalence of infection often approaches 100% in the adult age classes. Fig. 1, for example, records the prevalence of hookworm infections in various age classes of some rural communities in India, Taiwan, Iran and the Phillipines. The striking feature of such epidemiological surveys is the absolute abundance of intestinal helminths (where many individudls harbour more than one species), and the uniformity of infection throughout all segments of the community. The effect of such parasites on man is related to the burden of worms harboured and heavy infections of certain species often result in severe clinical symptoms (i.e. hookworm parasites). A newborn child in an endemic region of hookworm or *Ascaris* can expect to harbour worms for the majority of his or her life.

Despite their medical significance within the world today, very few attempts have been made to study the population biology of direct life cycle human helminths (Nawalinski, Schad & Chowdhury, 1978a). Indeed a feature of the literature associated with such infections is the complete absence of any research of a mathematical nature on the dynamical properties of infection within human populations. The only relevant work in a closely related area, namely that of veterinary epidemiology, is by Leyton (1968) and Tallis and Leyton (1969) on helminth population dynamics in vertebrate hosts. Indirect life cycle helminth infections of man, such as schistosomiasis, have received a great deal more attention, stimulated to a large.

TABLE 1 : Estimates of the number of people infected with various direct life cycle helminth parasites in different regions of the world in 1975 (data source Peters (1978)). (Figures in millions)

Parasite	Tropics and Subtropics				Temperate Zones			World Total
	Africa	Asia (excl. U.S.S.R.)	C. and S. America	Oceania	N. America	Europe (excl. U.S.S.R.)	U.S.S.R.	
Ascaris lumbricoides	159	931	104	1	5	39	30	1269
Hookworms (2 species)	132	685	104	2	3	2	4	932
Enterobius vermicularis	24	136	40	1	29	75	48	353
Trichuris trichiura	76	433	94	1	1	41	41	687

[In 1975 world population was approximately 3967 million United Nations (1976)]

extent by the pioneering work of MacDonald (1965).

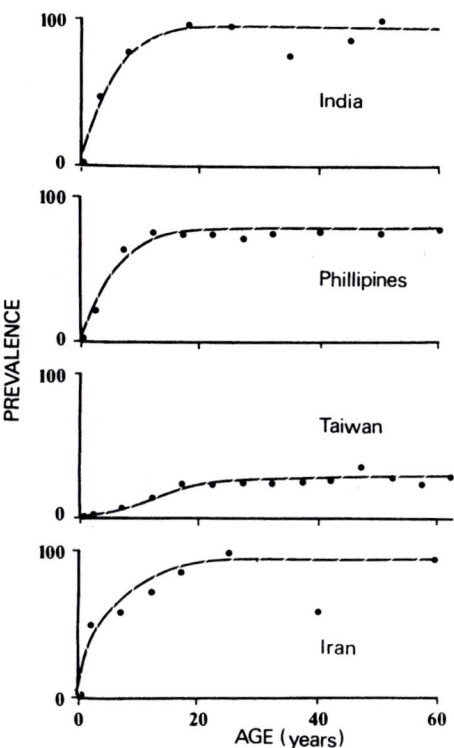

FIGURE 1 : The prevalence of hookworm infections in various age classes of human
populations.

Graph (a). *Ancylostoma duodenale* and *Necator americanus* infections in a
rural community in India (data from Chowdhury & Schiller (1968)).

Graph (b). *A. duodenale* infections in a rural community in the
Phillipines (data from Pesigan *et al* (1955)).

Graph (c). *N. americanus* infections in a rural community in Taiwan (data
from Hsieh (1970)).

Graph (d). *A. duodenale* and *N. americanus* infections in a rural
community in Iran (Gyorkos & Croll (1980) unpublished data).

This paper describes some preliminary work on the population dynamics of
directly transmitted helminths in which dynamical behaviour is explored by means of
simple mathematical models. The aim in model construction is to provide a theoretical basis for the exploration of population behaviour and the design of control

strategies. To this end, the paper is organised as follows. After a brief discussion of helminth life cycles, a mathematical framework is developed to describe the dynamics of directly transmitted infections. The general properties of this model are explored, where attention is focused on transmission thresholds and unstable breakpoints. Methods of predicting trends in the prevalence and intensity of infection within age structured populations are also considered. Next, the dynamics of hookworm infections are discussed and model predictions compared with two sets of data from India and Taiwan. The significance of seasonal climatic change and spatial heterogeneity are briefly considered. The final sections focus on an analysis of the effectiveness of various control methods and discuss future research needs.

The Life Cycles of Directly Transmitted Helminths

The life cycles of directly transmitted helminths contain many distinct developmental stages. These stages are identified by gross morphological features and by their respective habitats, either in the host, or in the external environment.

The developmental cycle of human hookworms, for example, begins with the production of eggs by mature female worms in the small intestine of the host. These pass to the exterior in the faeces and hatch to release a first stage, or L_1 larva. The larvae feed on bacteria and organic debris in the soil and moult once to produce the second stage or L_2 larvae, and then again to produce the third stage or L_3 infective larvae. The L_3 stage is responsible for host location and infection, gaining entry by either direct penetration via the skin (*Necator americanus*) or ingestion (*Ancylostoma duodenale*). Once inside the host a phase of migration occurs before the parasite reaches the small intestine where it undergoes two further moults during growth to sexual maturity (Muller, 1975). The complete life cycle of hookworm species therefore involves six distinct developmental stages, namely; the egg, L_1, L_2 and L_3 larvae and the immature and mature parasitic worms.

The overall reproductive success of the parasite during development through the life cycle will depend on the time spent in each developmental stage, the rates of mortality associated with these stages and the degree of reproduction achieved by each of them. In general, the ability to reproduce is restricted to the parasitic stages of directly transmitted helminths. An exception to this trend is shown by the nematode *Strongyloides stercoralis* which may undergo a phase of reproduction within both the host and the external habitat (Pampiglione & Ricciardi, 1972). It is important to note that reproduction by the parasitic stages does not <u>directly</u> increase parasite population size within the host, but involves the production of transmission stages, such as eggs or larvae, which pass into the external habitat usually via the alimentary tract.

The life cycles of all directly transmitted human helminths are basically of similar structure consisting of two principal populations, namely; the sexually mature parasitic worms and the free-living infective stages. The infective stage may not necessarily be a motile larval stage. Transmission of the nematode *Ascaris lumbricoides* and the tapeworm *Hymenolepis nana*, for example, is achieved by means of an egg which, when ingested by the appropriate host, hatches to release a larval parasitic stage.

The two principal populations clearly play a central role in determining over-all transmission success and hence parasite population growth and stability. The sexually mature worms are responsible for reproduction while the infective stages determine the rate at which new hosts are 'colonised'. Infection is basically a form of reproduction since it places the parasite in a habitat in which it is able to reproduce. The model development outlined in this paper centres on the mathematical description of the dynamics of the sexually mature worms and the free-living infective stages. A diagrammatic representation of the flow of parasites between these two populations is portrayed in Fig. 2. The biology of parasite development via the other stages in the life cycle will be reflected in the time delays and parasite mortalities associated with transmission between the two principal populations. In the context of disease epidemiology the parasitic population is clearly of central importance since the severity of clinical symptoms will usually be associated with the number of helminths harboured by an individual host. The collection of epidemiological data concerning direct life cycle helminths has thus been geared to the measurement of the prevalence (proportion of host population infected) and intensity (average worm burden per host) of infection within the human population (Fig. 1).

General Model Framework

The model outlined in this paper is based on a framework developed by Anderson and May (1978) and May and Anderson (1978). It consists of two coupled differential equations representing the dynamics of the sexually mature parasites within the host population and the free-living infective stages. The size of these two populations at time t is denoted by $P(t)$ and $L(t)$ respectively and it is assumed that the host population possesses a stable age distribution and is of constant size H.

The assumptions encorporated in the two equations of the model are as follows.

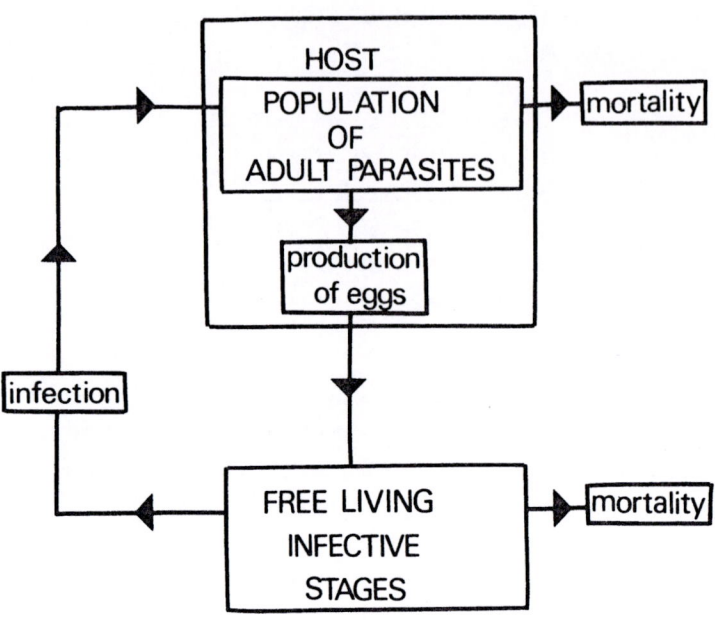

<u>FIGURE 2</u> : Diagrammatic flow chart of the populations and rate processes involved in the life cycles of directly transmitted helminths (see text).

1) The acquisition of mature parasites: host infection

It is assumed that hosts acquire parasites at a rate proportional to the density of hosts (H) times the density of infective stages (L) such that the net rate of acquisition is βHL where β is a transmission coefficient (see Bailey, 1975). Of those parasites acquired by an individual host only a proportion D_1 survive to reach sexual maturity. If the average time taken to develop to sexual maturity from the point of infection is T_1 time units, the proportion D_1 may be expressed as,

$$D_1 = \exp(-\mu_4 T_1) \tag{1}$$

where μ_4 represents the per capita instantaneous death rate of the immature parasites. The net rate of gain to the population of mature parasites is thus $\beta L(t-T_1)D_1 H$.

2) Parasite losses due to host mortality

Losses from the population of mature parasites result from host and natural parasite mortalities. Hosts are assumed to die at a per capita rate b such that the net loss of parasites due to such mortality is $bH \sum_{i=o}^{\infty} i \, p(i)$, where p(i) represents the probability that an individual host contains i parasites.

3) Natural parasite mortalities

The rate of natural parasite mortality is assumed to be dependent on the density of mature parasites within any given individual host. Quantitative information on the form and severity of density-dependent constraints on worm population growth within human hosts is at present limited. Some of the best evidence, concerning the existence of such responses, is provided by experimental work on dogs infected with the hookworm *Ancylostoma caninum*. The work of Krupp (1961), for example, clearly demonstrates that both hookworm fecundity and survival are dependent on the density of worms within the host (Fig. 3a and 3b). It appears probable that human helminths show similar population responses. Indeed, in the absence of such density-dependent regulatory mechanisms parasite population growth would be unconstrained and thus would either grow or decay exponentially. A striking feature of the epidemiology of human helminths (i.e. hookworm and *Ascaris*) is the remarkable degree of constancy in the prevalence and intensity of infection in endemic regions over many years. Such patterns imply the existence of tight regulatory constraints on parasite population growth. It seems likely that density-dependent worm fecundity and survival are responsible for these observed patterns. Patterns of the form shown in Fig. 3 may be generated by either competition for limiting resources within the gut of the host, or host responses (which may be immunological in nature) which increase in severity as parasite density rises (Anderson, 1976a; Anderson & Michel, 1977; Anderson & May, 1978; Wakelin, 1978; Mills, Anderson & Whitfield, 1979).

In the model developed in this paper density-dependent constraints are limited to parasite mortality for the sake of simplicity. It does appear likely, however, that parasite fecundity will also be functionally related to population density but experimental evidence concerning human infections is unavailable at present (Hill, 1926). In accord with the pattern recorded in Fig. 3b, the per capita rate of natural parasite mortality is assumed to be linearly related to parasite burden i, such that,

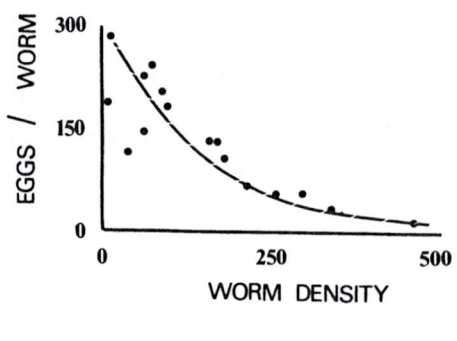

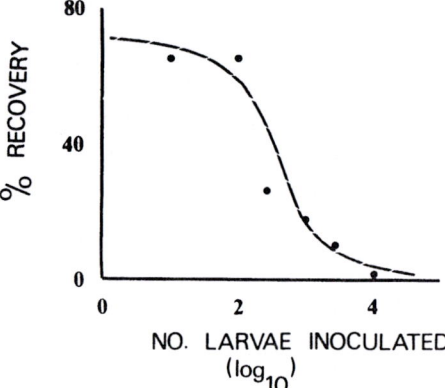

<u>FIGURE 3</u> : Density-dependent survival and fecundity in populations of the dog hook-
worm *Ancylostoma caninum* (data from Krupp (1961)).

    <u>Graph (a)</u>. The relationship between egg production per female worm per
gram of faeces and the total worm burden within the host.

    <u>Graph (b)</u>. The relationship between the percentage of the larval inoculum
to which the host was exposed, recovered after 2 months and the density
($\log_{10}$ scale) of the larval inoculum.

$$\mu(i) = \mu_1 + \alpha i \tag{2}$$

where $^1/\mu_1$ represents the expected life span of the mature parasites in the absence

of density-dependence and α is a coefficient measuring the severity of density-
dependent constraints on worm survival. As illustrated in Fig. 4, these assumptions
generate patterns broadly similar to those recorded for dog hookworm infections (Fig.
3b).

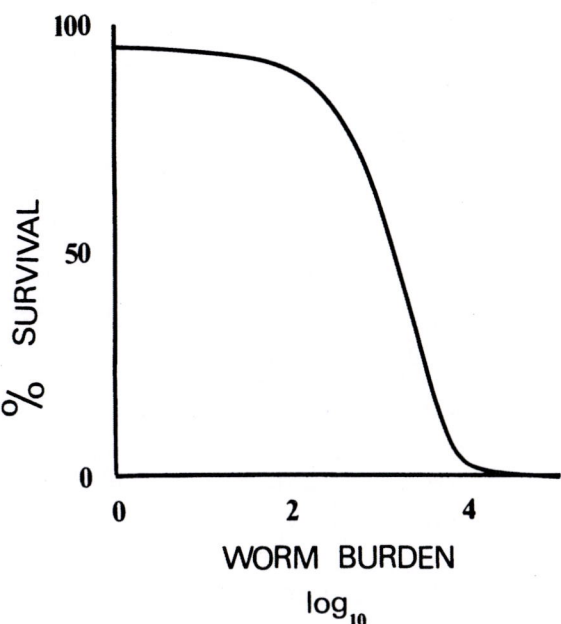

<u>FIGURE 4</u> : The form of the density-dependent survival function $\mu(i) = \mu_1 + \alpha i$, where the percentage survival of the worms after 60 days is plotted against initial worm burden (see text for details) ($\alpha = 7.0 \times 10^{-6}$, $\mu_1 = 7.83 \times 10^{-4}$).

The net rate of parasite losses due to such effects is therefore $H \sum\limits_{i=0}^{\infty} \mu(i)ip(i)$, where, as defined previously, $p(i)$ is the probability that a host contains i parasites.

4) The production of infective stages

Defining λ as the per capita rate of egg production by a mature female parasite, the net rate of egg production by P parasites (assuming a 1:1 sex ratio of males to females) will be $\frac{1}{2}\lambda P\emptyset$, where $\emptyset$ is the probability that any given female worm has been mated. This probability will clearly depend on both the statistical distribution of parasite numbers per host and the sexual habits of the helminth. In the case of hermaphroditic worms, for example, which are able to self-fertilize, the parameter $\emptyset$ is unity and the net rate of egg production is simply λP. The probability $\emptyset$ is certainly not unity in the case of dioecious species, such as hookworms, since the chance of an individual female worm being able to mate is dependent on the statistical distribution of parasite numbers per host. A more detailed treatment of the form of this mating probability will be given in a latter section. For the time being, we will assume that $\emptyset$ is some function of the mean number of parasites per host and the statistical distribution of parasite numbers.

Only a proportion D_2 of the helminth eggs produced in the host will survive to produce viable infective stages (either larvae or embrionated eggs). If the average time from egg release to the development of the infective stage is T_2 time units, the proportion D_2 may be expressed as

$$D_2 = \exp(-\mu_2 T_2) \tag{3}$$

where μ_2 represents the per capita death rate of the larval (or egg) stages during development to the infective state. The net rate of gain to the population of infective stages (L) is thus $\frac{1}{2}\lambda P(t-T_2)\emptyset D_2$.

5) Natural mortality of infective stages

The population of infective stages (whether larvae or eggs) will be subject to natural mortalities and if it is assumed that these occur at a per capita rate μ_3, then the net rate of loss is $\mu_3 L$. The expected lifespan of these infective stages is thus $1/\mu_3$.

6) Loss of infective stages due to host infection

Infective stages are also removed from the population as a consequence of host infection where the net rate of loss is βHL.

7) Model structure

The assumptions detailed in the preceeding sections give rise to the following differential equations for the populations of mature parasites (P(t)) and infective stages $(L(t))$,

$$dP/dt = \beta L(t-T_1)D_1 H - bH \sum_{i=o}^{\infty} i\, p(i) - H \sum_{i=o}^{\infty} \mu(i)\, i\, p(i) \qquad (4)$$

$$dL/dt = \tfrac{1}{2}\lambda\emptyset P(t-T_2)D_2 - \mu_3 L - \beta LH \qquad (5)$$

The Distribution of Parasite Numbers per Host

It is clear from the structure of eqns (4) and (5) that the dynamical behaviour of the population model is critically dependent on the nature of the statistical distribution of parasites within the host population.

Occasionally it is possible to make assumptions that permit this distribution to be deduced theoretically; its precise form depending on the number and type of population processes (i.e. birth, death and infection processes) encorporated in the model (Tallis & Leyton, 1969; Anderson, 1976b). Such an approach, however, is only feasible provided the structure of the model is relatively simple.

Hybrid models, which contain stochastic and deterministic components, have been used in the past to mimic the dynamics of helminth infections and to deduce the form of this distribution (see Nassell & Hirsch, 1973). Such models, however, invariably arrive at the conclusion that parasites are distributed randomly within the host population, since heterogenity between hosts, with respect to the rate at which they acquire infection, is excluded from model structure. The conclusion of randomness is far removed from reality; observed distributions of helminth parasites in human communities are invariably highly clumped or aggregated in form. The negative binomial probability model, a distribution defined by two parameters the mean and k (a parameter which varies inversely with the degree of aggregation or clumping), has proved to be a good empirical model of these observed patterns (Crofton, 1971; Anderson & May, 1978). As the parameter k tends to infinity this distribution collapses to the Poisson form, where parasites are independently randomly distributed.

A considerable simplication in model structure can be achieved by making a phenomenological assumption concerning this distribution based on a knowledge of observed patterns (Anderson & May, 1978; May & Anderson, 1979). In this paper it is assumed that the parasites are distributed in a negative binomial manner, with a characteristic degree of aggregation measured inversely by the parameter k. By the use of various statistical moments of the negative binomial distribution, namely;

$$\sum_{i=o}^{\infty} i\, p(i) \;=\; P/H \qquad \text{and}$$

$$\sum_{i=o}^{\infty} i^2\, p(i) \;=\; \frac{P^2\,(k+1)}{H^2 k} + \frac{P}{H}$$

eqns (4) and (5) (encorporating the density-dependent assumption defined in eqn (2)) can be expressed as

$$dP/dt \;=\; \beta L(t-T_1)D_1 H - (b+\mu_1)P - \alpha\frac{(k+1)P^2}{kH} \tag{6}$$

$$dL/dt \;=\; \tfrac{1}{2}\lambda\emptyset P(t-T_2)D_2 - (\mu_3+\beta H)L \tag{7}$$

Worm Pairing

The statistical distribution of parasite numbers per host also influences the liklihood of sexual mating between mature parasites. In addition the sexual habits of a given species are of obvious significance. As mentioned previously, hermaphroditic parasites, such as the human tapeworm *Hymenolepis nana* which is thought to be able to self fertilize, are unaffected by the frequency of mating encounters at low parasite densities. The majority of direct life cycle helminths of man, however, are nematode species which have separate sexes. In these cases the nature of worm pairing is of upmost importance in determining reproductive success. For example, it is important to establish whether the parasites are monogamous or polygamous, or whether a female needs to be mated once or a number of times to maintain viable egg production throughout her lifespan? Unfortunately our biological understanding of these problems is extremely limited at present. In the case of human hookworm species, current opinion is that the nematodes are polygamous where the presence of say 3 females and one male within a single host will result in all 3 females being fertilised.

Various workers have analysed the significance of parasite sexual habitats and the statistical distribution of parasite numbers per host to the form of the mating function $\emptyset$ (MacDonald, 1965; Leyton, 1968; Tallis & Leyton, 1969; Nassell & Hirsch, 1973; May, 1977). Table 2 lists various forms of the function $\emptyset$ given specific assumptions concerning mating behaviour and parasite distribution. A clearer picture of the relationship between the probability of a female worm being mated $\emptyset$ and the average burden of parasites per host is provided in Fig. 5.

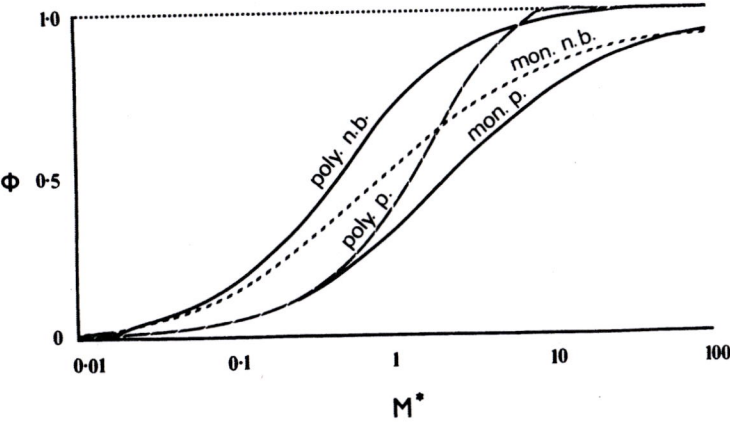

<u>FIGURE 5</u> : The relationship between the worm mating function ∅ and the mean worm
burden per host M* (plotted on a $\log_{10}$ scale). The various forms of the
function ∅ are detailed in Table 2 (see May (1977) for formal details of
derivation).

    <u>Poly. n.b.</u> = Polygamous worms distributed in a negative binomial manner
                where k = 0.34.

    <u>Poly. p.</u> = Polygamous worms randomly distributed (Poisson distribution).

    <u>Mon. n.b.</u> = Monogamous worm distributed in a negative binomial manner
                where k = 0.34.

    <u>Mon. p.</u> = Monogamous worms randomly distributed (Poisson distribution).

Irrespective of whether the parasites are monogamous or polygamous, worm
clumping is clearly advantageous with respect to the probability of mating, provided,
of course, that male and female worms are distributed together and not in an
independently clumped fashion (see May, 1977). This observation holds sound
intuitive sense and illustrates a major advantage of parasite aggregation to overall
transmission success, particularly under conditions of low average worm abundance

TABLE 2 : Worm mating functions (∅) (after May (1977)).

Type of reproduction	Function (∅)
1) Hermaphroditic, self fertilisation possible	$\emptyset = 1$
2) Dioecious (separate sexes), worms monogamous	
(a) Worm burden per host randomly distributed within the host population (Poisson distribution)	$\emptyset(M) = 1 - \dfrac{e^{-M}}{2\pi} \displaystyle\int_0^{2\pi} (1-\cos\theta)\, e^{-M\cos\theta}\, d\theta$
(b) Worm burden per host distributed in a clumped manner within the host (Negative binomial distribution, with parameter k)	$\emptyset(M,k) = 1 - \dfrac{(1-\gamma)^{1+k}}{2\pi} \displaystyle\int_0^{2\pi} \dfrac{(1-\cos\theta)}{(1+\gamma\cos\theta)^{(1+k)}}\, d\theta$ where $\gamma = \dfrac{M}{(M+k)}$
3) Dioecious (separate sexes) worms polygamous	
(a) Worm burden randomly distributed (Poisson distribution)	$\emptyset(M) = 1 - e^{-M/2}$
(b) Worm burden distributed in a clumped manner (Negative binomial distribution with parameter k)	$\emptyset(M,k) = \left[1 - \left(1 + \dfrac{M}{2k}\right)^{-1-k} \right]$

(Fig. 5). Fig. 5, also illustrates that polygamous habits are clearly beneficial to reproductive success when worm density is low. Under a regime of monogamy, even average worm burdens in the region of 100 parasites per host do not ensure that all females are mated and able to produce transmission stages (Fig. 5).

The main point to note from Fig. 5 is that reproductive success will be severely curtailed at low parasite densities, irrespective of the statistical distribution of parasites or whether they are monogamous or polygamous. As such the mating probability operates as a type of inverse density-dependence. Such mechanisms are unable to regulate parasite population growth, they simply decrease reproductive success at low densities. Only self fertilising hermaphroditic parasites are able to surmount these problems.

Time Scales

Before examining the dynamical properties of eqns (6) and (7) it is worth briefly considering (a) the relative time scales on which the dynamics of the various populations (i.e. $P(t)$ and $L(t)$) operate and (b) the relative magnitudes of the time delays (T_1 and T_2) involved in the helminth life cycles.

In the vast majority of cases the expected life span of the mature parasites is many orders of magnitude greater than that of the infective stage (whether larvae or eggs). In the case of the human hookworm *Necator americanus*, for example, adult worms are thought to have an expected life span of roughly $3\frac{1}{2}$ years (Hoagland & Schad, 1978; Nawalinski, Schad & Chowdhury, 1978a, 1978b), while the L_3 infective larval stage lives, under optimum conditions, for a few weeks (Sturrock, 1967; Muller, 1975). The dynamics of the mature parasite population ($P(t)$) thus operate on a much slower time scale relative to the dynamics of the infective stage population ($L(t)$) (May & Anderson, 1979). It is also relevant to note that the dynamics of both parasite populations operate on a much faster time scale than that of the human host. For instance, in many regions of endemic hookworm, human life expectancy is of the order of 50 years. It is thus not unreasonable to consider human density as a constant when examining the dynamics of the parasite populations over a period of say ten years (a time span relevant to the application and monitoring of control measures).

The developmental time delays T_1 and T_2 are also usually short in relation to the life span of the host and the mature adult parasites. For instances, in the case of *N. americanus* T_1 is approximately 42 days while T_2 is in the order of 5 days. These observations suggest that such time delays are unlikely to be of significance to the dynamics of the parasite populations if viewed over a period of several years. Specifically, they are unlikely to generate limit cycle behaviour under equilibrium conditions. This observation holds true for most direct life cycle helminths of man, but it is important to note that a few exceptions exist both with respect to the length of maturation delays and to the respective life spans of mature parasites and infective stages.

Dynamical Properties of the Model

An analytical solution of eqns (6) and (7) for arbitrary $\emptyset$ is not feasible. The qualitative dynamical behaviour can, however, be examined by the consideration of equilibrium properties. Such an approach is appropriate for the study of helminth disease in endemic regions where the prevalence and intensity of infection appear to be relatively stable through time.

First, some simplification of the structure of eqns (6) and (7) can be achieved by noting that the mean adult worm burden per host, M, is given by P/H. The model can thus be expressed in terms of M rather than P where,

$$dM/dt \;=\; \beta L(t-T_1)D_1 \;-\; (b+\mu_1)M \;-\; \alpha\frac{(k+1)M^2}{k} \tag{8}$$

$$dL/dt \;=\; \tfrac{1}{2}\lambda\emptyset M(t-T_2)\ HD_2 \;-\; (\mu_3+\beta H)L \tag{9}$$

By constructing isoclines in the L-M plane (setting dM/dt and dL/dt = 0) it can be seen in which directions the dynamical trajectories move in the various regions on this plane. Two general patterns of behaviour emerge. In the first, illustrated in Fig. 6a, the two isoclines intersect only at the origin, and all trajectories are attracted to M = 0, L = 0. In other words the parasite is unable to persist within the host population. In the second, illustrated in Fig. 6b, there are 3 points of intersection of the isoclines, corresponding to 2 stable points (at M = 0 and at M = M*), separated by an unstable point (at M = M_u). The directions of the trajectories in the various regions are as follows: points (i.e. initial values of M and L) originating to the left of the dashed line are attracted to the origin; points originating to the right of the dashed line are attracted to the point M* at which the parasite maintains itself in a stable endemic state within the human population.

The case illustrated by Fig. 6a corresponds to the population parameters of the parasite being below a transmission threshold, where the infection cannot be maintained. The case illustrated by Fig. 6b corresponds to the population parameters being above the transmission threshold and in this event there are two alternate stable states (one at L = 0, M = 0 and one at a finite value L*, M*). The dashed line in Fig. 6b, divides the L-M plane into the 2 point's respective domains of

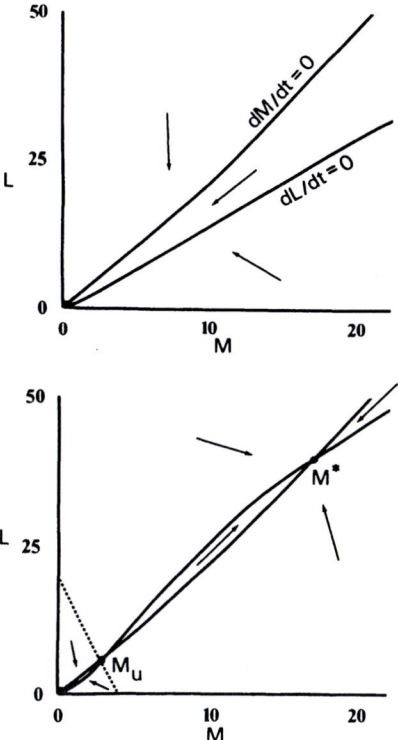

FIGURE 6 : The arrows indicate how the dynamical trajectories of L(t) and M(t) behave in the various regions into which the L-M plane is dissected by the
isoclines dL/dt = 0 and dM/dt = 0. The mating function ∅ represents a
polygamous parasite which is distributed in a negative binomial manner
with k = 0.34 .

Graph (a). This figure corresponds to the population parameters being
below the transmission threshold (R < 1), when the infection cannot maintain itself and all trajectories are attracted to the origin (L = M = 0)
(Parameter values, $b + \mu_1$ = 1, $\alpha(k+1)/k$ = 0.01, βD_1 = 0.5, $\frac{1}{2}\lambda HD_2$ = 1.5,
$\mu_3 + \beta H$ = 1.0, k = 0.34).

Graph (b). The parameter values are above the transmission threshold
(R > 1) and there are two alternative stable states (one at M*, one at
M = 0), each with its own domain of attraction. The dotted line indicates
the boundary between these two states which passes through the unstable
state M_u. When $\mu_3 \gg \mu_1$, this boundary becomes a vertical line through
the unstable point M_u and we can speak of the "breakpoint" at a worm load
M_u (see text) (Parameter values as for graph (a) except $\frac{1}{2}\lambda HD_2$ = 2.4).

attraction. The worm burden value M_u has been referred to as the *breakpoint* in the context of disease control (MacDonald, 1965).

The isoclines in Fig. 6b have been constructed on the assumption that the mating function $\emptyset$ corresponds to a polygamous parasite which adopts a clumped or aggregated distribution within the host population (see Table 2). One special case is worth noting, namely, that of hermaphroditic worms which are able to self-fertilise such as the human tapeworm *Hymenolepis nana*. In this case $\emptyset = 1$ and provided the parameters are above the transmission threshold, the isoclines intersect at 2 points (M = 0 and M = M*) corresponding to 1 stable point at M = M*. In other words the point M* is globally stable for all positive values of L and M. This pattern is displayed in Fig. 7b, while in Fig. 7a, the isoclines are drawn for the case where $\emptyset = 1$ and the parameters lie below the transmission threshold necessary for parasite maintenance. This special case makes clear that the existence of multiple stable states in the general case (Fig. 6) is a consequence of the mating function $\emptyset$ (May & Anderson, 1979).

Before examining the threshold concept in more detail it is possible to make some further general comments about the dynamics of the system. From eqns (8) and (9) it is clear that the characteristic dynamical response times of M(t) and L(t) are roughly $1/(\mu_1+b)$ and $1/(\mu_3+\beta H)$, respectively. In these two expressions the parameters μ_1 and μ_3 dominate and thus the responses times are approximately $1/\mu_1$ and $1/\mu_3$. As discussed previously, for the vast majority of direct life cycle helminth infections the expected life span of the infective stage $(1/\mu_3)$ is typically much shorter than that of the adult parasite $(1/\mu_1)$. Such circumstances correspond to $\mu_3 \gg \mu_1$. It follows that L(t) has a much faster response time than M(t), and the dynamical trajectories tend to become vertical lines in the L-M plane, parallel to the L-axis. In particular, the dashed "breakpoint" line in Fig. 6b straightens to a vertical line through M_u. In such cases (probably appropriate for most human helminth infections), we may effectively assume that the density of infective stages are essentially instantaneously adjusted to the stationary value L* for all values of M. Given that the time delays T_1 and T_2 are also short in relation to the expected life span of the adult worm $(1/\mu_1)$ the model can be reduced to a single dynamical equation for the variable M(t)

$$dM/dt = M\left[\frac{\frac{1}{2}\lambda\emptyset\beta D_1 D_2 H}{(\mu_3+\beta H)} - (b+\mu_1) - \alpha\frac{(k+1)M}{k} \right] \qquad (10)$$

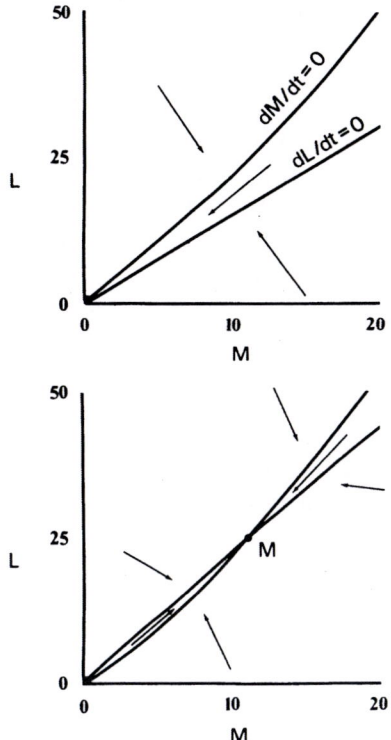

FIGURE 7 : The same as Fig. 6 except the mating function $\emptyset$ is for a hermaphroditic worm that is able to self fertilize ($\emptyset = 1$ for all values of M).

Graph (a). Parameter values below the transmission threshold (R < 1) (values as for graph (a) of Fig. 6).

Graph (b). Parameter values above the transmission threshold (R > 1) (values as for graph (a) except $\lambda HD_2 = 2.0$).

Transmission Thresholds:

the Basic Reproductive Rate of the Parasite

The precise manner in which the various population parameters determine whether or not the parasite is able to maintain itself within the host population ($M^* > 0$) can be easily seen from the structure of eqn (10). Essentially for parasite maintenance (the transmission threshold to be exceeded),

$$\frac{\frac{1}{2}\lambda\emptyset\beta D_1 D_2 H}{(\mu_1+b)\ (\mu_3+\beta H)} > 1 \qquad\qquad (11)$$

The left hand side of eqn (11) is often denoted by the symbol R, and termed the basic reproductive rate of the parasite (MacDonald, 1965; Anderson, 1980). The quantity R measures the average number of offspring produced by a mature female parasite which manage to successfully complete their life cycle and join the reproductive pool of mature parasites in the next generation. Clearly such a quantity, which measures reproductive success, must be greater than unity since an individual must at least replace itself in the next generation. Note that although R is often termed a reproductive rate (analogous to Fishers' net reproductive rate R_o in the contect of age structured single species populations (Fisher, 1930)), it is essentially a dimensionless quantity measuring reproductive success (or transmission success). The structure of eqn (11) clearly indicates that reproductive success is determined by the product of the rate of egg production times the rate of transmission, all divided by the product of the net rates of mortality in the population of adult parasites and infective stages. In other words eqn (11) is the rates of parasite gain divided by the rates of loss.

The concept of a basic reproductive rate is an important one which provides a unifying framework for the study of a wide class of infectious disease agents ranging from viruses to helminths (Dietz, 1976; Anderson, 1980). In particular, it forms a basis for the quantitative evaluation of the effects of various control options on the transmission success of a given disease. Clearly, a desired outcome is to reduce the value of R to below unity (i.e. below the transmission threshold shown in Figs. 6 and 7).

A further concept of significance to the epidemiology and control of infectious disease agents also emerges from eqn (11). By rearrangement it can be seen that for R to be greater than unity, host density H must be above some critical level H_T. Specifically,

$$H_T = \frac{(\mu_1+b)\mu_3}{\left[\frac{1}{2}\lambda\emptyset\beta D_1 D_2 - (\mu_1+b)\beta\right]} \qquad\qquad (12)$$

This condition is analogous to the classical threshold theorms derived, from models of viral and bacterial diseases, by Kermack and McKendrick (1927). In the case of direct life cycle helminths, H_T will typically be small due to the enormous reproductive capabilities of such parasites (λ very large). The frequency with which helminths persist endemically in low density human populations supports this prediction (CIBA, 1977).

If we represent the left hand side of eqn (11) by the symbol R we may rewrite eqn (10) as follows;

$$dM/dt = M\left[(R-1)(\mu_1 + b) - \alpha\frac{(k+1)M}{k} \right] \qquad (13)$$

Clearly the value of R will to a large extent determine the equilibrium intensity of infection M* within the human population. High levels of reproductive success will lead to high average worm burdens. In the special case where $\emptyset = 1$ (hermaphroditic self-fertilising worms) eqn (13) is of logistic form (Verhulst, 1838). The equilibrium average burden of parasites is simply,

$$M* = \frac{(R-1)(\mu_1 + b)k}{\alpha(k+1)} \qquad (14)$$

Furthermore, the prevalence of infection (proportion of host population infected) p* is

$$p* = \left[1 - (1 + \frac{M*}{k})^{-k} \right] \qquad (15)$$

As portrayed in Fig. 8, the intensity of infection M* rises linearly as R increases, while the prevalence of infection p* rapidly approaches an asymptote as the value of R increases beyond unity. The level of the asymptotic prevalence is determined by the statistical distribution of parasite numbers per host. For random distributions this asymptote is clearly 100% infection. As the degree of clumping or aggregation increases in severity (k gets smaller) the asymptotic prevalence becomes much smaller. In other words, irrespective of the degree of transmission success, the proportion of the population infected will never approach 100% if the worms are highly aggregated in their distribution.

In the more general case where $\emptyset \neq 1$, such as occurs for hookworms (which have separate sexes and are polygamous (see Table 2)), a more complex pattern emerges. As displayed in Fig. 9, the "transmission threshold" and "breakpoint" concepts emerge where, for a given value of R, two stable equilibria for M* can occur, separated by the unstable (dashed line) breakpoint equilibrium. It is important to note, however, that for values of μ_1, b, α and k in equation (13), characteristic of human helminth infections, the 'breakpoint' worm burden will typically be low. Specifically, for values of R of 1.1 and above, the breakpoint worm burden is less than one parasite

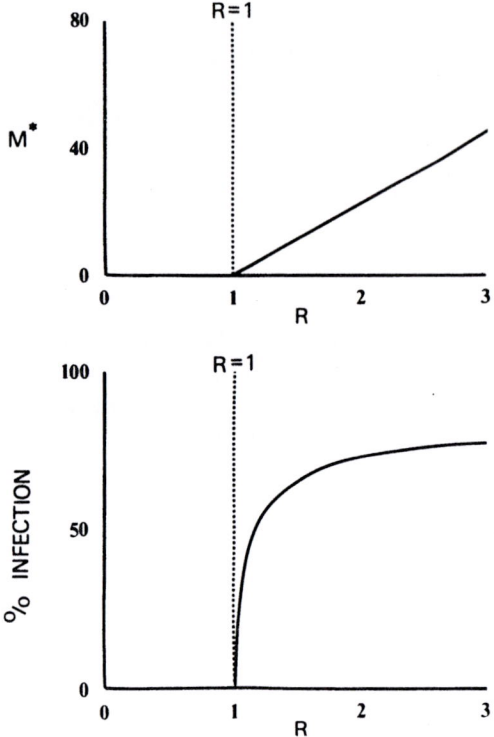

FIGURE 8 : The relationship between the mean intensity of infection (M*) (Graph (a))
and the prevalence of infection (p*) (Graph (b)) at equilibrium and the
basic reproductive rate of the parasite R (see eqns (14) and (15) in the
text) for a hermaphroditic parasite $\emptyset = 1$. The dashed vertical line
indicates the transmission threshold R = 1.

per host. The depressing conclusion to be reached from this observation is that the
stable equilibrium state M* > 0 (solid line) is effectively globally stable since
control measures would have to reduce the equilibrium worm burden to very low levels
before the system moves to the steady state M = 0 of parasite extinction.

Age Prevalence and Intensity Curves

Much epidemiological data of helminth infections in human communities is
collected in the form of the prevalence and intensity of infection in each of a
series of host age classes (see Fig. 1). Such data is often plotted in the form of

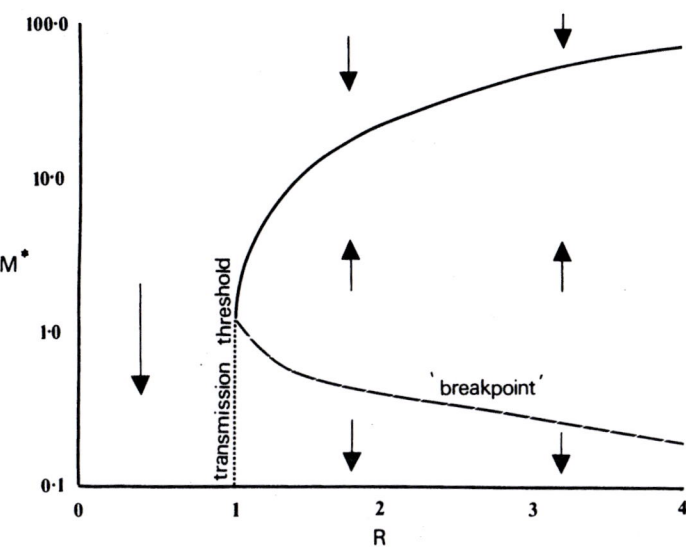

FIGURE 9 : The relationship between the equilibrium mean intensity of infection (M*) and the basic reproductive rate R for a polygamous parasite which is distributed in a negative binomial manner within the host population (k = 0.34). The dashed line indicates the unstable breakpoint M_u and the arrows denote the dynamical trajectories of the system following a perturbation from the two equilibrium states M* and zero. Below the transmission threshold, R = 1, the infection cannot be maintained (M* = 0). As the degree of worm clumping increases (k becomes smaller) the breakpoint line comes to lie closer to the horizontal axis and is thus less conspicuous (see May (1977)).

age-prevalence, or age-intensity curves which, at the point of sampling, provide a great deal of information concerning the sections of the community most at risk from infection and the overall magnitude of the problem of disease control.

The model defined by eqn (10) can be used to gain qualitative insights into the factors which determine the shape of these curves. Under conditions of a stable age distribution within a host population of constant size, the solution of eqn (10) yields the age-intensity curve. Specifically if $\emptyset$ = 1, then the mean intensity of infection at age a, M(a), is (the parameter K is determined by initial conditions),

$$M(a) = K\left[\exp\left[-(R-1)(\mu_1+b)a\right] + \frac{\alpha(k+1)}{k(R-1)(\mu_1+b)}\right]^{-1} \tag{16}$$

Eqn (16) describes a sigmoid curve which rises to the asymptotic equilibrium mean worm burden M* defined in eqn (14). The age prevalence curve can be obtained from the zero probability term of the negative binomial distribution with mean M(a) and parameter k, where the prevalence in age class a, p(a), is

$$p(a) = \left[1 - \left[1 + \frac{M(a)}{k}\right]^{-k}\right] \tag{17}$$

The prevalence of infection thus also rises to an asymptote, whoes level is determined by M* and the degree of worm clumping (k) within the host population.

In the case of dioecious parasites where $\emptyset \neq 1$, an analytic solution of eqn (10) for arbitary $\emptyset$ is not feasible. Numerical solutions can be obtained, however, and these provide insights into the factors which determine the shape of age-intensity curves. Clearly, for dioecious parasites, the rate of increase in the intensity of infection with host age, will be less rapid in the young age classes which harbour small worm burdens, as a consequence of low mating probabilities. Fig. 10 illustrates this point; the solid line denotes the age-intensity curve for a self-fertilising hermaphroditic species, while the dotted line represents the same curve for a dioecious polygamous species with identical population characteristics (i.e. the birth, death and infection rates are the same for both cases as is the clumping parameter k).

The Dynamics of Hookworm Infections

Of all the direct life cycle helminths of man, the most intensively studied are the two species of human hookworm, *Ancylostoma duodenale* and *Necator americanus* (Muller, 1975; Hoagland & Schad, 1978). These species often occur sympatrically over much of the Indian subcontinent and over much of the world, including parts of South America, the Far East and Africa. For example, in the Ganges region of West Bengal, 79% of the human population is infected with at least one species and 95% of this infected population harbours both species (Schad, 1971). Although the basic life history patterns of *N. americanus* and *A. duodenale* are well known, quantitative information on the many population parameters which control their epidemiology is

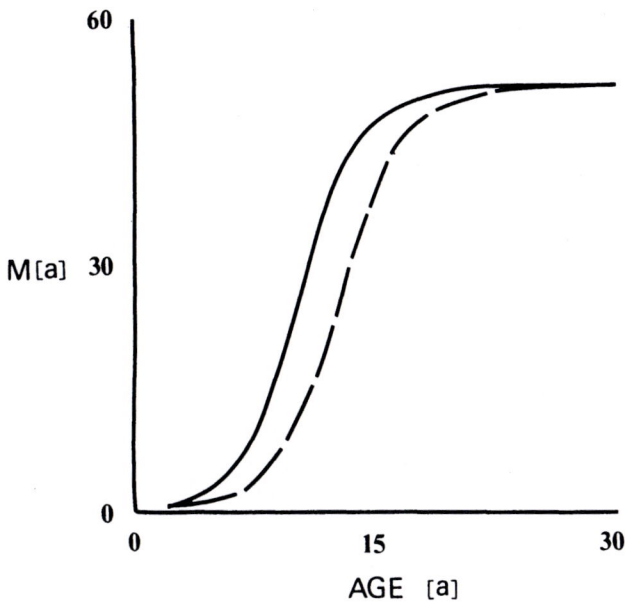

FIGURE 10 : The relationship between the average intensity of infection (M(a)) and
the age of the host (a) predicted by the model defined by eqn (13). The
solid line is for $\emptyset$ = 1 (eqn (16)) while the dashed line is for a polygamous parasite which is distributed in a negative binomial manner (k =
0.34) (numerical solution of eqn (13)). (The initial conditions were
defined at a = 2 years). Parameter values defined in Table 3.

extremely scarce (Hoagland & Schad, 1978). For instance, parameter estimates of the
various quantities which determine the value of R (eqn 11) are difficult to obtain
from the literature for any defined region of endemic disease.

This section concentrates on the epidemiology of *Necator americanus* in two
localities, namely one in India and the other in Taiwan, in an attempt to estimate
the magnitude of R from observed epidemiological parameters. The data bases for
this attempt are provided by the work of Nawalinski, Schad and Chowdhury (1978a & b)
in a rural community near Calcutta in India, and by the work of Hsieh (1970) in a
rural district of the Kaohsiung area of Taiwan.

Nawalinski *et al* (1978a & b) studied a community of 1-11 year old children plus
a proportion of the adult population, and recorded the prevalence and intensity of
infection in each age class. Age prevalence and intensity data for *N. americanus*
are recorded in Fig. 11. [These estimates were obtained from Table 2 of Nawalinski
et al (1978a) given that (a) children harboured approximately equal numbers of *A.
duodenale* and *N. americanus*, (b) the average sex ratio of male: female worms was 1:1,
(c) that 120 eggs/gram of faeces is the approximate daily egg output of one female
hookworm and (d) the worms are distributed in a negative binomial manner with the
age dependent clumping parameters (k) recorded in Fig. 12]. The human density per
square mile in this study area was approximately 1895 and life expectancy is assumed
to be in the region of 50 years. Data on egg production per female worm (λ), adult
worm life expectancy ($1/\mu_1$) and L_3 larval survival (μ_3) are available in the literature and these plus other parameter estimates (i.e. D_1, T_1, T_2) are recorded in
Table 3.

Information on the degree of aggregation of the hookworms within the host population can be obtained from the prevalence and intensity data (assuming 120 eggs/
gram of faeces = 1 female worm) recorded in Table 2 of Nawalinski *et al* (1978a).
This data is for overall hookworm infection; no distinction is made between *N.
americanus* and *A. duodenale*. Assuming that the worms are distributed in a negative
binomial manner eqn (17) can be used to obtain age-dependent estimates of the
clumping parameter, k, by means of an iterative method (Bliss & Fisher, 1953). These
estimates are recorded in Fig. 12a, from which it can be seen that the degree of
aggregation is most severe in the youngest age classes of hosts (k small) but
declines to reach an approximately constant level in the 8^+ age classes. The
average value of k in all 11 age classes is $\bar{k} = 0.34$ which reflects a fairly high
degree of worm clumping. This is probably a consequence of heterogeneity in social
habitats, particularly those concerned with defaecation and hygiene, in conjunction
with spatial aggregation in infective stage distribution. Such heterogeneity is
clearly most marked in the very young children. In the absence of any additional
information, it is assumed that the average k value estimated for the combined
distribution of both hookworm species is a rough approximation of the average k value
for the distribution of *N. americanus* alone.

With respect to the estimation of R, the basic reproductive rate of *N.
americanus* in this endemic region, no information is available on the parameters α
(measuring the severity of density dependent worm survival), β (the transmission
coefficient) and D_2 (the proportion of eggs that survive to produce infective larvae)
(see Table 3). Crude estimates of these parameters can be obtained by fitting age-
intensity curves (eqn (16)) and from the information that the equilibrium intensity
of infection (M*) in adults was roughly 51 *N. americanus* per individual (Nawalinski,

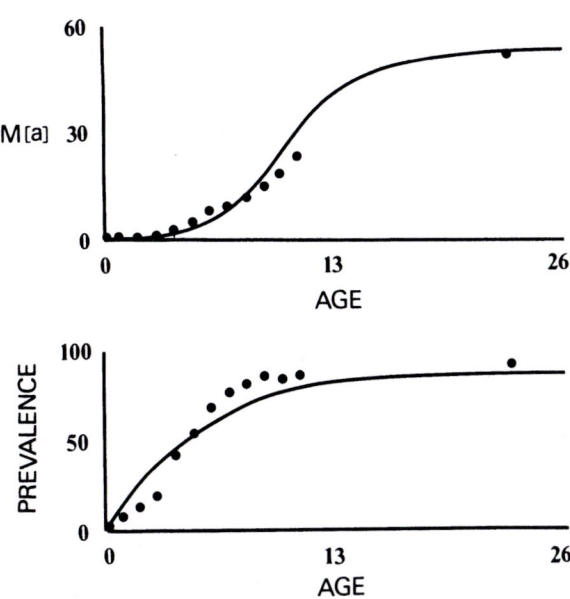

FIGURE 11 : Epidemiological data for *N. americanus* infections in a population of
children from a rural community near Calcutta in India (data from
Nawalinski *et al.*, 1978a & b).

Graph (a). The average worm burden per host in different age classes of
the population (age-intensity curve). Solid circles - observed data
(see text for details of estimation). Solid line - model prediction (eqn
(16)) fitted to observed data by non-linear least squares technique
($R = 2.7$; $\alpha = 7.0 \times 10^{-6}$).

Graph (b). The prevalence of infection in different age classes of the
population (age-prevalence curve). Solid circles - observed data.
Solid line - model predictions (eqn (17), $\bar{k} = 0.34$).

Schad & Chowdhury, 1978a & b). It must be noted that for a mean worm burden of 51,
the mating function $\emptyset$ for a polygamous species, irrespective of the degree of worm
clumping (the value of k) is approximately unity. Eqn (16) was fitted to the data
presented in Fig. 11a by means of a non linear least square method (Conway, Glass &
Wilcox, 1970) and estimates of R and α were obtained ($R = 2.7$, $\alpha = 7.0 \times 10^{-6}$/worm/
day). Given these estimates the predicted age-intensity (eqn (16)) and age-prevalence

TABLE 3 : Parameter estimates for *Necator americanus* in a rural community near Calcutta.

Parameter	Symbol	Value	Data Source
Human density per unit area	H	1895/sq. mile	Chowdhury & Schiller (1968)
Death rate of human host	b	0.000055/day	–
Human life expectancy	$1/b$	50 years	–
Death rate of mature worms	μ_1	0.000783/day	Hoagland & Schad (1978)
Mature worm life expectancy	$1/\mu_1$	3.5 years	Hoagland & Schad (1978)
Maturation time in the host (Adult worm prepatent period)	T_1	42 days	Payne (1924)
Proportion of infective larvae that penetrate the host which survive to maturity	D_1	0.1	Yanagisawa & Mizuno (1963)
Rate of egg production per female worm	λ	15,000/day	Nawalinski, Schad & Chowdhury (1978a, 1978b)
Maturation time from release of egg to the development of the L_3 infective larvae (Infective larvae prepatent period)	T_2	5 days	Muller (1975)
Proportion of eggs released into external habitat which develop through to the L_3 infective larval stage	D_2	?	–
Transmission coefficient	β	?	–
The product $\beta \times D_2$	βD_2	3.4365×10^{-10}	(This paper)

TABLE 3 : Continued.

Parameter	Symbol	Value	Data Source
Death rate of the L_3 infective larvae	μ_3	0.1955/day	Sturrock (1967)
Expected life span of L_3 larvae	$1/\mu_3$	5 days	Sturrock (1967)
Coefficient measuring the severity of density-dependent adult worm mortality	α	7.0×10^{-6} /worm/day	(This paper)
Parameter providing an inverse measure of the degree of clumping of worms with the host population (the negative binomial parameter k, averaged over all age classes)	k	0.339	(This paper)
Basic reproductive rate	R	2.721	(This paper)
Sex ratio males to females		1:1	Stoll (1923a)

(eqn (17) with k = 0.34) curves are recorded in Figs. 11a and 11b. The model provides reasonable qualitative predictions of the observed trends in prevalence and intensity. With respect to these predictions, it is important to note three points. First, the assumption that the mating function $\emptyset$ is unity is clearly a crude approximation. In the very young age classes, the mean worm burden is low and hence the value of $\emptyset$ will be considerably less than unity. Such effects, however, will not have a major influence on parameter estimation from the observed age-intensity curve for the following reason. For worm burdens greater than 3 parasites per host the value of $\emptyset$ lies between 0.9 and 1.0 (see Fig. 5). As illustrated in Fig. 11a, the vast majority of the population (individuals older than 4 years) harbour worm loads greater than this burden and as such, under equilibrium conditions, reduction in parasite egg output due to low density effects will be restricted to a minority of the total host population in this region of endemic hookworm infection.

The second point to note concerns the degree of worm clumping (measured inversely by the parameter k) in each age class of hosts (Fig. 12a). The use of an average value of k in eqns (16) and (17) is a crude approximation of the observed

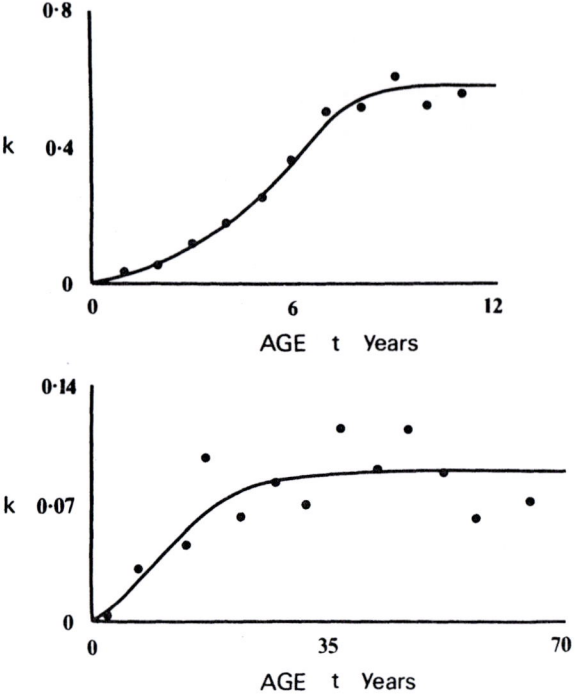

FIGURE 12 : The degree of aggregation of *N. americanus* (measured inversely by the negative binomial parameter k) in different age classes of the population.

    Graph (a). Data from the Indian community (Nawalinski *et al.*, 1978a & b). Average over all age classes $\bar{k}$ = 0.34.

    Graph (b). Data from Taiwan (Hsieh, 1970). Average over all age classes $\bar{k}$ = 0.077.

age-dependent patterns of worm clumping (Fig. 12a). In particular, the model fails to mimic the sigmoid rise in the prevalence of infection recorded in the observed data (Fig. 11b). This discrepancy between model behaviour and observed trends is principally a consequence of the use of an average k value. As illustrated in Fig. 13, the use of an average k value (k = 0.069) for the 1-3 year old children yields predictions which closely agree with the observed prevalences in these age classes. Similarly, the use of an average k value (k = 0.545) for the 6-11 year old children also yields good predictions for the prevalences in older children. A sudden change in the degree of worm clumping is observed around the ages of 4-5, where patterns of severe parasite aggregation in the very young children give way to lower degrees of aggregation in the older children. Many reasons, concerning behavioural patterns, could be suggested to explain these observations. In the absence of any quantitative data on behaviour, such suggestions, however, would be purely speculative. The main point to note is that the degree of worm clumping is markedly age-dependent. The inclusion of such effects in the framework of eqns (8) and (9) is clearly advisable in future work. The principal consequences of high degrees of clumping in very young children are to (a) reduce the impact of low average worm density on the mating probability $\emptyset$ and (b) to increase the severity of density-dependent worm mortality.

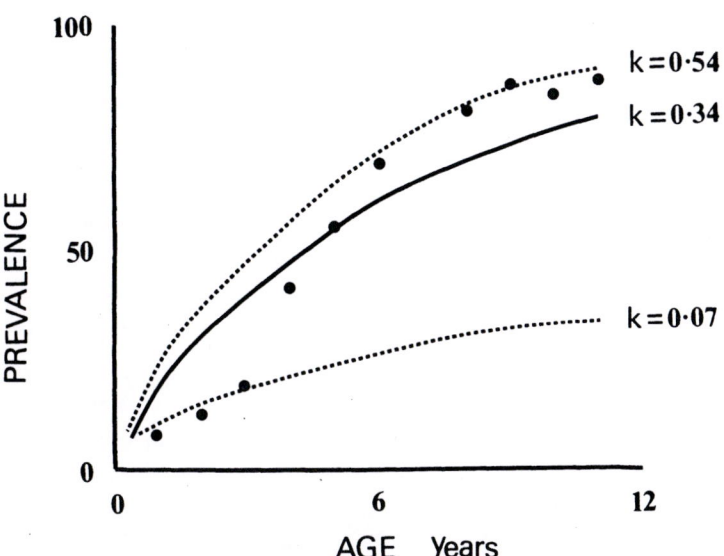

FIGURE 13 : The fit of the age-prevalence model to the data from India of *N. americanus* infections in a population of children (eqn (17)) for different values of the clumping parameter k. Top dashed line is for k = 0.54, the average k value for the 6-11 year old children. Solid line k = 0.34, the average over all age classes. Bottom dashed line is for k = 0.07, the average k value for the 1-3 year old children.

The _final_ point of significance concerning the estimation of parameter values from the Indian community data concerns the value of R, the basic reproductive rate of the parasite. The R value recorded for the Indian community (R = 2.7), suggests that the "breakpoint" between stable endemic disease and parasite eradication is an average worm burden per host (M_u in Fig. 6b) of approximately 0.3 worms per host (see Fig. 9). In other words to eradicate the parasite from this community, the average worm burden in the whole population (given that the average degree of worm clumping is still k = 0.34) must be reduced by control measures, to less than 0.3 worms per host. This result argues that the 'breakpoint' concept is of little value to disease control in this community since the region of attraction of the stable equilibrium state of parasite extinction is extremely small (i.e. 0-0.3 worms/host). In contrast, the region of attraction to the state of stable endemic disease is very large (i.e. 0.3-51-∞ worms/host) and thus this state is effectively globally stable.

The data recorded by Hsieh (1970) for a community in a rural district of Taiwan, can also be used to obtain a crude estimate of R for _Necator americanus_. The age-prevalence and age-intensity data of Hsieh (1970) for _N. americanus_ infections are portrayed in Fig. 14. [The prevalence data was obtained from Table 3 of Hsieh (1970). The intensity data was estimated from the observations recorded in Table 4 of the same paper, assuming (a) that 120 eggs/gram of faeces is the approximate daily output of one female worm and (b) that the degree of worm clumping (measured by k) in each age class was the same for _N. americanus_ and _A. duodenale_]. The degree of worm aggregation in each age class of hosts is recorded in Fig. 12(b) where k values were estimated from the age prevalence and intensity data displayed in Fig. 14. It is interesting to note that the degree of clumping of _N. americanus_ in the Taiwan community is much more severe than that recorded in the Indian community (Fig. 12a). A point of similarity between the two patterns is the marked difference in worm aggregation in the young children when compared with older children and adults. An average k value, $\bar{k}$, is used (average overall age classes) to estimate the parameters R and α ($\bar{k}$ = 0.077). Using fitting procedures identical to those described for the data from the Indian community (given that the average worm burden of _N. americanus_ in adults was roughly 6.2 worms/host) an R value of approximately 1.5 is obtained (it is assumed that the life expectancy of the adult worms ($1/\mu_1$) and their hosts ($\frac{1}{b}$) is identical in both the Indian and Taiwan communities). The density dependent parameter α is estimated as $\alpha = 5.0 \times 10^{-6}$, a value which is in close agreement with that recorded for the Indian community.

The fit of eqns (16) and (17) (encorporating these parameter estimates (R = 1.5, $\alpha = 5.0 \times 10^{-6}$, k = 0.077)) to the observed age-prevalence and age-intensity data is portrayed in Figs. 14a and b. The model again provides a reasonable qualitative prediction of the observed trends. The low R value recorded for the Taiwan community

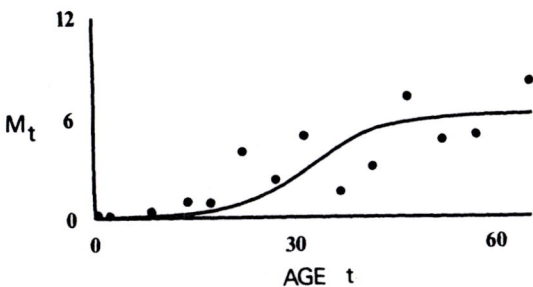

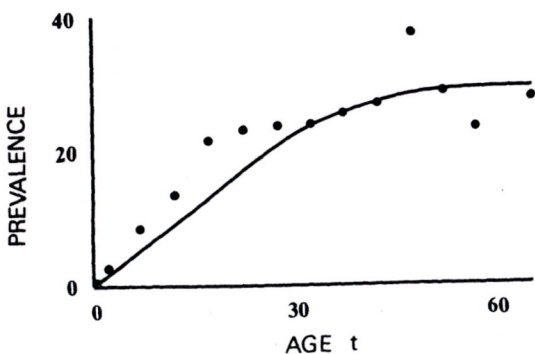

FIGURE 14 : The same as Fig. 11 except representing the data for *N. americanus* infections in Taiwan (Hsieh, 1970) (see text for details).

> Graph (a). Age-intensity curve. Solid circles - observed data (see text for details of estimation). Solid line - model predictions (eqn (16)) fitted by non-linear least squares technique (R = 1.5, α = 5.0 x 10^{-6}).

> Graph (b). Age-prevalence curve. Solid circles - observed data. Solid line - model predictions (eqn (17), $\bar{k}$ = 0.077).

clearly reflects the low average worm burden observed in each age class of hosts.

Seasonal changes in parameter values

In regions of endemic hookworm infection, many of the parameters which determine the magnitude of the basic reproductive rate of the parasite, R, will be subject to seasonal variation due to changes in climatic and host behavioural factors. Time dependence in any of the population parameters may, in principle, produce seasonal changes in the prevalence and intensity of infection. Such patterns have been recorded by Nawalinski *et al* (1978a & b) in the Indian community discussed in the preceeding section. These authors recorded a loss of worms during the post-monsoon dry period and a gain of parasites during the pre-monsoon and monsoon seasons in various age classes of children. As recorded in Fig. 12, however, a net gain of parasites occurred on a year to year basis which gave rise to an increase in the intensity and prevalence of infection with age.

Seasonal changes in the value of R may be due to (a) changes in host behaviour during the various seasons of the year, influencing the rate of contact with infective stages (the parameter β); (b) changes in host diet altering worm survival or reproduction (the parameters μ_1, α and λ); (c) the prevailing climatic conditions (temperature and rainfall) influencing the survival of the infective L_3 larvae (the parameter μ_3) and (d) climatic conditions altering the maturation time of the L_3 larvae (T_2 in eqn (3)) and the survival of the eggs and non-infective larvae (μ_2 in eqn (3)) (the composite parameter D_2).

The last two factors ((c) and (d)) will be of major significance. The survival potential of the infective larvae is very sensitive to changes in soil temperature and moisture content. For example Augustine (1923a) demonstrated that, under field conditions, the expected life spans of larvae ($1/\mu_3$) maintain in moist soil under conditions of dense shade, moderate shade and direct sunlight were 12.4, 8.5 and 0.8 days respectively. In the laboratory Augustine (1923b) also demonstrated the direct effects of temperature where the expected life span of the larvae was 28.7 days when maintained at $16^{\circ}C$ but only 14.6 days when maintained at $27^{\circ}C$. Soil moisture content is also critical; larval survival is optimum when the soil is moist but neither too dry nor too water logged. Larval survival in water covered soils is poor, whether in conditions of dense shade, light shade or direct sunlight ($1/\mu_3$ = 2.0, 5.4 and < 1 days respectively (Augustine, 1923a)).

The proportion of eggs that survive to produce L_3 larvae is also critically dependent on the prevailing conditions of soil moisture and temperature. The rate of larval development (the developmental period T_2) is optimum at around $25^{\circ}C$ - $35^{\circ}C$ in moist conditions (T_2 approximately 5 days). If temperatures are below $17-20^{\circ}C$ the ova and larvae of *N. americanus* cease development and death rapidly follows (Muller, 1975). *A. duodenale* is able to develop at slightly lower temperatures than *N. americanus* and is thus found in some temperate regions of the world.

Aside from the direct effects of temperature and moisture on larval or egg survival, climatic conditions can influence development in the free-living habitat in other ways. Rainfall, for example often breaks up faecal material and in doing

so improves the chances of larval survival (Docherty, 1926). For example, Stoll
(1923b) demonstrate that the proportion of ova (eggs) that survive to reach the L_3
larval stage was much lower when culture took place in pure faecal material (D_2 =
0.005) when compared with charcol culture media (D_2 = 0.175). Heavy rainfall, however, may have a detrimental effect by its action in washing larvae from the soil
and in creating water logged soil conditions (Cort, Payne & Riley, 1923; Augustine,
1923a & b).

Soil type and structure, with respect to water retention properties, is clearly
of importance to egg and larval development and survival. As recorded in Table 4,
fine sandy soils appear to be optimum. This table lists the values of D_2 (eqn 3)
recorded for larval development in various types of soil in Porto Rico and Alabama,
U.S.A. (Stoll, 1923b; Augustine & Smillie, 1926). Fine sandy soils are optimum
because of the poor survival properties of the L_2 and L_3 larvae in soils which have
a tendency to become water logged (i.e. clay soils). In summary, therefore the
infective potential of eggs released into a habitat (the parameters D_2 and μ_3) will
be optimum under conditions of warmth, shade, moisture and light sandy soils. These
four factors are major determinants of the global distribution of hookworm
infections.

In the vast majority of regions of endemic hookworm, the value of R will fall
below unity during certain periods of the year as a consequence of unsuitable
climatic conditions for egg and larval survival, and development. Often, the value
of R may be below unity for the majority of the year, transmission being restricted
to short periods of high temperatures and adequate rainfall (Augustine, 1926). For
parasite persistence in a defined region, the period during which R falls below unity
must be less than the maximum life span of any one stage in the paraistes life cycle.
For hookworm infections, where the expected lifespan in man of *N. americanus* is
roughly 3.5 years and that of *A. duodenale* approximately 1 year, seasonal changes in
R which lead to a value of less than unity during certain seasons, will be of little
significance to the overall persistence of the parasite from year to year. Seasonal
changes in R will only be important if they lower the average worm burden per host
below the 'breakpoint' level (M_u). This appears unlikely, unless R is only just
above unity during the optimum seasons for parasite transmission in a defined habitat
(i.e. the equilibrium worm burden M* is low).

The model development outlined in earlier sections is of value in exploring the
dynamics of the parasite on a year to year basis since the estimation of the parameter R, is based on the equilibrium endemic distribution of intensity and prevalence
of infection within the host population, and not on season to season changes within
any one year. The parameter components of the measure R, and R itself, must thus be
regarded as average yearly values for a defined habitat.

TABLE 4 : The influence of soil type on the development of hookworm eggs through to the infective larval state.

Soil type	The proportion of ova that develop to the L_3 state (D_2)
a) Porto Rico; Stoll (1923b)	
Loam	0.25
Sand	0.28
Humus	0.67
Clay	0.02
b) Alabama, U.S.A.; Augustine & Smillie (1926)	
Fine sand	0.39
Sandy loam	0.38
Fine sandy loam	0.22
Shale loam	0.09
Silt loam	0.07
Silty clay loam	0.05
Clay	0.06
	0.03

Spatial factors

The dependence of parasite development in the free-living habitat and infective larval survival, on soil type and the prevailing conditions of shade or sunlight, suggest that the spatial distribution of infective stages in a defined habitat will be highly heterogeneous. The principal cause of such heterogeneity will of course be related to the defaecation habits of the human population. However, each site in which faeces are deposited will differ with respect to soil type and conditions of shade and moisture. It appears highly probable that the high degree of contagion or clumping of the adult worms observed within human populations (see Fig. 12) is predominantely caused by heterogeneity in human movement patterns within a defined region and the respective spatial distribution of infective larvae. Recent studies of the influence of spatial distribution of infective stages on the dynamics of host infection (Keymer & Anderson, 1979) suggest that such heterogeneity has a marked impact on the frequency distribution of parasites per host. Parasite clumping can be induced by random distributions of infective stages, due to differences in host behaviour, but aggregated spatial patterns greatly increase the degree of parasite aggregation within the host population (Keymer & Anderson, 1979). If data were available, interesting comparisons could be made between the degree of adult parasite aggregation within the host population and the degree of spatial heterogeneity in infective stage distribution in various habitats.

The control of hookworm infections

Control of hookworm infection is at present based on two approaches which are often used concomitantly in endemic regions.

1) A range of chemotherapeutic agents are available which when administered to an infected person cause the expulsion and death, of a proportion of the worm burden (the proportion killed is dependent on the dosage level and frequency) (Muller, 1975).

2) Improvements in sewage disposal facilities, and the general level of hygiene within a population, are obvious forms of control of a parasitic agent whose transmission stage leaves the host in the faeces. Education is clearly an important component of such methods and is also of value in persuading people to wear shoes to prevent contact with the infective larvae.

Within the model defined by eqn (13) chemotherapy acts to increase the death rate of adult worms in a density independent manner, if applied randomly within the human population. For example, if we treat a proportion g of the population per year, and this treatment kills a proportion h of their individual worm burdens, then assuming the proportion g harbour on average the mean worm burden M, then the extra death rate applied to the worm population by chemotherapy, c (defined/year/worm) is given by

$$c = -\ln(1 - gh) \qquad (18)$$

Equation (13) therefore becomes

$$dM/dt = M\left[(R-1)(\mu_1+b) - c - \alpha\frac{(k+1)M}{k}\right] \qquad (19)$$

and the new basic reproductive rate $\hat{R}$ is

$$\hat{R} = \frac{\tfrac{1}{2}\beta\lambda\emptyset HD_1 D_2}{(\mu_1+b+c)\ (\mu_3+ H)} \tag{20}$$

For hookworm eradication ($\hat{R} < 1$) the required death rate c induced by chemotherapy is thus given by

$$c > (R-1)\ (\mu_1+b) \tag{21}$$

The proportion g of the population which must be treated to achieve this goal can be derived from eqns (18) and (21) where

$$g > \left[1 - \exp\left[(1-R)\ (\mu_1+b)\right]\right]/h \tag{22}$$

For a chemotherapeutic agent which is 80% effective, the value of g for the Indian community near Calcutta with an R value of 2.7 is approximately 0.5. In other words the treatment of 77% of the population every year should lead to disease eradication. This result is encouraging, but it is important to note two points. First, the preceeding analysis of hookworm dynamics suggests that the equilibrium worm burden is essentially globally stable. It is thus unrealistic to attempt to reduce M below the breakpoint by a short intensive application of chemotherapy since once treatment stops the worm burden will return to its previous endemic level. The approach adopted in eqns (18)-(22) attempts to reduce transmission below the threshold level (see Fig. 9), rather than below the breakpoint, but control measures must still be applied continuously over very many years if eradication is to be achieved. As long as adult parasites persist in the community such that the mean worm burden is above the breakpoint, cessation of control measures will result in a slow return to the endemic levels that existed prior to control (the survival or persistence of the infective larvae is of little consequence due to their short expected lifespans when compared with that of the adult parasite). Some improvement in the likely efficiency of chemotherapy on a long term basis could be achieved by the intensification of application during periods of the year when the basic reproductive rate of infection, R, is at a minimum (i.e. dry cool periods).

An alternative method of application of chemotherapy is to simply treat the most heavily infected members of the community (assessed by means of faecal egg counts). Since worm distribution is highly clumped such action will be extremely effective in rapidly lowering the average worm burden, since it acts as a density-dependent regulatory mechanism. However, such treatment must again be continued until the average worm burden falls below the breakpoint (which for the Indian community is close to zero, M_u = 0.3).

The reduction of transmission below the transmission threshold (Fig. 9) where R < 1, can be achieved by improvements in sanitation, education and hygiene. Such methods have clear advantages if they are permanent in nature (i.e. sewage disposal facilities), since once introduced if adhered to they are likely to achieve rapid results. For the Indian community, a 63% decrease in transmission efficiency would result in the eradication of infection. A sound policy would be to combine chemotherapy with programmes to improve sanitation and levels of hygiene in an integrated approach to control. The principle stumbling block to successful control by this means is clearly the availability of economic resources.

Vaccination against human hookworm is a potential method of control for the future, since effective vaccines have been developed over the last decade for dog hookworms (*Ancyostoma caninum*). These vaccines are based on gamma irradiated L_3 larvae (Miller, 1978; Clegg & Smith, 1978). Although effective, these canine vaccines have a short shelf life and thus at present are not accepted as a viable economic proposition by pharmaceutical companies (chemotherapeutic agents are more profitable since they have to be applied repeatedly!) (Miller, 1978). It appears likely, however, that a human vaccine could in theory be developed, although developmental costs and safety regulations concerning the use of prophylatic agents make this unlikely in the near future.

It is possible to consider the likely effectiveness of a vaccine within the model framework defined by eqn (13). If a proportion g of the population is vaccinated per year (where vaccination is centred on the young children; the 'susceptible' individuals), and the vaccine provides effective protection for $^1/v$ years, then the new basic reproductive rate $\hat{R}$ is given by

$$\hat{R} = R\left[1 - \frac{g}{v}\right] \tag{23}$$

Here the quantity $\frac{g}{v}$ represents the proportion of the population "protected" at any one point in time. For the eradication of infection clearly $\hat{R}$ < 1, which gives

$$g > \left[1 - \frac{1}{R}\right]v \tag{24}$$

If the vaccine provides protection for only a limited period of time ($\frac{1}{v}$ small) the proportion g must be high and vica versa. These notions are displayed in Fig. 15a for R = 2.7.

A general relationship between the proportion of the population that must be protected at any one time, p, (where $p = \frac{g}{v}$), and the parameter R is displayed in Fig. 15b. For the Indian community (Fig. 11), this figure suggests that 63% of the population must be protected to eradicate *N. americanus* while in the Taiwan community the equivalent figure is 35% (Fig. 14).

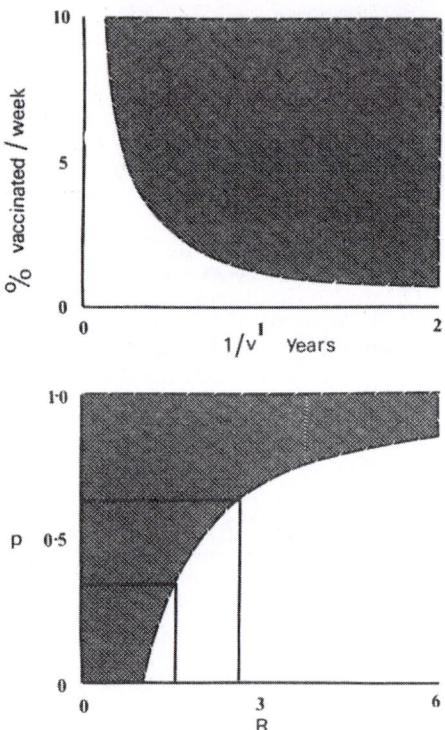

FIGURE 15 : Graph (a). The relationship between the proportion of the population vaccinated per week (g) and the duration of protection provided by the vaccine ($\frac{1}{v}$ years) (see eqn (24) in text). The shaded region denotes a sufficient degree of vaccination for the eradication of the parasite (R = 2.7).

Graph (b). The relationship between the proportion of the population that must be protected at any one point in time ($p = \frac{g}{v}$) for parasite eradication and the basic reproductive rate of the parasite R (eqn (24)). The shaded region denotes parasite eradication. The solid vertical and horizontal lines denote the values of R and p for the Taiwan and Indian communities (R = 1.5 and R = 2.7, respectively).

The preceeding discussion is hypothetical in the absence of an effective human vaccine, but it serves to illustrate the potential of such a method of control, particularly if the duration of protection provided is long ($\frac{1}{v}$ large).

CONCLUSIONS

The basic framework of the model developed in this paper (eqns (8) and (9)) can be adapted to mimic the dynamics of a wide range of direct life cycle helminth parasites of man. Broadly speaking, the general dynamical properties will be fairly robust to changes in biological detail, induced by variations in life cycle structure. Transmission thresholds and unstable breakpoints will still emerge as the central concepts governing the dynamics of parasitic infection.

Improvements in model structure are clearly required, however, since the work described in this paper represents a preliminary attempt at the exploration of the dynamics of this class of parasitic infections. With respect to hookworm, it appears likely that the rate of production of eggs (λ) is related to the burden of parasites harboured by an individual host (Hill, 1926). The inclusion of additional density-dependent constraints will therefore be necessary and will introduce added complexity into the dynamics of such models. It is unlikely, however, that such effects will raise the level of the 'breakpoint' (the unstable worm burden M_u) since this is largely set by the sexual mating habits of the worm concomitant with its statistical distribution within the host population. As such the inclusion of density-dependent reproduction will not invalidate the conclusion that the observed equilibrium level of infection is probably effectively globally stable in most regions of endemic hookworm disease.

Other refinements required include some representation of age dependency in the degree of worm clumping and an exploration of the impact of seasonal changes in R on the long terms dynamics of the parasite.

Refinements in model structure are to some extent secondary to a more fundamental requirement, namely; the need for quantitative data concerning the many rate processes which control the epidemiology of such helminth infections. As noted by Nawalinski *et al* (1978a) up to 1978 only four accounts of longitudinal studies (surveys over a period of years) among populations exposed to natural reinfection with hookworms have been published (this total includes their own study in 1970). The position is similar, or worse, for other direct life cycle helminth infections. There is thus an urgent need for more quantitative epidemiological studies of such disease, both of a horizontal and longitudinal nature. Experimental work is also required to measure specific biological parameters, such as infective stage survival under varying climatic conditions, the severity of density dependent constraints on adult worm survival and reproduction and the nature of sexual reproduction.

In parallel with such work, statistical methods must be developed to enable parameters, such as the basic reproductive rate R, to be accurately estimated from observed age-prevalence and age-intensity data. Measurement of the quantity R is clearly of central importance to the design and implementation of control methods (see eqns 22 and 24).

Mathematical models which mimic the dynamics of parasitic infections can clearly be of considerable practical as well as theoretical value. They provide precise guidelines concerning the type of data that must be collected if one is to first understand the factors which govern the persistence and stability of the parasite population. They may then be used, in conjunction with such data bases, to predict the level of control required in a defined habitat for either parasite eradication, or the reduction of the mean worm burden below the level which induces clinical symptoms. The construction of a robust, and practically useful, mathematical framework for the study of the dynamics of such diseases will require a close degree of collaboration between epidemiologists, mathematicians and statisticians in future research.

REFERENCES

ANDERSON, R.M. (1976a). Dynamic aspects of parasite population ecology. In: *Ecological Aspects of Parasitology*. (Ed. by C.R. Kennedy). Ch. 21. North Holland, Amsterdam.

ANDERSON, R.M. (1976b). Some simple models of the population dynamics of eucaryotic parasites. *Mathematical Models in Medicine*. (Ed. by J. Berger, W. Bühler, R. Repges and P. Tautu). pp. 16-57. *Lecture Notes in Biomathematics* 11, Springer-Verlag, Berlin.

ANDERSON, R.M. (1980). Strategic models for the control of infectious disease agents. In: *The Management of Pest and Disease Systems*. (Ed. by G.R. Conway). (in press)

ANDERSON, R.M. & MAY, R.M. (1978). Regulation and stability of host parasite population interactions: I Regulatory processes. *J. Anim. Ecol.* 47: 219-249.

ANDERSON, R.M. & MICHEL, J.F. (1977). Density dependent survival in populations of *Ostertagia ostertagi*. *Int. J. Parasitol.* 7: 321-329.

AUGUSTINE, D.L. (1923a). Investigations on the control of hookworm disease. XVI Variation in length of life of hookworm larvae from the stools of different individuals. *Am. J. Hyg.* 3: 127-136.

AUGUSTINE, D.L. (1923b). Investigations on the control of hookworm disease. XXIII Experiments on the factors determining the length of life of infective hookworm larvae. *Am. J. Hyg.* 3: 420-443.

AUGUSTINE, D.L. (1926). Studies and observations on soil infestation with hookworm in southern Alabama from October 1923 to September 1924. *Am. J. Hyg.* 6: 63-79.

AUGUSTINE, D.L. & SMILLIE, W.G. (1926). The relation of the type of soils of Alabama to the distribution of hookworm disease. *Am. J. Hyg.* 6: 36-62.

BAILEY, N.T.J. (1975). *The Mathematical Theory of Infectious Diseases*. (2nd Edition) Griffith, London.

BLISS, C.I. & FISHER, R.A. (1953). Fitting the negative binomial distribution to biological data and a note on the efficiency of fitting of the negative binomial. *Biometrics* 9: 176-200.

CHOWDHURY, A.B. & SCHILLER, E.L. (1968). A survey of parasitic infections in a rural community near Calcutta. *Am. J. Epidemiol.* 87: 299-312.

C.I.B.A. Foundation Symposium No. 49 (1977). *Health and Disease in Tribal Societies*. Elsevier, Amsterdam.

CLEGG, J.A. & SMITH, M.A. (1978). Prospects for the development of dead vaccines against helminths. *Advances in Parasitology* 16: 165-218.

CONWAY, G.R.; GLASS, N.R. & WILCOX, J.C. (1970). Fitting non-linear models to biological data by Marquardt's algorithm. *Ecology* 51: 503-508.

CORT, W.W.; PAYNE, G.C. & RILEY, W.A. (1923). Investigations on the control of hookworm disease. XXVIII A study of a heavily infected group of people on a sugar and coffee estate in Porto Rico, before and after treatment. *Am. J. Hyg.* 3: 85-110.

CROFTON, H.D. (1971). A quantitative approach to parasitism. *Parasitology* 62: 179-194.

DIETZ, K. (1976). The incidence of infectious diseases under the influence of seasonal fluctuations. In: *Mathematical Models in Medicine*. (Ed. Berger, J.; Bühler, W.; Repges, R. and Tautu, P.). *Lecture Notes in Biomathematics* 11: 1-15.

DOCHERTY, J.F. (1926). Hookworm infestation and reinfestation in Ceylon. A study of high incidence with a moderate degree of infestation. *Am. J. Hyg.* 6: 160-171.

FISHER, R.A. (1930). *The genetical theory of natural selection*. Clarendon, Oxford.

HILL, R.B. (1926). The estimation of the number of hookworms harboured, by the use of the dilution egg count method. *Am. J. Hyg.* 6 (suppl.): 19-41.

HOAGLAND, K.E. & SCHAD, G.A. (1978). *Necator americanus* and *Ancylostoma duodenale*: Life history parameters and epidemiological implications of two sympatric hookworms of humans. *Expt. Parasitol.* 44: 36-49.

HSIEH, H.C. (1970). Studies on endemic hookworm: I. Survey and longitudinal observations in Taiwan. *Jap. J. Parasit.* 19: 508-522.

KERMACK, W.O. & McKENDRICK, A.G. (1927). Contributions to the mathematical theory of epidemics. *Proc. Roy. Soc.* A, 115: 700-721.

KEYMER, A.E. & ANDERSON, R.M. (1979). The dynamics of infection of *Tribolium confusum* by *Hymenolepis diminuta*: the influence of infective stage density and spatial distribution. *Parasitology* 79: 195-207.

KRUPP, I.M. (1961). Effects of crowding and of superinfection on habitat selection and egg production in *Ancylostoma caninum*. *J. Parasitol.* 47: 957-961.

LEYTON, M.K. (1968). Stochastic models in populations of helminthic parasites in the definitive host: II. Sexual mating functions. *Math. Biosci.* 3: 413-419.

MacDONALD, G. (1965). The dynamics of helminth infections, with special reference to schistosomes. *Trans. Roy. Soc. Trop. Med. Hyg.* 59: 489-506.

MAY, R.M. (1977). Togetherness among schistosomes: its effects on the dynamics of the infection. *Math. Biosc.* 35: 301-343.

MAY, R.M. & ANDERSON, R.M. (1978). Regulation and stability of host parasite population interactions: II. *J. Anim. Ecol.* 47: 249-267.

MAY, R.M. & ANDERSON, R.M. (1979). Population biology of infectious diseases: Part II. *Nature* 280: 455-461.

MILLER, T.A. (1978). Industrial development and field use of the canine hookworm vaccine. *Advances in Parasitology* 16: 333-342.

MILLS, C.A.; ANDERSON, R.M. & WHITFIELD, P.J. (1979). Density-dependent survival and reproduction within populations of the ectoparasitic digenean, *Transversotrema patialense* on the fish host. *J. Anim. Ecol.* 48: 383-399.

MULLER, R. (1975). *Worms and Diseases*. Heineman, London.

NASELL, I. & HIRSCH, W.M. (1973). The transmission dynamics of schistosomiasis. *Can. Pure Appl. Maths.* 26: 395-453.

NAWALINSKI, T.; SCHAD, G.A. & CHOWDHURY, A.B. (1978a). Population biology of hookworms in children in rural West Bengal. I. General parasitological observations. *Am. J. Trop. Med. Hyg.* 27: 1152-1161.

NAWALINSKI, T.; SCHAD, G.A. & CHOWDHURY, A.B. (1978b). Population biology of hookworms in children in rural West Bengal. II. Acquisition and loss of hookworms. *Am. J. Trop. Med. Hyg.* 27: 1162-1173.

PAMPIGHONE, S. & RICCIARDI, M.L. (1972). Geographic distribution of *Strongyloides fülleborni* in humans in tropical Africa. *Parassitologia* 14: 329-338.

PAYNE, F.K. (1924). Investigations on the control of hookworm disease. XXXI. The relation of the physiological age of hookworm larvae to their ability to infect the human host. *Am. J. Hyg.* 3: 584-597.

PESIGAN, T.P.; FOROOQ, M.; HAIRSTON, N.G.; JAUREQUI, J.J.; GARCIA, E.G.; SANTOS, A.T.; SANTOS, B.C. & BESA, A.A. (1953). Studies on *Schistosoma japonicum* infection in the Philippines. I. General considerations and epidemiology. *Bull. Wld. Hlth. Org.* 18: 345-455.

PETERS, W. (1978). Medical Aspects: Comments and Discussion II. In: *The Relevance of Parasitology to Human Welfare Today*. (Ed. by A.E. Taylor and R. Muller). Symposium of the British Society for Parasitology 16. Blackwell Scientific Publications. Oxford.

SCHAD, G.A. (1971). The ecology of interacting populations of man and hookworms in rural West Bengal. *Report of the John Hopkins Center for Medical Research and Training* 1969-1970: 5-24.

STOLL, N.R. (1923a). Investigations on the control of hookworm disease. XVIII. On the relation between the number of eggs found in human faeces and the number of hookworms in the host. *Am. J. Hyg.* 3: 103-117.

STOLL, N.R. (1923b). Investigations on the control of hookworm disease. XVII. A quantitative study defining a point of breakdown of hookworm eggs cultured in faeces, and its association with intense acidity. *Am. J. Hyg.* 3: 137-155.

STURROCK, R.F. (1967). Hookworm studies in Tanganyika (Tanzania): The results of a series of surveys on a group of primary school children and observations on the survival of hookworm infective larvae exposed to simulated field conditions. *E. Afr. Med. J.* 44: 142-149.

TALLIS, G.M. & LEYTON, M.K. (1969). Stochastic models of populations of helminthic parasites in the definitive host: I. *Math. Biosci.* 4: 39-48.

WAKELIN, D. (1978). Immunity to intestinal parasites. *Nature* 273: 617-620.

UNITED NATIONS (1976). *Demographic Yearbook 1975*, United Nations, New York.

VERHULST, P.F. (1838). Notice sur la loi que la population suit clans son accroissement. *Corresp. Math. Phys.* 10: 113-121.

YANAGISAWA, R. & MIZUNO, T. (1963). On the infection mode of hookworm. *Medical Culture* S(1): 112-118.

EPIDEMIOLOGIC MODELS OF BACTERIAL DISEASES

B. Cvjetanović

Institute of Immunology, Rockefellerova 10,
41000 Zagreb, Yugoslavia

The author reviewed epidemiological models of major bacterial
diseases - tetanus, typhoid, cholera, cerebrospinal meningitis, diphtheria and pertussis - which have been fully described[1]. These models
have been constructed with the practical purpose to enable the study of
public health interventions, such as immunization on the natural course
of the infection.

The complexity of the epidemiological processes on one end and the
requirements for the assessment of the impact of control measures under
a variety of specific situations renders difficult rigorous mathematical
solutions of these complex situations. The models therefore were conceived essentially as simulation models and therefore called rather
"epidemiological" than mathematical ones. However, the core of these
models is a mathematical one.

Epidemiological models are based on the natural history of the dynamics of the specific infections in the population. An infection is
conceived as a structured flow of population through epidemiological
states (or class) such as the incubation, the illness, the carrier
state etc. in strict sequence and direction and at precise time intervals. The population is thus at any time distributed in various epidemiological classes. The transfer of individuals from one class to another
is regulated by the transfer coefficients.

The incidence of infection and illness, respectively, is determined
by transfer factor from the healthy class of ill individuals. In fact,
the incidence rate is regulated by the "force of infection", which is an
expression of totality of various factors which bring about a certain
frequency of infection in real life. In some diseases model solutions
are obtained by strict mathematical, analytical methods. The nature of
the dynamics of some disease and/or of the problems related to their
control are suitable for deterministic approach, while in other diseases
and epidemic situations stochastic methods seem to be more relevant.

Simulation of the effects of the disease control programmes is conceived as an interference at a specific point and specific time interval
of the natural course of an infection. When certain control measures,
such as immunization, are systematically applied, the actual situation

thus produced can be taken as baseline in the study of the effects of an additional specific control measure. Simultaneous or alternative application of various control measures can be studied this way.

With the essential characteristics of the contemplated programme, e.g. (a) immunization schedule (including age and vaccine composition and efficiency)and (b) coverage, on hand, the effect of such programme on disease(s), resulting incidence and changes in epidemiological classes over a certain period of time can be simulated. Furthermore, simulated effects of various coverages and schedules can be compared and the one which suits best selected, in line with the actual epidemiological situation, available resources and constraints. For example, the effect of several different immunization schedules with DPT vaccine on whooping cough and diphtheria in European countries was assessed. The models have shown definite advantages of certain immunization schedules in the control of whooping cough in particular, which is borne out by actual data in European countries.

The model on typhoid was used in search for most effective and least expensive control programme in various countries. Similarly other models have been used in field practice. The model simulations were able to bring also to light inadequacies of certain control programmes.It therefore seems reasonable to examine new programmes first by means of the models, as simulations with the models are quick and cheap, and finding errors in Public Health practice takes a long time and costs much.

The models proved useful in determining the advantages and disadvantages of various control programmes based on sanitation or chemoprophylaxis of various mixes of these and other measures. The effectiveness, the costs and health and economic benefits of various alternatives were assessed. This proved useful in public health practice in decision-making processes on the selection of an appropriate control strategy.

Explorations of long-term trends and feasibility of disease eradication has also been done with these models.

The epidemiological models have been shown in public health to be useful in the planning of control programmes and their evaluation. They permit assessment of their cost-effectiveness and health and economic benefits and thus permit a more effective use of available resources and formulation of optimal control programmes in given circumstances.

The use of the models is feasible wherever modest computer facilities exist and is relatively simple and inexpensive. Therefore, they should be more often utilized by the managers of communicable diseases in order to obtain best results with available resources.

Models besides their use in the search of solutions of practical
public health problems provide also the means for a better understanding of the dynamics of epidemic process and the underlying mechanism of
the long term trends.

Explorations with the typhoid model have brought to light two unknown epidemiologic features of this infection, namely: (a) self-limiting
mechanism of disease when certain threshold level of incidence is reached
and (b) the dependence of disease trends on the population dynamics.
These two features, discovered while modelling typhoid fever, deserve
to be mentioned in view of their practical implications in the planning
of typhoid control and to demonstrate the contribution which mathematical
modelling can make to the advancement of the epidemiology of this and
other diseases.

The basic feature of an epidemic such as is the one caused by
S.typhi is the propagation of the infection from infectious persons to
susceptibles. The basic epidemic process in a fixed period of time can
be presented as follows:

The number of new infections (cases)		Number of infect- ious persons in the population		Force of infection		Proportion of susceptible persons
	=		x		x	

Force of infection (RI) which is an expression of all factors which
determine the transmission of infection from an infectious person to
the susceptibles regulates the epidemic process in the population (divided into 10 epidemiological classes of our typhoid model), namely
the transfers of the infection from infectious classes $(x_3 x_4 x_6 x_7)$ to
the susceptible (x_1).

The following are the classes (x) and daily rates of exits (P) in
our model:

x_1 susceptible   RI $\dfrac{x_3 + x_4 + x_6 + x_7}{x_T}$

x_2 incubating non infectious

x_3 incubating infectious   PI

x_4 sick infectious   PS

x_5 sick noninfectious

x_6 temporary carrier   PC

x_7 permanent carrier

x_8 resistant (1 year)   PR1+PR2

x_9 resistant (10 years)

x_{10} typhoid deaths

Coefficients of transfer (R) from one class to another (e.g. $R_{1,2}=$
= transfer from class x_1 to class x_2) are derived from the epidemiolo-

gical evidence and the force of infection (RI) from actual incidence
of the disease. Accordingly the mathematical relationship between the
10 classes which are interrelated in strict time sequence and direction of the flow of epidemic process is expressed in the following system
of 10 equations (The rates are calculated on daily basis and symbols
x_1, x_2 etc. represent the number of persons in each class at the given
moment.)

$$\Delta x_1 = - (x_3 + x_4 + x_6 + x_7)\,(x_1/x_T)RI +$$
$$(x_4 R_{4,1} + x_5 R_{6,1})PS + x_6 R_{6,1}PC +$$
$$x_8 R_{8,1}PR_1 + x_9 R_{9,1}PR_2 + x_7 PB -$$
$$x_1\,(PD - dx_{10}/x_T)$$
$$\Delta x_2 = R_{1,2}\,(x_3 + x_4 + x_6 + x_7)\,(x_1/x_T)RI +$$
$$x_3 R_{3,2}PI - x_2\,(PI + PD - dx_{10}/x_T)$$
$$\Delta x_3 = R_{1,3}(x_3 + x_4 + x_6 + x_7)\,(x_1/x_T)RI +$$
$$x_2 R_{2,3}PI - x_3\,(PI + PD - dx_{10}/x_T)$$
$$\Delta x_4 = (x_2 R_{2,4} + x_3 R_{3,4})PI + x_5 R_{5,4}PS -$$
$$x_4\,(PS + PD - dx_{10}/x_T)$$
$$\Delta x_5 = (x_2 R_{2,5} + x_3 R_{3,5})\,PI + x_4 R_{4,5}\,PS -$$
$$x_5\,(PS + PD - dx_{10}/x_T)$$
$$\Delta x_6 = x_4 R_{4,6}PS - x_6(PC + PD - dx_{10}x_T)$$
$$\Delta x_7 = x_6 R_{6,7}PC - x_7(PD - dx_{10}x_T)$$
$$\Delta x_8 = (x_4 R_{4,8} + x_5 R_{5,8})PS + x_6 R_{6,9}PC -$$
$$x_8(PR_1 + PD - dx_{10}/x_T)$$
$$\Delta x_9 = x_8 R_{8,9}PR_1 - x_9(PR_2 + PD - dx_{10}/x_T)$$
$$\Delta x_{10} = (x_4 R_{4,10} + x_5 R_{5,10})PS$$

where $x_T = \sum_i x_i$

Self-control of typhoid is a logical consequence of its dynamics
as defined in our model. The size of the epidemiological classes has
almost a linear relationship to the reciprocal of the force of infection (RI). The reason for this inverse proportionality is a logical consequence of the model and is due to the fact that the typhoid mortality
rate is small in comparison with overall death rate. Were the typhoid
mortality exactly equal to zero ($R_{4,10}=R_{5,10}=0$) then assuming a constant
population size (Death rate = Birth rate) and a stable stationary
endemic situation where the number of individuals in each class remains
constant - the proportion of susceptible individuals (x_1/x_T) would be
strictly inversely proportional to RI. The model shows that stable
endemicity can be established only if RI remains above a certain critical value. Assuming constant class sizes the critical value for daily
force of infection RI is 0.0017. When RI falls below above value
typhoid fever is extinguished slowly by itself. What happens is that
the permanent carriers slowly die out from natural causes while their
replenishment from new infections decreases because of the low force
of infection. Thus the reservoir of infection is depleted and the
infection eradicated by its own intrinsic mechanisms. We have shown on
the examples of trends of typhoid in developed countries that this is
not only our mathematical theory but that this process has begun in a

number of countries. This is as far as we know the only example of theoretical basis of self-control and eradication of an infection. This both from the theoretical and practical points of view is an important contribution of the mathematical models to the understanding of the dynamics of typhoid permitting long term projections.

However, in the study of actual situations in some countries the assumed basis for self-control which is a stable population is not met. The population dynamics has an important effect on the fragile equilibrium which depends on RI in the stable population. Therefore it is evident that the host population dynamics should be closely studied together with the dynamics of the parasite as they are not only interrelated, as this is obvious, but the population dynamics has much more profound effect on typhoid dynamics than has ever been suspected before the model was constructed.

The above is only one, selected example among many of the valuable contributions which mathematical modelling can give to the development of the theoretical basis for understanding the epidemiological processes and then to the use of thus gained knowledge in the public health practice.

In conclusion it seems that there is ample evidence indicating that in modern epidemiology mathematical models not only have their place but that they are an indispensable tool for a proper study of the dynamics of infection in a quantitative and meaningful way.

REFERENCES

Cvjetanović,B., Grab,B. and Uemura,K. Dynamics of Bacterial Diseases,
Epidemiological Models and their Use in Public Health. Bull. Wld Hlth
Org., Suppl.No.1,   56; 1978

STRATEGIC PLANNING MODELS FOR RUBELLA VACCINATION PROGRAMMES

E.G. Knox

Health Services Research Centre, Department of Social Medicine,
University of Birmingham,
Birmingham B15 2 TJ. U.K.

There is a class of epidemiological model which contains both biological and operational components. Such models are directed towards problems of health-care planning, where the rational design and development of a service demands a planning tool which responds not only to operational considerations (e.g. queuing, manpower constraints, etc.), but which predicts the effects of biological uncertainties (e.g. natural history of disease, response to vaccine etc.) and of the human problems of implementation (e.g. responsiveness, compliance etc.).

The examination reported here is in this class. It is directed towards a particular question. The question is: what is the best way of deploying Rubella vaccine in order to minimise the occurrence of Congenital Rubella Syndrome (CRS) ?

Existing Solutions

Two approaches have been adopted in different parts of the world. In the UK and in other European countries the adopted policy is to vaccinate adolescent girls. In the USA the policy is to vaccinate both boys and girls in the pre-school years. Both policies are supplemented by additional vaccination at other ages, but the main component of the policy is as stated above. In the first case the objective is to provide personal protection while leaving Rubella to spread without serious interruption. In the second policy the objective is to provide herd immunity, as much through the suppression of the transmission of the virus as through the personal protection which (in time) it also provides.

So far as can be ascertained the decisions were reached on intuitive grounds, without detailed computation. The problem is to decide which of them, or which alternative scheme, is likely to give the best results. In order to answer this question two models were constructed. The first is a fairly simple mathematical model representing a 'steady-state' in a uniform population. The second is more complex, taking account of population heterogeneity, and of serial changes both in policy and in response, and can be used to determine intermediate, as well as long-term steady-state, outcomes.

STEADY STATE MODEL

This model is a simple mathematical one and depends upon a number of strictly unwarranted simplifications.   That is, we suppose the existence of a homogeneous population of fixed size, unstratified with respect to virus exposure, the women giving birth to infants at a fixed 'average' age; deaths also occur at a fixed average age and   at   steady rate, matching the steady rate of births.   The natural virus spreads at an even rate, in a non-epidemic manner, and results in a pattern of exponential decline with age of the proportion of Rubella-susceptible women.

The proportion of susceptibles (s) at age t is given by the formula
$$s = e^{-at} \ldots\ldots\ldots \qquad\qquad 1$$
..... where a is the rate of transmission, and of attrition of the susceptibles.

We can fit this curve to the real population with reasonable approximation if we know the proportion of susceptibles at a given age, through the use of the inverse form of the above formula, in order to calculate a.   Thus:
$$a = \log_e (1/s) \quad /t \ldots\ldots\ldots \qquad\qquad 2$$

We can also use this model to calculate an index of the incidence of CRS.   The incidence is proportional to the decline in the numbers of susceptible women at two ages separated by a period of about 2 months.   Not all exposed infants are affected, not all survive to delivery, and not all are diagnosed.   We must therefore multiply the results of this calculation by a factor p to produce a realistic estimate of incidence (i).
$$i = p \, (e^{-ab} - e^{-a \, (b + g)}) \ldots\ldots\ldots \qquad\qquad 3$$
..... where b is the mean age of the mother at the birth of the child and where g is the length of the susceptible period expressed as a fraction of a year.

At this point we can introduce vaccination at a chosen age and at a chosen level of efficacy. By efficacy, in this context, we imply a combination of the proportion of girls who accept the vaccination offer, multiplied by the proportion in whom efficacious levels of immunity are produced.   The result is a downward step in the exponential curve of the declining susceptibles. However, the value a is reduced by this process to a degree which depends both upon the age of the offer, and upon the efficacy.   We thus have to recalculate the curve, recalculate the step, recalculate the curve.....until a new curve, complete with step, stabilises.   At this point we can recalculate the incidence of CRS and , by comparing with the value for an unvaccinated population, calculate the effectiveness of the programme. (In keeping with widely used practice we retain the term efficacy as a measure of the performance of a procedure; and effectiveness as a measure of the performance of a service). A series of experiments was carried out, using this model, and results (relative to an unvaccinated CRS incidence standardized to 1.0) are given in Fig. 1.

These results show that provided an efficacy/uptake value of 70 percent or more can be obtained, the vaccination of pre-school children of both sexes gives a better long-term (steady-state) result than does the vaccination of adolescent girls at comparable efficacy levels. However, if efficacy/uptake values of less than 70 percent are the best that can be obtained, then for given efficacy levels, the vaccination of adolescent girls gives the best results.

FIG. 1

EFFICACY/EFFECTIVENESS RELATIONSHIPS

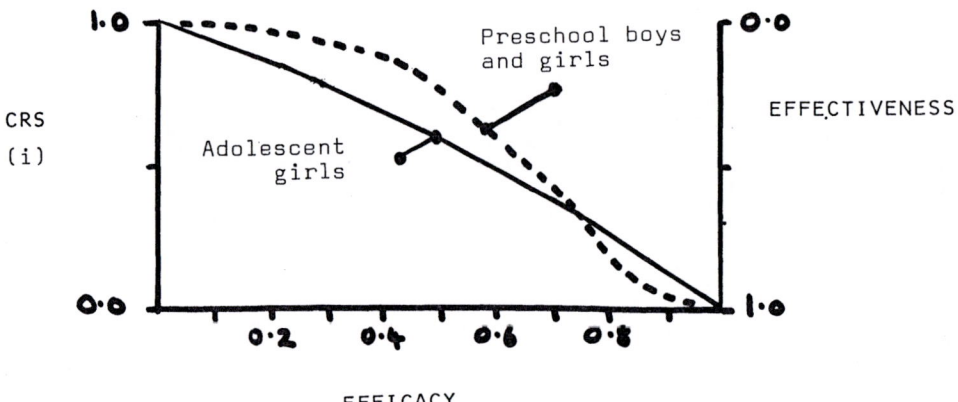

EFFICACY

DYNAMIC MODEL

In this model we add some of the complications of real life.   That is, there are facilities for
the entry of the real distribution of maternal age-at-delivery; for the specification of
population strata in which the average value of a is loaded in different layers; for the
specification of spontaneous secular changes in a, for example a continuing decline ; for a
decay-rate in artificial vaccine-immunity; and for an interaction between wild-virus infection
and vaccine-immunity which boosts the immunity level from a labile to a permanent state.
The experimenter may also change his policy (ages and sexes) in successive years, and enter
changing estimates of efficacy/uptake.   The outcomes, likewise, are given year by year, and
characterize the period of transition towards the steady states indicated in the simpler model.

The steady state model made little demand upon the computer except for simple calculations,
and the iterative procedure for stabilising the relationship between vaccination and the
modified value for the attrition parameter.   By contrast, the dynamic model requires computer
simulation.   The initial 'setting-up' of an age-distributed cross-sectional image of the
population is based upon a negative exponential curve, as previously, but the process thereafter
takes place in successive annual steps.   At each step a proportion of the susceptibles becomes
infected and is transferred to the class of 'natural immunes'.   The proportion depends upon the
value of a.   The value of a is then recalculated for the subsequent year, in proportion to the
number of cases occurring during the current year, and subsequently modified in the light of
any specified secular changes.   Vaccination procedures are carried out at specified ages, with
specified efficacies, resulting in transfers from the 'susceptibles' to the class of 'vaccine-
immune'.   Vaccine-immunes infected with wild-virus are transferred to the class of 'natural-
immunes': (this movement can be suppressed).   A proportion of the 'vaccine-immunes' reverts
to the class of 'susceptibles', according to the input 'decay' parameter.   Everyone is aged one
year, a cohort of elderly persons dies, and a new cohort is born.   Finally, the number of cases
of CRS is accumulated across the age-at-delivery distribution, and the result is printed.

A range of simulation experiments was undertaken.   They included experiments with no
vaccination, with the U.K. system of vaccination, with the USA system of vaccination, and with
combined systems;   each of these was repeated for a range of efficacy levels and a series of
decay rates, (including no decay), and the interaction with wild virus was studied.   Finally,
the effects of superimposed spontaneous 'secular trends' of the attrition parameter (a) were
investigated.

Results of Experiments

Vaccination of adolescent girls gave a relatively uncomplicated result. Steady states were reached in about 25 years, and half the ultimate achievement was attained within about 10 years. As with the simple model, effectiveness at steady state was almost linearly proportional to efficacy. Steady state incidences for the dynamic model were about about 0.8 of the incidences for the simple model. The difference was chiefly due to the introduction of an extended distribution of age-at-delivery. The outcomes of the dynamic model can be regarded as the most accurate.

Vaccination of boys and girls in the pre-school period gave a more complicated result. The initial rate of decline of CRS was quicker, and for high efficacies the steady states were achieved in 14-20 years and the halfway point in about 7 years. However, the relationship with efficacy was non-linear - as was also seen in the simple model. The pattern of the non-linearity was, however, complex and the results of low efficacies were unexpected. Thus, for efficacies below about 60 percent the subsequent history of CRS in the population became unstable, rebounding to a peak 20 to 30 years after the initiation of the scheme. This probably stems from a movement of girls who at the beginning of the scheme were aged between 2 and 10 years and who had not yet had Rubella; nor were they vaccinated against it. They were exposed to wild-virus at much lower levels than would have otherwise existed and this resulted in the passage of a large number of susceptibles into the reproductive age groups. At high levels of efficacy this does not matter, but for lower levels there is still sufficient wild virus passing in the population to infect a substantial number. A selection of results is shown in Fig. 2.

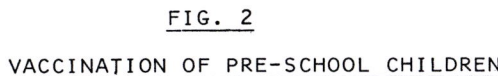

FIG. 2

VACCINATION OF PRE-SCHOOL CHILDREN

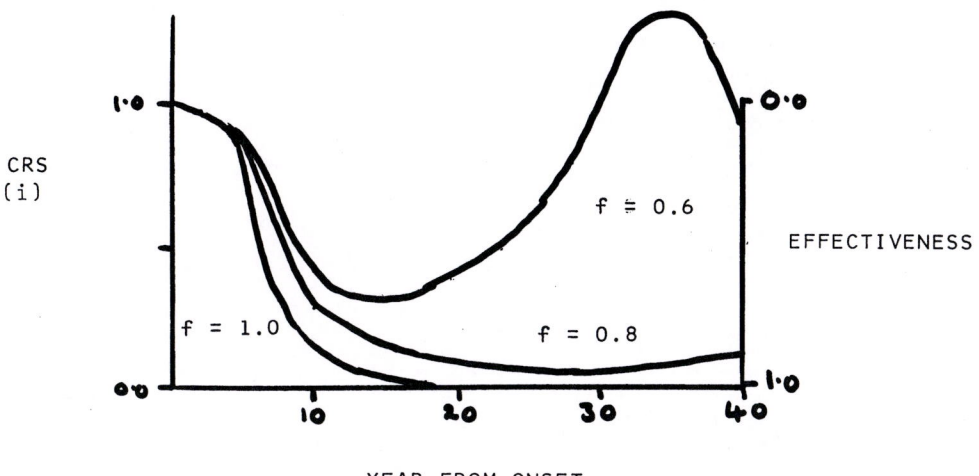

CRS (i)

EFFECTIVENESS

f = 0.6

f = 1.0

f = 0.8

YEAR FROM ONSET

f = EFFICACY

Combined systems of vaccination in pre-school children and adolescent girls ameliorated this dependency upon high efficacies and uptakes. That is, efficacies of 0.6 attained at two ages avoided the dangers of severe rebound.

Decay rates, for vaccine immunity, of one percent and two percent, were next investigated. In the case of adolescent vaccination this resulted in a substantial degradation of effectiveness which was, however, partially amerliorated by wild virus interaction. For example, a two percent per annum decay rate without the wild virus interaction resulted in an ultimate deficit of effectiveness of 43 percent. The wild virus interaction reduced this to 32 percent.

The effect of decay upon programmes of pre-school vaccination was more dramatic. Decay rates as small as 1 percent threw otherwise effective programmes into severe rebound. Moreover, the modifying effects of the wild-virus boost interaction were much smaller than in the other scheme because of the low level of wild virus. These experiments show that an accurate appraisal of rates of decay for vaccine-induced immunity is much more critical for a herd immunity plan, than it is for a personal immunity plan. Combined-age vaccination schemes were also critically sensitive to small decay rates, and failed to provide the levels of insurance, here, that they did in the case of low uptakes.

The effects of 'spontaneous' secular changes in the attrition parameter were greater than had been expected. Without vaccination the incidence of CRS rose steeply in response to a 1 percent per annum decline in $\underline{a}$, increasing by more than 60 percent over a period of 40 years. For a 2 percent per annum decline the increase was about 150 percent. These experiments imply that vaccination programmes which simply hold the incidence of CRS steady, must not necessarily be regarded as totally unsuccessful.

DISCUSSION

The general validity of these models is arguable mainly on prior grounds, but several features of their outputs confirm their utility as predictive and planning tools. The first is a reasonable quantitative match between the outcomes of the dynamic model, without vaccination, and observations of incidence obtained in the L K. Thus, a postulated 2 percent per annum secular decline in the attrition parameter (a) leads to a calculation that 0.30 per thousand fetuses are currently exposed to maternal infection within a postulated susceptible period of 0.1 years. If we suppose, on the basis of field studies, that about one third of the fetuses survive to term and exhibit CRS, then our model predicts an absolute incidence of about 0.1 per thousand births. Ascertained cases in the L K in the period 1970-73 suggest a true incidence of about 0.08 per thousand births. (1,2,3).

The exponential decline of susceptibility with age results in the prediction that the incidence will be especially high in young mothers and in first infants. This phenomenon has in fact been observed. (4). The model also predicts that the vaccination of adolescent girls will result not only in a decline in the proportion of susceptibles in young women, but, because of a reduction in the attrition parameter, an increasing proportion of susceptibles in young men. This has also been observed. (5). Finally, the predictions of rebound look very much as if they will be borne out in the USA. Since the introduction of pre-school vaccination the incidence of Rubella has declined in the early age groups but recent studies show it to be increasing in adolescents and early adult life. (6).

The practical implications are that countries which have already adopted adolescent female vaccination, and which have already progressed some way along its rather sluggish response curve, would be safer to persist with their policy. By contrast, countries which have adopted pre-school vaccination, and which have achieved uptakes of less than 75 percent, need to take quite urgent action in their adolescents and young adult female populations if they are to avoid the risk of severe secondary epidemics. Finally, as soon as we can be reassured, on the basis of experience, that vaccine-immunity is stable and declines at rates substantially less than 1 percent per annum, both policies might profitably be transmuted into combined programmes covering both pre-school children and adolescents. All proposed policy changes, however, should be investigated through simulation methods such as those described above, before they are implemented.

REFERENCES

1. Knox, E.G. Strategy for Rubella Vaccination , Int. Jnl. of Epid. 1980 (In press)

2. Sheppard S., Smithells R.W., Peckham C.S., and Marshall W.C., National Congenital Rubella Surveillance , 1971-75; Health Trends 1977, 9: 38-41.

3. Dudgeon J.A., Peckham C.S., Marshall W.C., and Smithells R.W., National Congenital Rubella Surveillance Programme . Health Trends 1973, 5: 75-79.

4. Marshall W.C., Peckham C.S., Dudgeon J.A., Sheppard S., Smithells R.W., and Weatherall J.A., Parity of Women Contracting Rubella in Pregnancy . Lancet 1976, 7971: 1231-1233.

5. Clarke M., Schild G.C., Boustred J., and Seagroatt V., Effect of the Rubella Vaccination Programme on the Serological Status of Young Adults in the UK . Lancet 1, (8128) 1979. 1224-1226.

6. Hayden G.F., Modkin J.F., and Witte J.J., Current Status of Rubella in the United States 1969-75; J. Inf. Dis. 1977, 185: 337-340.

THE CYBERNETICS OF BIOLOGICAL MACROMOLECULES

Jeffries Wyman

C.N.R. Center for Molecular Biology, Istituto di
Chimica Biologica, The University, Rome, Italy

Introduction

It used to be said, in accordance with Newtonian philosophy, that every-thing in this world of ours is in some degree related to everything else. And I suppose that at a macroscopic level, the same may still be maintained, although to be sure there are macroscopic situations, as in the case of evolution, where chance, or apparently chance, events, come into play. Nowhere is this interdependence of macroscopic events more apparent than in living organisms, whose very name stems from recognition of their high degree of organization; and nowhere in the organism is this more evident than in the polyfunctional macromolecules of which it is composed. Here the interrelated events to a large extent involve and depend upon the specific binding of smaller molecules which may be regarded as ligands. These may be such simple inorganic substances as proton, oxygen, CO_2, phosphate or other ions, which react with specific sites in the macromolecule, as in the respiratory proteins; or they may be more complex substances such as hormones and neurotrans-mitters or even another macromolecule. The interactions may involve the successive binding of molecules of a given ligand by a set of sites specific for that ligand, or the binding of different ligands by their several sites. In the one case we speak of the interactions as homotropic, in the other as heterotropic; both types are associated with phenomena of cooperativity and anticooperativity. Not only do these linkage effects, as they are called, involve the interdependence of the binding of small ligands by a given macromolecule (as in the case of O_2 and proton or phosphate binding by hemoglobin), but they also involve the con-trol of reactions between macromolecules. Thus whenever a given reaction involving macromolecules leads to an uptake or release of a given ligand, then owing to a dif-ference between the binding of that ligand by the different macromolecular species involved, the equilibrium constant will be a function of the activity of the ligands. This applies equally to polymerization or simple conformational change, and indeed, in polyphase systems, to the distribution of a macromolecule between the several

phases. It is basic to the phenomena of macromolecular assembly.

In this paper we give a brief account of these linkage phenomena as they

show up under equilibrium, steady state, and transient conditions. The simplest case

is that of a one phase system which exists in a state of thermodynamic equilibrium,

and we begin with that.

A One Phase System at Equilibrium

In this case we know that the total energy E is uniquely determined

by values of the total volume V , total entropy S , and total amount X of each of

n components: $\quad E = E(S, V, X_1, \cdots X_n)$

From this the temperature T , pressure p , and the chemical potential μ of each

component are obtained as the corresponding first partial derivatives:

$$T = \frac{\partial E}{\partial S} \; , \quad p = -\frac{\partial E}{\partial V} \; , \quad \mu_i = \frac{\partial E}{\partial X_i} \tag{1}$$

It is to be noticed that E has one particularly important property: if

each of the variables ($S, V, X_1, \cdots X_n$) is multiplied by a factor α , E

is multiplied by the same factor. This means that E is first order homogeneous in

these variables. It follows that each of the above derivatives is O order homo-

geneous in the same variables--its value is independent of the size of the system.

These derivatives are said to be intensive, as distinct from S , V , and the $X's$,

which are extensive.

From Equation (1) we can, by equating cross derivatives, obtain a vari-

ety of linkage relations such as

$$\frac{\partial \mu_i}{\partial X_j} = \frac{\partial \mu_j}{\partial X_i} \quad , \quad \frac{\partial \mu_i}{\partial S} = \frac{\partial T}{\partial X_i} \tag{2}$$

Such relations serve to reduce the number of experimental quantities required to describe the system, and often make it possible to substitute an easier measurement for another more difficult one.

The list of such linkage relations as (2) may be greatly increased by application of a set of Legendre transformations to the energy function to obtain a corresponding set of new functions, or potentials, in which one or more of the extensive variables is replaced by a corresponding intensive one. For example, one such transformation would be to $\phi = E + pV - TS - \mu_1 X_1 = \phi(p, T, \mu_1, X_2, \ldots)$ which has the property that $d\phi = V dp - S dT - X_1 d\mu_1 + \mu_2 d X_2 + \cdots$ and yields a variety of new linkage relations such as

$$\left(\frac{\partial X_1}{\partial X_2}\right)_{p,T,\mu_1,\cdots} = -\left(\frac{\partial \mu_2}{\partial \mu_1}\right)_{p,T,X_2\cdots} \tag{2.1}$$

It will be seen that these potentials occur in pairs of opposites, with one exception. Owing to the fact that the energy is first order homogeneous its opposite, in which all the extensive variables are replaced by corresponding intensive ones, vanishes identically. That this should be so is obvious from physical considerations, for it is clear that, from the values of p, T, and the chemical potentials μ of the components of a system, nothing can be inferred as to its absolute size.

In view of this it is convenient for many purposes to choose one of the components as a reference component, and express the energy and all the extensive variables of which it is a function as amounts per unit of reference component ($1,2$.) This is possible because of the first order homogeneous property of the energy. It reduces the number of independent variables by one and gives us a function, the "normalized" energy, whose opposite _does_ exist, and to which all possible Legendre transformations are applicable. These transformations form a group, of order 2^{n+2-1} and having the symmetry of an $n+2-1$ dimensional rectangle, which is isomorphic with the group of potentials which it generates. From this group all possible link-age relations applicable to the normalized system may at once be obtained. The op-posite of the energy normalized with respect to the amount of any one of the chem-ical components is, except for sign, the same as what has been called the binding potential and denoted by $\varLambda$, the Russian L , for linkage. It has the property that

$$\frac{\partial \varLambda}{\partial \mu_i} = \bar{X}_i = \frac{\partial \varLambda}{RT \delta \ln x_i} \tag{3}$$

where X_i is the activity of component i and $\bar{X}_i$ is its amount per unit of reference component (macromolecule). Similarly $\partial \varLambda / \partial T = \bar{S}$ and $\partial \varLambda / \partial p = -\bar{V}$

From this, by equating cross derivatives, we obtain such linkage relations as

$$\frac{\partial \bar{X}_i}{\partial \mu_j} = \frac{\partial \bar{X}_j}{\partial \mu_i} \quad , \quad \frac{\partial \bar{S}}{\partial \mu_i} = \frac{\partial \bar{X}}{\partial T}$$

By introducing another member of the group, e.g.

$$\varLambda' = \varLambda - \bar{X}_2 \mu_2 = \varLambda'(T, p, \mu_1, \bar{X}_2, \mu_3, \cdots)$$

for which
$$d\varLambda' = \bar{S} dT - \bar{V} dp + \bar{X}_1 d\mu_1 - \mu_2 d\bar{X}_2 + \cdots$$

and again taking account of the equality of cross derivatives we obtain

$$\left(\frac{\partial \bar{S}}{\partial \bar{X}_2}\right)_{T, p, \mu_1, \cdots} = -\left(\frac{\partial \mu_1}{\partial T}\right)_{p \mu, \bar{X}_2, \cdots} \tag{3.1}$$

as the analogue of 2.1 applicable to the normalized system.

An example of the power of this approach is provided by one of the com-ponents of trout hemoglobin (Hb Trout I) (3). The oxygen binding curves of this hemo-globin measured at two temperatures and fixed pH are of the form shown in Fig. 1. If

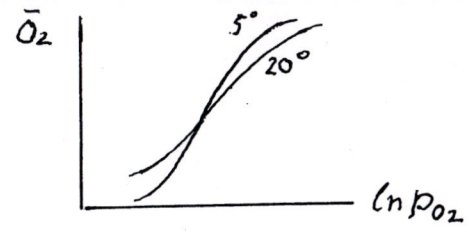

we multiply both sides of 3.1 by T and introduce the re-lation $RT d \ln p_{O_2} = d\mu_{O_2}$

we obtain $\left(\dfrac{\partial \bar{H}}{\partial \bar{O}_2}\right)_{T,pH} = -RT^2\left(\dfrac{\partial \ln p_{O_2}}{\partial T}\right)_{\bar{O}_2,pH}$ where $\bar{H}$ denotes heat content per

heme equivalent. When applied to the results shown in Fig. 1 this tells us at once

that there is a change of sign in the heat of oxygenation of the four site molecule

from a negative to a positive value as the reaction proceeds. This surely reflects

some profound change in the macromolecule accompanying ligation. The subject of li-

gand induced changes in the state of a macromolecule as a basis of linkage will be

discussed in the next section. In order to prepare the way for it we pause to con-

sider the effect of the ligands on the equilibrium constant for the reaction involv-

ing several macromolecules.

It is easily shown, by comparison with the Gibbs-Duhem equation, that

Π is equal to minus the chemical potential of the reference component expressed as

a function of the intensive variables p , T , and the chemical potentials μ of

each of the ligands. This provides the basis for a general formulation of the equi-

librium constant for a reaction involving a set of macromolecules. Take the simple

case of the reaction $A \to B$. For this reaction we can write

$$\Pi_B - \Pi_A = -\Delta G_0 = RT \ln K$$

K being the equilibrium constant. Consequently

$$K = K_0 \, e^{(\Pi_a - \Pi_A)/RT}$$

(4)

where K_0 is a constant depending on the choice of standard states. Since the two

$\Pi's$ are functions of p , T , and the chemical potentials of all the ligands, e-

quation (4) embodies the dependence of the equilibrium constant for the macromolecular

reaction on all these quantities. Written in differential form

$$RT\, d\ln K = d\Pi_B - d\Pi_A = (\bar{S}_B - \bar{S}_A)\, dT - (\bar{V}_B - \bar{V}_A)\, dp + \sum (\bar{X}_{iB} - \bar{X}_{iA})\, d\mu_i$$

(5)

it becomes an immediate source of the vant Hoff equation for the reaction as it occurs at constant p and constant values of the chemical potentials of the ligands; alternatively it shows how K varies with the activity of a given ligand in accordance with the difference between the binding of that ligand by two macromolecules. Furthermore, introducing the equality of the cross derivatives, it shows how the heat of the reaction varies with the chemical potentials of the ligands··and provides other similar relations. It is, in particular, applicable to the case where a macromolecule exists in several different forms (or conformations) which differ in their binding properties for their ligands. Likewise, if we treat entropy (and heat) as ligands, it governs the effect of temperature on thermal transitions of a macromolecule such for instance as the melting of DNA (4). More generally it applies to polymerization, or to such reactions as the reversible combination of an antigen with its antibody, or finally to macromolecular assembly. A good example of the last is provided by certain of the haemocyanins which consist of disparate subunits whose association is sensitive to various ions and to oxygen (5).

Linkage Mechanisms

Up to now our discussion has been purely phenomenological. Like all thermodynamic analyses it has had nothing to say about mechanism, that is, about the molecular basis for the various linkage effects. Moreover, due to its complete generality, it has not distinguished true binding, governed by mass law relations, from binding represented by activity effects. Indeed in borderline cases it is hard to do so. Sometimes, to be sure, there are specific and obvious spectral changes associated with the/binding of a ligand, as in the case of oxygen binding by the respiratory proteins; also there may be NMR signals associated with the binding of specific ions. But this is by no means always the case, and more often than not we lack, as it were, the necessary"spectacles" to distinguish between the two.

Why is it, in the case of true binding, that the presence of a molecule of ligand at one site in a large molecule should affect the probability of the binding of another molecule of ligand, the same or different, at another site, perhaps very far away? Sometimes of course this may be due to gross electrostatic effects, as in the case of proton binding by a large polybasic acid such as a protein. But this cannot be an explanation of the positive homotropic cooperativity observed in many respiratory proteins and enzymes. Nor can such cooperativity be explained on the basis of the instability of free radicals as in the case of the <u>nearly</u> two step oxidation of many small organic molecules such as the quinones.

It has now been fairly well established that the explanation of a great variety of linkage effects involving often widely separated sites in large molecules is to be found in ligand linked changes in the physical state of the macromolecule. Such changes may be purely conformational, without change of molecular weight, or they may involve aggregation or dissociation. In the former case, which is the simpler one to deal with, they are called allosteric; in the latter, polysteric. Conceptually the picture is extremely simple, based on the general principle that whenever to a macromolecular system at equilibrium a given ligand is added, the equilibrium will shift in such a way as to favor the forms which have the higher affinity for the ligand. This immediately provides a qualitative explanation of why homotropic interactions al-show positive cooperativity   whereas the heterotropic ones can be either positively or negatively cooperative (6).

The concept may be made more precise by introduction of the relations given above for the effect of a ligand on an equilibrium involving macromolecules. This is particularly simple in the case of an allosteric system where the macromolecule exists in a number of different conformations $1, 2, \dots t$. In this case the amount of ligand X bound per macromolecule is given by

$$\bar{X} = \frac{M_1 \bar{X}_1 + M_2 \bar{X}_2 + \cdots M_t \bar{X}_t}{M_1 + M_2 + \cdots M_t}$$

where each M denotes the concentration of macromolecule in a particular conformation. From this, by assuming the activity of each form of the macromolecule to be proportional to M and writing the equilibrium constant for the transformation from conformation 1 to conformation i as $K_{1i} = (K_{1i})_0\, e^{(\Pi_i - \Pi_1)/RT}$ and $\bar{X}_i$ as $\partial \Pi_i / \partial \mu_x$ we obtain

$$\bar{X} = \frac{e^{\Pi_1/RT}\,\partial\Pi_1/\partial\mu_x + (K_{12})_0\, e^{\Pi_2/RT}\,\partial\Pi_2/\partial\mu_x + \cdots (K_{1t})_0\, e^{\Pi_t/RT}\,\partial\Pi_t/\partial\mu_x}{e^{\Pi_1/RT} + (K_{12})_0\, e^{\Pi_2/RT} + \cdots (K_{1t})_0\, e^{\Pi_t/RT}}$$

$$= \frac{\partial \ln[\, e^{\Pi_1/RT} + (K_{12})_0\, e^{\Pi_2/RT} + \cdots (K_{1t})_0\, e^{\Pi_t/RT}]}{\partial \mu_x}$$

$$= \frac{\partial \ln (\, v_{10}\, e^{\Pi_1/RT} + v_{20}\, e^{\Pi_2/RT} + \cdots v_{t0}\, e^{\Pi_t/RT})}{RT\,\partial \ln x}$$

where the $v_0's$ denote the mole fractions of the macromolecule in the various conformations in the absence of ligand, (or where the ligand is in some specified standard state). From this, taking account of the relation $\partial \Pi/\partial \mu_x = \bar{X}$ applicable to the whole system, we obtain as binding potential for the whole macromolecule the expression

$$\Pi/RT = \ln \sum_i e^{\Pi_i/RT}$$

(6)

Here Π is a function of p, T, and the chemical potentials μ of all the ligands;

when differentiated partially with respect to any one of these it gives the value of the corresponding extensive variable expressed per unit of reference component (macromolecule). (It should be noted that when we differentiate with respect to temperature the factor RT is to be treated as a constant. This is due to the fact that the activities, which enter into the mass law, are defined independently of the temperature.)

Except for the approximation involved in taking the activity of each form of the macromolecule as proportional to its concentration, Equation 6 is quite general and applies equally to true binding or to binding associated with activity effects or to a combination of the two. When we limit ourselves to true binding, say of ligand X at constant p and T, the equation may be expressed in a more readily applicable form. If we assume that in each conformation there are q_i independent sites and that the binding to each is described by a simple mass law equation, then

$$\bar{X}_i = \frac{k_{i1} X}{1 + k_{i1} X} + \cdots \frac{k_{it} X}{1 + k_{it} X} = \frac{\partial \Pi_i}{\partial \mu_x} = \frac{\partial \Pi_i}{RT \partial \ln X}$$

and integration gives

$$\Pi_i = RT \ln \left(1 + k_{i1} X\right)\left(1 + k_{i2} X\right) \cdots \left(1 + k_{iq_i} X\right)$$

As a result Equation 6 becomes

$$\Pi = RT \ln \sum_i \left(\nu_{i0} \left(1 + k_{i1} X\right)\left(1 + k_{i2} X\right) \cdots \left(1 + k_{iq_i} X\right)\right.$$

$$(7)$$

We have only to differential this with respect to $\mu_x = RT \ln x$ to get the total binding of X per macromolecule. If we further assume, as in the so called MWC model, that there are only two (quarternary) conformations and that the sites in each are identical, then Equation 7 becomes

$$\pi = RT \ln \left(V_{10} (1 + k_r x)^q + V_{20} (1 + k_R x)^q \right) = RT \ln \left((1 + k_r x)^q + L_0 (1 + k_R x)^q \right) \tag{8}$$

where $L_0 = V_{20} / V_{10}$

In this special case it follows from Equation 8 that the binding curve (X vs $\ln x$) is at every point steeper than a simple titration curve. More generally, quite apart from the shape of the curve, it is clear that the total free energy of binding is always reduced as a result of the allosteric transitions, which we might describe as a progressive yielding of the macromolecule to the ligand.

It will be seen that the expansion of the sum in Equation 7 always gives rise to a polynomial. This may or may not be factorable into subpolynomials with real positive coefficients (no others are physically acceptable). If it is completely factorable into first degree factors the allosteric macromolecule will be indistinguishable in terms of functional binding from a simple molecule with q independent sites. In this case the binding curve (normalized to a single site) can nowhere be steeper than a simple titration curve; contrariwise, if at any point the curve is steeper than a simple titration curve, we know at once that the polynomial is not completely factorable and that there are site interactions. A "prime" factor (with real positive coefficients) may be interpreted in terms of a set of interacting sites. The question of the factorability of the binding polynomial has been the subject of much discussion. It takes one back to the nineteenth century algebra of Cayley and Sylvester (7).

When we take account of the presence of other chemical ligands the poly-

nomial will include other activities, one for each ligand. Here again the concept
of factorability comes in. If this mixed polynomial is factorable into separate
polynomials, one for each ligand, it means of course that the ligands are independent.
Otherwise they will be either positively or negatively linked.

The behavior of various hemoglobins and some other macromolecules has
been exhaustively studied, both kinetically and under conditions of equilibrium, in
accordance with these concepts. In the case of human hemoglobin (HbA) the oxygen
binding curve at fixed pH can be surprisingly well accounted for on the basis of the
simplest allosteric model--the MWC model with only two conformations in each of which
the four oxygen combining sites are the same and independent, and the existence of
two such quarternary conformations has been confirmed by Xray crystallography. In
HbA, however, studies of the influence of other ligands, particularly proton, when
analyzed in terms of the allosteric model, suggest that there must be additional allosteric effects local to each of the four subunits (the 2α and 2β chains). It
is an easy matter to expand the formal relations developed above to take account of
such a situation and indeed to generalize Equation 6 to include a hierarchy of nested
conformational changes, one inside the other. To do this we have only to write Equation 6 as
$$\Pi/RT = \ln \sum v_{io} e^{\Pi_i/RT}$$
and express each Π_i/RT in the same way. Upon continuing the process we
have an expression which is reminiscent of Mandelbrot's geometrical concept of fractals
("scaled fractals"), patterns which look the same seen under any degree of magnifica-
tion.

From a teleological point of view heterotropic interactions, as a basis
of regulation and control at a molecular level, are of the greatest importance, particularly in enzymes, and the allosteric mechanism which makes them possible must be
regarded as a major development in macromolecular evolution. Homotropic interactions

too, represented in the steepening of the binding curve for a given ligand, say oxygen in the case of the respiratory proteins, can be of great value in transport phenomena. The steepness of a binding curve is limited by the number of sites in the macromolecule, or in its subunits. In the case of some of the larger hemocyanins and some of the giant invertebrate hemoglobins, the number of sites may exceed 100, and the steepness of the binding curve may be very great. Closer consideration, however suggests that these superlarge molecules do not change confromation as a unit, but exist in constellations of sites forming more or less independent allosterically functioning subunits (8). A possible reason for this might be a kinetic one; the relaxation time associated with a conformational change would be expected to increase with the size of the unit (think of the effect of size on the rotary diffusion constant of a macromolecule) and if it were too great it might impair the efficiency of the circulating vehicle of transport. There are indications that in the kinetics of the oxygenation of the hemocyanins the conformational change is rate limiting, just the opposite of what is found in hemoglobin (9).

Polysteric and Polyphasic Linkage

When we come to polysteric linkage, involving the ligand linked association or dissociation of a macromolecule, the underlying principles remain the same, but the formalism is more complex, and it is no longer possible to formulate the binding potential in terms of a single polynomial like that given above ((0,11). A type case is provided by human hemoglobin. Under non-physiological conditions, namely at very high dilution, this hemoglobin undergoes an oxygen linked dissociation into dimers ($\alpha\beta$ subunits) and the tetramer-dimer equilibrium gives rise to much the same cooperativity of oxygen binding as the normal allosteric change (12). In sickle cell hemoglobin (HbS), which is the cause of the genetic disease known as sickle cell anemia in man, a similar polysteric linkage is greatly magnified and moved up into the physiological range. When HbS above a certain critical concentration is deoxygenated it polymerizes to form elongated aggregates which have been likened to microtubules, and which distort the cells in such a way as to impede their free passage through the capillaries. This extreme instance of a polysteric phenomena, which really amounts to a ligand controlled phase change, generates a large amount of cooperativity of oxygen binding, in itself not detrimental, indeed rather the reverse. In the present connection, however, it is of interest primarily as an example of the way in which a ligand can serve as a mechanism of control for the formation of a subcellular structure as a new phase--at almost every level a living cell is to be thought of as a polyphasic system. Thus to the phenomena of allosteric and polysteric linkage we may add that of polyphasic linkage.

Linkage Under Steady State Conditions

Thus far we have limited the discussion to linkage under conditions of equilibrium where the principles of classical thermodynamics are applicable. True equilibrium however is rare in biological systems.More commonly such systems exist in a steady state or a transient state. This is true of all functioning enzymes, and even the circulating blood, when looked at as a whole, is to be regarded as representing a steady state (13). Seen from the outside, superficially, a steady state may be hard to distinguish from an equilibrium state, but in terms of the governing equations there is all the difference in the world between them. In the case of a steady state there are no potentials to rely on, and the resulting powerful reciprocal linkage relations described above are lacking. As a result we are left alone with the kinetic equations. In a large number of cases of biological interest these will be first order, and in what follows we limit ourselves to such.

Consider a simple allosteric system in which a macromolecule exists in two conformations T and R in each of which it can combine with a ligand X at a single site. Then there will be four possible states of the molecule which can be

represented by a square and which we designate by 1,2,3,4. If we limit ourselves to

$$(1) \; T \; \underset{k_{-2}}{\overset{k_2}{\rightleftarrows}} \; TX \; (2)$$

$$k_1 \Big\Updownarrow k_{-1} \qquad k_{-3} \Big\Updownarrow k_3$$

$$(4) \; R \; \underset{k_4}{\overset{k_{-4}}{\rightleftarrows}} \; RX \; (3)$$

one step transitions, the system will be described by the 8 kinetic constants $k_1, \cdots k_{-4}$, as shown, and if we denote the activity

(concentration) of the ligand by X we have the four kinetic equations

$$
\begin{aligned}
\dot{T} &= -(k_2 X + k_{-1})T \;+\; k_{-2} TX \;+ O\; RX \;+\; k_1 R \\
\dot{TX} &= \quad k_2 X T \;-(k_{-2}+k_3) TX \;+\; k_{-3} RX \;+ O\cdot R \\
\dot{RX} &= \qquad O \cdot T \;+\; k_3 TX \;-(k_4+k_{-3}) RX + k_{-4} X R \\
\dot{R} &= \quad k_{-1} T \;+ O \cdot TX \;+\; k_4 RX \;-(k_1 + k_{-4} X) R
\end{aligned}
\qquad (9)
$$

where dot denotes time derivative. It will be seen that these equations provide for

the conservation of the macromolecule. Moreover, if X is held constant they are

linear, and it can be shown that their solution involves 3 relaxation times given by

the roots λ of the secular equation

$$
\left|
\begin{array}{cccc}
[-(k_2 X + k_{-1}) - \lambda] & k_{-2} & O & k_{-4} \\
k_2 & [-(k_{-2}+k_3)-\lambda] & k_{-3} & O \\
O & k_3 & [-(k_4+k_3)-\lambda] & k_{-4} X \\
k_{-1} & O & k_4 & (-[k_1 + k_{-4} X] - \lambda
\end{array}
\right| = 0
\qquad (10)
$$

one of the roots being O. In this simple case a full solution is possible and it can

be shown that there is a unique critical point asymptotically stable in the large.

That is, there is a steady state which will always be approached regardless of the

starting point. Provided the velocity constants satisfy the condition of the micro-

scopic balance, namely that the product of those pointing clockwise round the square

be equal to that ofthose pointing counterclockwise, this steady state will be a true
equilibrium. But when this condition is not fulfilled certain unexpected things can
happen and in the steady state there will be a circulation of the macromolecule round
the equare in one direction or the other depending on the values of the constants.
The amounts of the various forms of the macromolecule are proportional to the cofactors of the elements of the top row of the matrix obtained from Equation (9) and the
binding curve of even a one site macromolecule may show cooperativity or anticooperativity (14).

When other conformations and other ligands (for each of which there may
be more than one site) are present, the number of governing equations is increased
by one for each new form of the macromolecule, and the square will be replaced by a
multidimensional cube. But the principles illustrated by the simpler case remain the
same. There will always be a steady state, unique and asymptotically stable in the
large. The number of relaxation times involved in the approach to this steady state
will be one less than the number of different forms of the macromolecule. The amounts
of the various forms in the steady state will be proportional to the cofactors of the
elements of the first row of the now enlarged matrix obtained from the governing
equations, and thus there will be a linkage between the binding of the various ligands
and at the same time the conformation of the macromolecule will be controlled by the
various ligand activities. Microscopic balance now depends on equality of the clockwise and counterclockwise products of the constants round each face of the cube; and
in the absence of such balance there will be a circulation of the macromolecule round
the edges of the cube as in the simpler two dimensional case. Under these conditions
the macromolecule can act as a free energy transducer (14).

Free Energy Transduction

Suppose the macromolecule is an enzyme for which there are two substrates X and Y which are released by the enzyme in the forms X' and Y' as indicated in Figure 2.

$$
\begin{array}{ccc}
& (1) & (2) \\
M+Y' \underset{}{\overset{}{\rightleftharpoons}} MY & \overset{k_2}{\underset{k_{-2}}{\rightleftharpoons}} & MXY \\
k_1 \Big\uparrow \Big\downarrow k_{-1} & & k_{-3}\Big\uparrow \Big\downarrow k_3 \\
M & \overset{k_{-4}}{\underset{k_4}{\rightleftharpoons}} & MX \rightleftharpoons M+X' \\
(4) & & (3)
\end{array}
$$

(In this simple example there is no need to consider a conformational change. The presence of a second ligand plays the same role.) Provided the activities of the substrates X and Y and their products X' and Y' are maintained at constant non equilibrium values the kinetic equations will be linear and there will be a steady state in which there is a circulation of the enzyme round the square, clockwise or counterclockwise in accordance with whichever of the reactions $MX \to M+X'$ and $MY \to M+Y'$ is master, i.e. whichever involves the greater free energy change. Thus the free energy derived from one reaction is used to drive the other. All this may be formulated more precisely if desired by writing down the equations in detail. It will then be seen how the addition of the constants for the side reaction destroys the condition of microscopic balance, assuming it to be obeyed in their absence (14).

The Existence of a Steady State When the Equations are Non Linear

Often, and in fact generally, the first order kinetic equations will not be strictly linear. This will be so in polysteric systems and whenever the activities of the ligands are not maintained at strictly constant values. Under these conditions the problem of establishing whether or not there is a steady state, unique and asymptotically stable, as in the linear case, becomes vastly more complicated. To be sure, if all the constants satisfy the condition of microscopic balance the physical principles of thermodynamics tell us that the system will surely come to thermodynamic equilibrium; but otherwise the question remains open. In the latter case there is no secular equation and the possibility of some kind of limit cycle cannot be ruled out. However the problem has been rigorously dealt with, and the existence of a steady state, with all the implications which it carries, has been established in the case of a simple but not unrepresentative model system (15). This system was suggested by consideration of the visual system involving rhodopsin which undergoes a series of photochemical reactions in the presence of light. It may be represented by the following scheme

$$
\begin{array}{ccc}
(1) & \xrightarrow{\;k_2\;} & (2) \\
MN & \underset{k_{-2}}{\rightleftharpoons} & MNX \\
k_1 \Big\uparrow \Big\downarrow k_{-1} & & k_{-3} \Big\uparrow \Big\downarrow k_3 \\
(4)\; M+N & \underset{k_4}{\overset{k_{-4}}{\rightleftharpoons}} & M+NX \;(3)
\end{array}
$$

in which MN stands for the intact macromolecule composed of a protein moiety N which has one site for a ligand X of activity (concentration) x, and a prosthetic group M, which does not combine with X.

The kinetic equations for this scheme are the following:

$$
\dot{MN} = -(k_2 x + k_{-1}) MN + k_{-2} MNX + 0 \cdot M \cdot NX + k_1 M \cdot N
$$

$$
\dot{MNX} = k_2 x \cdot MN - (k_{-2} + k_3) MNX + k_{-3} M \cdot NX + 0 M \cdot N
$$

$$
\dot{NX} = 0 \cdot MN + k_3 \cdot MNX - (k_{-3} M + k_4) \cdot NX + k_{-4} X \cdot N
$$

$$
\dot{N} = k_{-1} MN + 0 \cdot MNX + k_4 \cdot NX - (k_1 M + k_{-4} X) M
$$

$$
(11)
$$

It will be seen that these equations satisfy the condition of conserva-
of the macromolecule. At the same time they are subject to the constraints

$$M + MN + MNX = C_M$$
$$MN + MNX + N + NX = C_N \tag{12}$$
$$X = C_X - MNX - NX$$

where C_M is half the total number of subunits and C_X is the total amount of ligand. From the first and second equations (12) it follows that $M = N$
which shows that it would be redundant to include an equation for $\dot{M}$.

The proof for the existence of a steady state even in this simple case
is difficult and involved, and the reader is referred to the original paper (15).
It is noteworthy, however, that in the special case where the constants satisfy the
condition of microscopic balance, the existence of a unique steady state asymptotically stable in the large follows immediately from the laws of thermodynamics, which
may themselves be regarded as existence theorems based on experience. Thus physical
principles here provide the solution of what would seem to be a purely mathematical
problem. Clearly it would be of interest to see how far the above model system could
be expanded without destroying the proof. In view of what has just been said, it
might be conjectured that in any system where, in the special case that the kinetic
constants satisfy microscopic balance, there is thermodynmaic equilibrium, there will,
even in the absence of microscopic balance, be a unique and globally stable critical
point.

Transients

The foregoing analysis has been limited to macromolecular systems either
in thermodynamic equilibrium or in a steady state. When we attempt to extend it to
transient states, involving an approach either to equilibrium or to a steady state,
we are confronted by a far more difficult problem. Indeed when the kinetic equations
are non linear and we cannot even be sure that they admit of a solution in the large,

and where in any case there is no secular equation, it would seem to be wholly beyond us. Nevertheless under limited conditions, especially when the equations are
linear, much can be deduced from them, and much has indeed already been learned from
experimental studies of the transient behavior of respiratory proteins and enzymes
as they relax either to equilibrium or to a steady state. Most of these experiments
have been carried out either by the temperature jump or the stopped flow method under
conditions where the equations can be treated as linear.

　　There has recently been given a rigorous analysis, within the framework
of the preceding discussion, of relaxation in three particularly simple model systems in which the equations are linear and allow of exact solution with the aid of
the generating function technique (16). Each of these models represents a variant
of the original two state concerted model of Monod, Wyman and Changeux, which can be
represented by the ladder shown in Figure 2. Here the arms correspond to the two
conformational states T and R of the macromolecule and the rungs to the allosteric
transitions between the different liganded forms. Here we give only the briefest out-

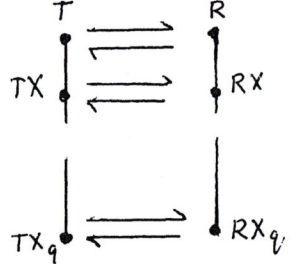

line of what was done.

　　In accordance with the original MWC model it was assumed throughout that in each conformation the sites
were identical and independent, hav-
ing the same velocity and equilibrium constants. In the first model one conformation was eliminated, so that the kinetic ladder was reduced to one side. In the second model the structural velocity constants, corresponding to the rungs of the
ladder, were assumed to be all the same, independent of the degree of ligation. This
corresponds to the most extreme departure from microscopic balance and it gives a
set of eigen values of fairly simple form although the probability of site occupancy

becomes a rather complicated function of time. In the third model the velocity of either the "on" reactions or the "off" reactions were supposed to be negligible, so that either the combination or dissociation of ligand was irreversible. This corresponds to many of the experiments made with the stopped flow technique, and the model, quite apart from its inherent interest, is useful in providing a starting point for dealing with the general case by successive approximations in which we progressively eliminate irreversibility, starting from either end. Altogether, in spite of the highly limited nature of the models involved, this analysis is useful in the light it throws on the concept of transients.

Conclusion

In this brief account I have endeavored to develop the concept of linkage, both homotropic and heterotropic, which is so fundamental at every level of organization in living systems in terms of macroscopic concepts. In doing this I have focused attention on a macromolecule, or set of interacting molecules, in the presence of a set of ligands as representing the middle ground from which one may proceed either upwards or downwards in scale.Three cases have been considered, namely when the system is in thermodynamic equilibrium,in a steady state,or in a transient state;and the analysis has been developed to cover three possible model systems,allosteric,polysteric, polyphasic.Metaphorically one can think of a macromolecule as a community of interacting ligands, of which the solvent is an important member, linked through the macromolecule and interacting with it, and of larger systems as communities of interacting macromolecules. Thus such diverse phenomena as the Bohr effect or phosphate effect in respiratory proteins, the regulation of enzymes by activators and inhibitors, the interaction of antigen and antibody, macromolecular assembly, neurotransmission, are brought under one roof. In this picture everything hangs on the existence of a steady state, defined by the ligands, towards which, as towards a goal, the system is re-

laxing, without perhaps ever reaching it before it changes, or about which it is
fluctuating whenever, as is often the case, the energy of transition from one state
to another is of the order of kT. The times involved in the relaxations will vary
enormously, from picoseconds to seconds, depending on the size of the elements involved, whether assemblies of macromolecules, or the smallest parts of a single macromolecule. One is reminded once again of the concept of scaled fractals and white
noise, and if there were correlations between the fluctuations, as has been suggested (7), the white noise might be converted into Brownian noise, and further, and
this might provide a clue to the riddle of the enzymes--why it is that such large
and complex molecules are required to perform what is often such a simple task, for
example, the hydration of carbondioxide by carbonic anhydrase.

References
1. Wyman, J. (1965) J. Mol. Biol. 11, 631-644.
2. Wyman, J. (1975) Proc. Nat. Acad. Sci. U.S.A. 72, 1464-1468.
3. Wyman, J., Gill, S.J., Noll, L., Giardina, B., Colosimo, A. and Brunori, M.(1977) J. Mol. Biol. 109, 195-205.
4. Wyman, J., Gill, S.J. and Colosimo, A, (1979) Biophys. Chem. 10,363-369.
5. van Driel, R. and van Bruggen, E.F.J. (1974) Biochemistry 13, 4079-4083.
6. Bardsley W.G. and Wyman J. (1978) J. Theor.Biol. 72, 373-374.
7. Bardsley W.G. and Waight, R.D. (1978) J. Theor. Biol. 72, 321-372.
8. Colosimo, A., Brunori, M. and Wyman, J. (1974) Biophys. Chem. 2, 338-344.
9. van Driel, R., Kuiper, H.A., Antonini, E.and Brunori, M. (1978) J. Mol. Biol. 121, 431-439.
10. Colosimo, A;, Brunori, M. and Wyman, J. (1976) J. Mol. Biol. 100,47-57.
11. Woolfson, R. and Bardsley W.G. (1980 in press) J. Mol. Biol. 136.
12. Thomas, J.O. and Edelstein, S.J. (1972) J. Biol. Chem. 247, 7870-7884.
13. Wyman, J. (1978) Atti della Accad. Naz. Lincei, Roma, Serie VIII   LXIV,409-413.
14. Wyman, J. (1975) Proc. Nat. Acad. Sci. U.S.A. 72,3983-3987.
15. Fichera, G., Sneider, M.A. and Wyman, J. (1977) Atti della Accad. Naz. Lincei, Roma, Serie VIII vol. XIV, 1-27.
16. Phillipson, P.E. and Wyman, J. (1980) Biopolymers (In press).
17. Careri, G., Fasella, P. and Gratton, E. (1979) Ann. Rev. Biophys. Bioeng. 8, 19-97.

A PATTERN FORMATION MECHANISM

AND ITS APPLICATION TO MAMMALIAN COAT MARKINGS

J.D. Murray,
Mathematical Institute,
University of Oxford,
England.

1. Introduction

This paper is in a general sense concerned with biological pattern formation but more specifically with the development of the pre-patterns for mammalian skin markings.

Until Wolpert's (1969) seminal paper on positional information and the pattern of cellular differentiation the general area of pattern formation in developmental biology was rather neglected. He was concerned with spatial differentiation and how genetic information can be translated to give specific patterns of cellular differentiation. His model, developed further by him and his co-workers in subsequent papers, essentially assigns positional information to cells which subsequently develop pattern according to certain rules. In a more recent paper Lewis et al. (1977) consider the interpretation of gradients in positional information. They consider a simple kinetic model for a gene product, which exhibits positive feedback and threshold effects and relate the solution behaviour to a background gradient of a diffusible morphogen.

To date most developmental fields found experimentally are of the order of 1 mm or about 100 cell-diameters in length. Here we anticipate fields which are larger than these, which we consider to operate on the relatively large integument of embryos at an early stage in their development. We propose here a model mechanism for generating the pre-pattern for observed mammalian skin markings.

There are several books specifically on animal colouration such

as those by Fox and Vevers (1960), Bagnara and Hadley (1973), which
is mainly concerned with colour change in animals, and Searle (1968)
on comparative genetics of animal colouration. The latter hypothesized that a reaction-diffusion mechanism might be responsible for
mammalian coat colour.

It is generally accepted that developmental pattern and specifically colour patterns in mammals are genetically determined but
the actual mechanism of this pattern formation is not known. We
suggest that a reaction-diffusion mechanism could be responsible
for most of the colouration patterns. That a single mechanism could
suffice for this has also been suggested independently by Findlay
(1978) from his work with zebra and giraffe. Bard (1977) proposed
that a single mechanism, as yet unknown, is responsible for the stripe
pattern of the zebra.

Mammalian colouration is due to melanin in the epidermis and
is present in pigment cells called melanocytes which derive from
embryonic neural crest material from where they migrate (diffuse)
as melanoblasts with genes determining which cells become melanoblasts. In colour regions melanocytes undergo mitotic division
providing a continous turnover of melanin. According to McLaren
(1976), in her definitive work on mammalian chimaeras, colours mark
the areas where melanoblasts exists and can move about freely. On
the other hand, Bagnara and Hadley (1973) suggest from evidence on
mice that melanoblasts can migrate into white areas but do not differentiate. In any event there is no doubt that the epidermal distribution of melanocytes is not uniform and by inference, their
precursors.

From graft experiments it seems that melanogenesis is caused
or related to the availability of some substrate. In the model
mechanism proposed below in effect we use such a concept in the

form of some (genetically controlled or triggered) negative or
positive melanogenesis inhibitor which affects the governing reactions
in a realistic pattern formation way.

The essentials of melanogenesis is given by the Raper-Mason
theory [see, for example, Nicolaus (1968)] in which tyrosine, a
precursor of melanin, is oxidized to DOPA in the presence of the
enzyme tyrosinase. Further oxidations result in polymerisation to
melanin.

In spite of the wide variety of epidermal patterns in vertebrates there is a paucity of detailed experimental work. Important
work on mice has been done by Mayer (1967) and Mintz (1967, 1971).
A critical survey of chimaeric mice is given in the book by McLaren
(1976) including a detailed discussion of lateral striping that was
found by Mintz (1967) in a series of experiments in which she obtained
allophenic (chimaeric) mice by aggregating pairs of genotypically
different embryos at the cleavage stage. Lateral striping was
frequently found when black and white genotypes were used. Mintz
(1967) on the basis of her experiments suggested that the patterns
in chimaeric mice were non-random. Lateral striping is a natural
consequence of our mechanism if the geometry is appropriate at the
time of laying down of the pre-pattern. Wolpert and Gingell (1970)
suggested the patterns could be random. The conclusions of the
research presented below indicate a certain randomness but in which
there are limits to the allowed (random) number of stripes.

Reaction-diffusion models have been proposed for generating
spatial patterns in ecology: see, for example Okubo (1979) for a
survey. In connection with slime mould aggregation a chemotactic
reaction-diffusion system has been developed with considerable
success: see the survey article by Segel (1976). Another notable
application of a reaction-diffusion type of theory is that by

Meinhardt and Gierer (1974: see earlier references there) on hydra. The model they use is phenomenological and not specifically derived from a specific practical mechanism. A pedagogical discussion of some practical applications of reaction-diffusion systems among other things is given in the book by Murray (1977). Recent published lecture notes by Fife (1979) give a comprehensive survey of the more important mathematical results that have accrued over the past decade.

The extensively studied Belousov-Zhabotinskii reaction is a practical mechanism which exhibits oscillatary behaviour and spatial patterns in the form of waves of chemical concentration. A simple introduction to the system is given by Murray (1977) with a more detailed survey by Tyson (1976). Experimentally Winfree (1974: see also 1978 for a more recent general discussion) has demonstrated many of the dramatic features of this reaction.

The main mathematical results from the analysis in this paper relate to the predictability of finite amplitude spatial pattern from the linearized theory. In one (space) dimension, Mimura and Murray (1978a) considered a model predator-prey system which could be driven unstable by diffusion in the Turing (1952) sense. They thought that this could be a possible contributing factor to observed planktonic patchiness in the sea. They found that linear theory predicted a fastest growing unstable mode. Numerical computation of the finite amplitude structure from the full nonlinear equations showed that the linear theory gave an accurate qualitative prediction of the ultimate heterogeneous structure. Mimura and Murray (1978b) showed that the same situation obtained for the Seelig (1976) mechanism. What is shown below is that in two (and higher) dimensional domains the finite amplitude structure bears no (obvious) relation to the fastest growing linearly unstable mode. The finite amplitude heterogeneity depends on the initial conditions and of course the boundary conditions.

Although, for given initial conditions, the finite amplitude structure was unique small variations in the initial conditions resulted in quite different spatial patterns in that the distribution was different although the general qualitative overall character was similar. This inevitably leads to a certain randomness in the final spatial patterns obtained from reaction-diffusion mechanisms. This is a positive aspect from the point of view of a mechanism for animal coat patterns which exhibit, within the same species, a randomness but in general only within certain bounds. For example, all leopards are spotted but the distribution of the spots is unique to each animal.

This two-dimensional domain behaviour probably has a bearing on the reaction-diffusion theory proposed by Kauffman et al. (1978) for the regular patterns clonal lines found in the wing disc of Drosophila.

In the following Section 2 we describe an experimental situation which is the basis of our illustrative model mechanism while in Section 3 we demonstrate the pattern formation process, essentially a Turing type diffusive domain heterogeneity. In Sections 4 and 5 we discuss the role of geometry and the application of the results to specific animal markings.

2.   SUBSTRATE INHIBITION REACTION-DIFFUSION MODEL MECHANISM

The melanin production process is very complicated and it is premature here to try and model the specific reaction mechanism. This is not our main purpose since we are concerned with pre-pattern. We thus have in mind a mechanism for generating, say, one of the necessary reactants in melanogenesis. We consider a fairly general system which has certain key features common to many practical substrate inhibition reaction mechanisms.

The generally highly efficient role of enzymes in enzyme catalyzed systems frequently allows a multi-species mechanism to be reduced to one with fewer species by using the fact that many of the reactions involving the enzymes are effectively at equilibrium. The model substrate-inhibition reaction mechanism proposed by Seelig (1976) is a detailed case to point: it is a practical example of the general class taken here and it demonstrates a realistic reduction from a multi-species system to a tractable two-species one. We consider a mechanism which also reduces to a two-species system; it has been studied experimentally by Thomas (1976). It suffices to demonstrate many of the observed structural patterns in animal markings even though we discuss only a few of the vast number of spatial structures possible. We thus hypothesize that reaction-diffusion mechanisms can produce practically all of the observed colour patterns on animals and is therefore a possible universal mechanism for the laying down of the pre-pattern for coat markings in animals.

Melanogenesis involves the precursor tyrosine which combines with the melanocytes to produce melanin. Critical to this process is the presence of the enzyme tyrosinase. We propose for the main features of the pre-pattern formation (almost certainly before the arrival at the epidermal surface of the melanoblasts) a multi-species mechanism which reduces to a two species system, for S and A say, which involves substrate inhibition, with S a substrate of higher molecular weight than the cosubstrate A . One of the species could be associated for example with the critical tyrosinase or the tyrosine.

We consider the species to diffuse on a two-dimensional surface on which they also react with a given rate: the experimental arrangement of Thomas (1976) has a surface on which the enzyme catalyst is immobilized. The specific Thomas-scheme has the enzyme uricase immobilized on an artificial membrane in which uric acid and oxygen can diffuse and react under the enzyme catalyzed reaction

$$\text{uric acid} + \text{oxygen} \xrightarrow{\text{uricase}} \text{allontoïn} + \text{other products}$$
$$\text{(S)} \qquad \text{(A)} \qquad \text{(E)}$$

where S and A denote the concentrations of the substrate, uric acid, and the cosubstrate oxygen respectively. The reaction and diffusion take place on a membrane of thickness L_2 (of the order of 50 μ) above which there is an inactive membrane of thickness L_1 through which S and A diffuse from a reservoir maintained at constant concentrations S_0 and A_0 . The lateral dimension of the membrane is L.

The reaction-diffusion equation governing each species is of the form

$$\frac{\text{time rate}}{\text{of change}} = \frac{\text{flux of species}}{\text{to surface (F)}} - \frac{\text{reaction}}{\text{rate (G)}} + \frac{\text{diffusion}}{\text{on surface}}$$

Denoting the active ocncentrations of the two species by S and A the system we take is thus generally of the form

$$\frac{\partial S}{\partial t} = F_S(S) - G_S(S,A) + D_S \nabla^2 S = U(S,A) + D_S \nabla^2 S,$$

$$\frac{\partial A}{\partial t} = F_A(A) - G_A(S,A) + D_A \nabla^2 S = V(S,A) + D_A \nabla^2 A,$$

$$(1)$$

where D_S and D_A are diffusion coefficients, $\nabla^2 S$ and $\nabla^2 A$ represent diffusion, F_S and F_A the externally supplied flux terms while G_S and G_A the rate of loss due to reaction. The functions $U(S,A)$ and $V(S,A)$ defined by (1) are the overall reaction rates.

The type of reaction involved is most easily seen by the general form of the curves $U(S,A) = 0$, $V(S,A) = 0$ on the S-A plane; these are the reaction isoclines or null reaction lines. Figure 1 illustrates typical reaction isoclines of the kind we consider. The inhibition is indicated in the $U(S,A) = 0$ isocline by the S-like shape.

The uniform steady state for the mechanism is where the two isoclines intersect since there the overall rates $U(S,A)$ and $V(S,A)$ are both zero, that is at P in Figure 1. The reaction parameters determine whether or not there are 3 or 1 steady states: the former occurs with $V(S,A) = 0$ like the dashed line in Figure 1.

Under typical experimental conditions the reaction rate G for the Thomas (1976) scheme is

$$G = V_M AS/(K_M + S + S^2/K_S) \qquad (1)$$

where V_M, K_M and K_S are constants with K_S related to the inhibition. The diffusional fluxes F_S, F_A of S, A through the inactive layer from the reservoir to the active layer are proportional to $D_S'(S_0-S)$ and $D_A'(A_0-A)$ respectively, where D_S', D_A' are the diffusion coefficients of S and A in the inactive layer.

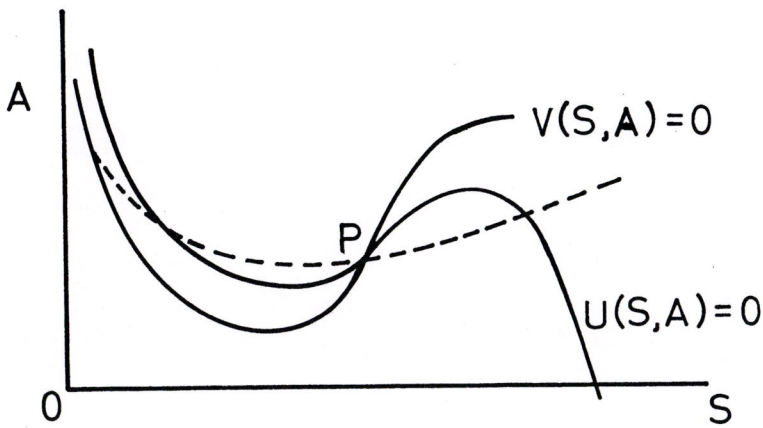

Figure 1

Illustrative reaction rate forms for the two species S and A. U(S,A) = 0 exhibits typical substrate inhibition. Steady states are solutions of   U(S,A) = 0 = V(S,A): there can be 1 or 3 steady states.

With D_S, D_A the diffusion coefficients in the active layer the governing reaction diffusion equations are then

$$\left.\begin{array}{l} \dfrac{\partial S}{\partial t} = \dfrac{D_S'}{L_1 L_2} (S_0 - S) - \dfrac{V_M AS}{(K_M + S + S^2/K_S)} + D_S \nabla^2 S, \\[4mm] \dfrac{\partial A}{\partial t} = \dfrac{D_A'}{L_1 L_2} (A_0 - A) - \dfrac{V_M AS}{(K_M + S + S^2/K_S)} + D_A \nabla^2 A, \end{array}\right\} \qquad (2)$$

where ∇^2 is the Laplacian (diffusion) operator.

For convenience, we write (2) in nondimensional form by introducing the following dimensionless variables:

$$\left.\begin{array}{l} s = S/K_M, \quad a = A/K_M, \quad \nabla*^2 = L^2 \nabla^2, \quad t* = tD_S/L^2 \\[2mm] \alpha = D_A'/D_S', \quad \beta = D_A/D_S, \quad K = K_M/K_S, \\[2mm] \gamma = L^2 D_S'/L_1 L_2 D_S, \quad \rho = L_1 L_2 V_M K_M/D_S' \end{array}\right\} \qquad (3)$$

Substituting these into (2) and dropping the asterisks on $\nabla*^2$ and $t*$ for convenience the governing system is then

$$\frac{\partial s}{\partial t} = g(s,a) + \nabla^2 s, \quad \frac{\partial a}{\partial t} = f(s,a) + \beta \nabla^2 a, \qquad (4)$$

where

$$\left.\begin{array}{l} f(s,a) = \gamma[\alpha(a_0 - a) - \rho F(s,a)], \\[2mm] g(s,a) = \gamma[s_0 - s - \rho F(s,a)], \\[2mm] F(s,a) = sa/(1+s+Ks^2), \end{array}\right\} \qquad (5)$$

where β, ρ, α, γ and K are positive constants.

The non-dimensional form of the reaction rates f and g has γ as a multiple of both f and g and so can be considered as a size scale parameter. It could be incorporated into the length scale and time scale by writing γt for t and $\frac{1}{\gamma} \nabla^2$ for ∇^2. We

370

specifically retain it as in (5) so that for a given geometry of typical dimension ℓ we obtain a larger or smaller similar geometry by simply varying γ . <u>The size of the domain is proportional</u> to $\sqrt{\gamma}$.

With s representing a substrate with high molecular weight compared with a this means that the ratio of the diffusion coefficients $\beta = D_A/D_S$ is greater than 1. The constant K in (5) is the <u>inhibition</u> parameter, with the larger inhibition corresponding to a larger K . The α, ρ, a_0 and s_0 are constants related to the experimental arrangement.

For our purposes the main parameters are β, γ and the inhibition factor K with only the latter being involved in the form of the reaction isoclines and the position and number of the uniform steady states here the positive solutions $(\tilde{s},\tilde{a})$ of $f(s,a) = 0 = g(s,a)$. The reduction or increase in the inhibition parameter K is considered to be controlled genetically.

3. PATTERN FORMATION MECHANISM

We require a mechanism which can respond differentially to stimuli in such a way that homogeneity gives way to heterogeneity. The mechanism (4) with (5) can give rise to steady state two-dimensional spatial structures if the parameters lie in appropriate ranges. The heterogeneous structure is the final result of diffusion driven instability of the uniform steady state in a Turing (1952) sense. That is, the uniform steady state $(\tilde{s},\tilde{a})$, given by the single solution of

$$f(\tilde{s},\tilde{a}) = 0 = g(\tilde{s},\tilde{a}) \tag{6}$$

is stable to small homogeneous perturbations but is unstable to small heterogeneous perturbations in concentration about $(\tilde{s},\tilde{a})$. The role of diffusion is critical and drives the instability. We follow the procedure described pedagogically by Murray (1977).

Appropriate boundary conditions for (4) and (5) are zero flux ones on the boundary, (or alternatively periodic conditions if the surface is cylindrical) that is

$$\underset{\sim}{n}.\nabla s = 0 = \underset{\sim}{n}.\nabla a \quad \text{for} \quad \underset{\sim}{r} \in B \tag{7}$$

where $\underset{\sim}{r}$ is the space variable, B is the boundary of the reaction-diffusion domain ∇ is the gradient operator, and $\underset{\sim}{n}$ the unit normal to B.

Linearizing (4) about the steady state and for convenience introducing the following matrix and vector quantities:

$$W = \begin{pmatrix} s - \tilde{s} \\ a - \tilde{a} \end{pmatrix}, \qquad D = \begin{pmatrix} 1 & 0 \\ 0 & \beta \end{pmatrix}$$

$$M = \begin{pmatrix} m_{11} & m_{12} \\ m_{21} & m_{22} \end{pmatrix} = \begin{pmatrix} \dfrac{\partial g}{\partial s} & \dfrac{\partial g}{\partial a} \\ \dfrac{\partial f}{\partial s} & \dfrac{\partial f}{\partial a} \end{pmatrix}_{\tilde{s},\tilde{a}}$$

(8)

the linearized problem (4) with the zero flux conditions (7) becomes

$$\frac{\partial w}{\partial t} = Mw + D\nabla^2 w, \qquad n.\nabla w = 0, \quad r \in B. \tag{9}$$

Let the eigenvalues for the geometry of interest be k^2, that is the eigenvalues of

$$\nabla^2 W + k^2 W = 0, \qquad n.\nabla W = 0, \quad r \in B. \tag{10}$$

Writing

$$w(r,t) = e^{\lambda t} W(r,t) \tag{11}$$

and using (10), (9) gives the eigenvalues λ as solutions of the quadratic equation

$$|M - k^2 D - \lambda I| = 0$$

namely

$$\lambda^2 + \lambda[-(m_{11} + m_{22}) + k^2(1 + \beta)] + h(k^2) = 0,$$

$$h(k^2) = \beta k^4 - (m_{11}\beta + m_{22})k^2 + (m_{11}m_{22} - m_{12}m_{21})$$

(12)

We require the conditions such that when spatially homogeneous perturbations about $(\tilde{s},\tilde{a})$ are present the system is stable but not when the perturbations are spatially heterogeneous. That is w in (11) has $R\ell\lambda < 0$ when diffusion effects are not present but at least one λ exists with $R\ell\lambda > 0$ when they are: in this way the steady state is diffusionally unstable.

In the absence of diffusion   the eigenvalues λ satisfy, from (12) with $k^2 = 0$

$$\lambda^2 + \lambda(-(m_{11} + m_{22})) + (m_{11}m_{22} - m_{12}m_{21}) = 0.$$

Since $R\ell\lambda < 0$ this means the parameters in f and g in (5) are such that

$$m_{11} + m_{22} < 0, \quad m_{11}m_{22} - m_{12}m_{21} > 0 \tag{13}$$

with the m's from (8).

When diffusion effects are present $k^2 \neq 0$ and the λ are given by (12). We now wish to find conditions that $R\ell\lambda > 0$ for at least one eigenvalue. Since $-(m_{11} + m_{22}) + k^2(1 + \beta) > 0$ because of (13) the only way a positive eigenvalue can exist is if $h(k^2) < 0$ in (12). From the second of (13) and (12) this can only happen if $(m_{11}\beta + m_{22}) > 0$. Since, from (13), $m_{11} + m_{22} < 0$ this means we must have $\beta \neq 0$, that is s and a must have different diffusion coefficients.

Finally the necessary and sufficient conditions for diffusion driven instability of the system (4), (5) and (7) are

$$\left[\frac{\partial g}{\partial s} + \frac{\partial f}{\partial a}\right]_{\tilde{s},\tilde{a}} < 0, \quad \left[\frac{\partial g}{\partial s}\frac{\partial f}{\partial a} - \frac{\partial g}{\partial a}\frac{\partial f}{\partial s}\right]_{s,a} > 0$$

$$\left[\beta\frac{\partial g}{\partial s} + \frac{\partial f}{\partial a}\right]_{\tilde{s},\tilde{a}} > 0, \quad (\Rightarrow \beta > 1), \tag{14}$$

and at least one postive eigenvalue k^2 exists such that

$$h(k^2) = \beta k^4 - \left[\beta\frac{\partial g}{\partial s} + \frac{\partial f}{\partial a}\right]_{\tilde{s},\tilde{a}} k^2 + \left[\frac{\partial g}{\partial s}\frac{\partial f}{\partial a} - \frac{\partial g}{\partial a}\frac{\partial f}{\partial s}\right]_{\tilde{s},\tilde{a}} < 0. \tag{15}$$

This determines a critical β, β_c, such that $h(k^2) = 0$ for some $k^2 > 0$.

From the inequality (15) the unstable eigenvalue k^2 must satisfy

$$\frac{1}{2\beta}\left\{(\beta\,\frac{\partial g}{\partial s} + \frac{\partial f}{\partial s}) - \left[(\beta\,\frac{\partial g}{\partial s} + \frac{\partial f}{\partial a})^2 - 4\beta(\frac{\partial g}{\partial s}\frac{\partial f}{\partial a} - \frac{\partial g}{\partial a}\frac{\partial f}{\partial s})\right]^{1/2}\right\}_{\tilde{s},\tilde{a}}$$

(16)

$$< k^2 < \frac{1}{2\beta}\left\{(\beta\,\frac{\partial g}{\partial s} + \frac{\partial f}{\partial a}) + \left[(\beta\,\frac{\partial g}{\partial s} + \frac{\partial f}{\partial a})^2 - 4\beta(\frac{\partial g}{\partial s}\frac{\partial f}{\partial a} - \frac{\partial g}{\partial a}\frac{\partial f}{\partial s})\right]^{1/2}\right\}_{\tilde{s},\tilde{a}}$$

For each k^2 satisfying (16) the corresponding unstable eigenvalue λ ($R\ell\lambda > 0$) is given by (12).

In one-dimensional domains, that is (10) is $d^2W/dx^2 + k^2\underset{\sim}{W} = 0$, $d\underset{\sim}{W}/dx = 0$ for $x = 0$, $x = a$, the linear fastest growing eigensolution, that is the one with the largest $R\ell\lambda > 0$, tends to indicate the final finite amplitude state: see Mimura and Murray (1978). In two-dimensions this is no longer the case.

For the rectangular geometry $0 \le x \le a, 0 \le y \le b$ the eigenfunction problem (10) is

$$\left. \begin{array}{l} \dfrac{\partial^2\underset{\sim}{W}}{\partial x^2} + \dfrac{\partial^2\underset{\sim}{W}}{\partial y^2} + k^2\underset{\sim}{W} = 0 \\[2em] \dfrac{\partial\underset{\sim}{W}}{\partial x} = 0 \quad \text{on} \quad x = 0, a, \quad \dfrac{\partial\underset{\sim}{W}}{\partial y} = 0 \quad \text{on} \quad y = 0, b \end{array} \right\}$$

(17)

the solutions of which are

$$\underset{\sim}{W}(x,y) = \sum_{m,n} \underset{\sim}{A}_{mn} \cos\frac{n\pi}{a}x \cos\frac{m\pi}{b}y$$

(18)

where $\underset{\sim}{A}_{mn}$ are constants and m, n integers with the eigenvalues k^2 given by

$$k^2 = k^2_{mn} = \frac{m^2\pi^2}{b^2} + \frac{n^2\pi^2}{a^2} \quad .$$

(19)

With f and g from (5) substituted into (16), with k^2 from (19), the result is the inequality.

$$\gamma[X-Y] < \pi^2\left(\frac{n^2}{a^2} + \frac{m^2}{b^2}\right) < \gamma[X+Y] \tag{20}$$

where X and Y are functions of the parameters α, ρ, β, a_0, s_0, and K given by

$$\left.\begin{aligned} X &= -\frac{1}{2\beta}[\beta + M(\tilde{s},\tilde{a}) + \alpha + N(\tilde{s},\tilde{a})] \\[2mm] Y &= \frac{1}{2\beta}\{[\beta + M(\tilde{s},\tilde{a}) - \alpha - N(\tilde{s},\tilde{a})]^2 + 4M(\tilde{s},\tilde{a})N(\tilde{s},\tilde{a})\}^{1/2} \end{aligned}\right\} \tag{21}$$

where

$$M(\tilde{s},\tilde{a}) = \left[\frac{\beta\rho a(1-Ks^2)}{(1+s+Ks^2)^2}\right]_{\tilde{s},\tilde{a}} \quad , \quad N(\tilde{s},\tilde{a}) = \left[\frac{\rho s}{1+s+Ks^2}\right]_{\tilde{s},\tilde{a}}$$

with $\tilde{s},\tilde{a}$ the solutions of the algebraic equations (6). Note that $\tilde{s},\tilde{a}$ do not depend on the scale factor γ which only appears as a multiplicative factor in the inequality (20).

For the tapering cylindrical geometry the eigenvalue problem in the coordinate system r, θ and z is

$$\frac{1}{r^2}\frac{\partial^2 W}{\partial\theta^2} + \frac{\partial^2 W}{\partial z^2} + k^2 W = 0, \frac{\partial W}{\partial z} = 0 \quad \text{at} \quad z = 0, \ell$$

with W necessarily periodic in θ . The solutions are of the form

$$W(\theta,z,r) = \sum_{m,n} B_{mn} \cos n\theta \cos \frac{m\pi}{\ell} z$$

where the B_{mn} are constants and the eigenvalues k^2 are

$$k^2 = k^2_{mn} = \frac{m^2\pi^2}{\ell^2} + \frac{n^2}{r^2} . \tag{22}$$

Again, with f and g from (5) and k^2 from the last equation (16) gives

$$\gamma[X-Y] < \frac{n^2}{r^2} + \frac{m^2\pi^2}{\ell^2} < \gamma[X-Y] \tag{23}$$

with X, Y from (21). Here the local radius r of the cylinder is simply a parameter but it plays a critical role in the surface pattern obtained.

The inequality (16) depends on the geometry only through the specific form of the eigenvalues k^2. With f and g as in (5) we can thus evaluate the range of unstable eigenvalues k^2.

In the following sections we discuss the consequences of the diffusion driven instability as it applies to problems related to animal markings.

4.   SPATIAL PATTERNS AND THE EFFECT OF GEOMETRY AND SCALE

What follows holds for all reaction mechanisms which can be diffusionally driven unstable.   For clarity we shall be specific and consider the reaction-diffusion mechanism (4) with (5) with the parameters such that the uniform steady state is typically equivalent to P in Figure 1.   This steady state is taken to be stable to homogeneous perturbations in the concentrations about (š,ã) but can be diffusionally driven unstable by small heterogeneous pertur-bations if the ratio of diffusion coefficients $\beta = D_A/D_S$ is sufficiently greater than 1.   As shown above the critical value β_c , for which the system is unstable for $\beta > \beta_c$, depends on the para-meter values and most importantly on the geometry while the pattern which evolves depends also on the scale.

A direct measure of scale is the parameter γ which for given geometries also has a critical bifurcation value γ_c for the exist-ence of spatial structures, all other parameters being kept fixed. In Section 5 it will be seen that it plays a critical role in the patterns obtained.   The linear scale of the reaction-diffusion domain, which for our interests is the integument of foetuses or parts of it like legs and tail, backs (excluding the belly) is proportional to $\sqrt{\gamma}$.

To demonstrate some important points we consider here the two simple geometries discussed above: (i) a rectangular domain $0 \le x \le a$, $0 \le y \le b$ where x,y are Cartesian coordinates and a,b are constants as in Figure 2 and (ii) the surface of a tapering cylinder of radius r_0 at $z = 0$ and r_1 at $z = \ell$ as in Figure 4 below.

Consider the domain in Figure 2 with no flux of either species from it. Thus the concentrations $s(x,y,t)$ and $a(x,y,t)$ are governed by (4) and (5) and must satisfy the zero flux boundary conditions.

The time development of small perturbations about the steady state are given by

$$u(x,y,t) = s(x,y,t) - \tilde{s}, \quad v(x,y,t) = a(x,y,t) - \tilde{a} \; .$$

The solutions for u and v from Section 3 can be written in the form of a sum of terms (eigenfunctions) like

$$e^{\lambda_{mn} t} \cos \frac{n\pi}{a} x \cos \frac{m\pi}{b} y \qquad\qquad (23)$$

where the λ_{mn}, the eigenvalues, depend on a, b and the integers m and n. For example the solution u is of the form

$$u(x,y,t) = \sum_{m,n} U_{mn} e^{\lambda_{mn} t} \cos \frac{n\pi}{a} x \cos \frac{m\pi}{b} y \qquad\qquad (24)$$

where $\sum_{m,n}$ denotes the sum over all integer pairs m, n and the U_{mn} are constants. If $\lambda_{mn} > 0$ for at least one integer pair m, n then as time t increases the magnitude of u increases exponentially which means the steady state is unstable. If $\lambda_{mn} < 0$ for all m,n then $u, v \to 0$ and so the steady state is stable.

Each term in (24) is a mode or eigensolution and represents a specific spatial pattern on the rectangle in Figure 2 and depending on the sign of λ_{mn} either grows or decays with time. Denoting by shading $u > 0$, that is $s > \tilde{s}$, Figure 2 illustrates the eigen-solution for various pairs m, n.

Consider now the time development of the solution (24) and the subsequent spatial patterns. On a linear basis, the largest $\lambda_{mn} > 0$

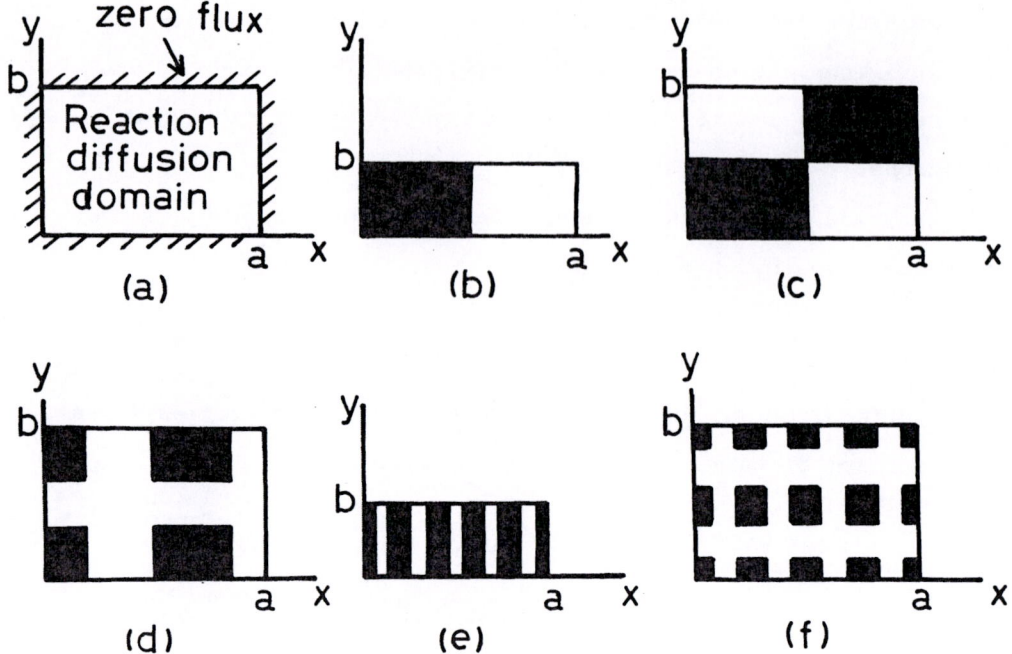

Figure 2

Rectangular reaction-diffusion domain showing simple (linear) patterns with dark/white representing concentrations greater/less than the steady state $\tilde{s}$, from equation (23): (b) $m = 0$, $n = 1$, (c) $m = 1 = n$, (d) $m = 2$, $n = 3$, (e) $m = 0$, $n = 10$, (f) $m = 4$, $n = 8$.

determines which is the dominant spatial pattern. Figures 2(b) and

(e) have m = 0 and so (23) is essentially only one dimensional.

If the dominant λ_{mn} corresponds to one of these then the linear

time developing pattern is essentially one-dimensional and is indic-

ative of the final pattern obtained from the numerical solution of

the full nonlinear system (4) with (5) and the same boundary conditions

(7) almost irrespective of initial conditions. It is possible, even

for quasi-one dimensional domains, to obtain patterns which are not

those predicted by linear theory if the initial conditions are chosen

appropriately.

   If the dominant eigenfunction is genuinely two-dimensional as in

Figure 2 (d) and (f), then the full nonlinear spatial pattern is not

in general predicted by the linear analysis: it depends on the initial

conditions and the nonlinearities in the reaction scheme. What was

found numerically was that small random variations in the initial

conditions gave qualitatively similar spatial patterns. Since we have

coat patterns in mind this is consistent with the individual detailed

patterns in animal coat markings.

   For the system (4) with (5) and the rectangular domain in

Figure 2 we found above that the integer pair m and n which result

in unstable eigenfunctions that is positive eigenvalues λ_{mn} , must

satisfy (20).

   To be specific if we take one of the parameter sets used below,

namely $\alpha = 1.5$, $\rho = 13$, $s_0 = 102$, $a_0 = 77$, $K = 0.1$ then the steady

state from (6) is $\tilde{s} = 8$, $\tilde{a} = 14$. The system (4) with (5) is

diffusionally unstable for $\beta \geq 4.6$. With $\beta = 5$ the unstable modes

have integer pairs satisfying, from (20),

$$0.036 \, \gamma < \frac{n^2}{a^2} + \frac{m^2}{b^2} < 0.115 \, \gamma \ . \tag{25}$$

The roles of the scale parameter, domain size and shape can now be clearly seen.

Suppose we take $\gamma = 1$ and the rectangular domain in Figure 2(a) with $a = 3$ and $b = 1$ say. Then from (25) the unstable eigensolutions (23) have m and n values which satisfy $0.036 < n^2/9 + m^2 < 0.115 \gamma$. Thus the only unstable mode has $m = 0$, $n = 1$ namely that illustrated in Figure 2(b). It is also the final steady state obtained from the full nonlinear system. If the domain size is now increased by a factor of 2 then a and b are doubled or alternatively γ increased to $\gamma = 2^2 = 4$ and the unstable modal values from (25) are $m = 0, n = 2$. Thus for a given domain, it is clear that size can be varied by changing γ .

If we now choose $\gamma = 10$ then from (25), $0.36 < n^2/9 + m^2 < 1.15$ which admits several modal configurations namely (i) $m = 1, n = 0$ or (ii) $m = 0, n = 2$ and $n = 3$. These give corresponding eigenvalues $\lambda_{mn} > 0$ the largest of which determines the dominant solution which bifurcates from the uniform steady state and in this quasi one-dimensional situation evolves into a similar modal configuration even in the nonlinear case and is thus similar to the predator-prey situation of Mimura and Murray (1978a).

As γ increases the number of unstable eigensolutions increases with genuine two-dimensional modes among them. It is not surprising that, as the nonlinear effects become progressively more important, interaction between the growing modes is no longer determined by the linear solutions and the final configuration is, at the current state of mathematical development, unpredictable from the linear bifurcation solutions. As mentioned above the final steady state depends on the initial conditions.

From (25) and in general from (20) it is clear that if one of the dimensions is sufficiently small, b say, then all $m \geq 1$ are necessarily excluded from the range of unstable modes. The problem

is then a one-dimensional eigenfunction problem with m = 0 and
n^2/a^2 satisfying (20). In this case the pattern produced, both
linear and nonlinear, is a series of transverse stripes typically
illustrated in Figure 2(e). As b increases, for a fixed a , the
possibility of genuine two-dimensional patterns increases.

We now relate this behaviour to Mintz's (1967) stripe patterns
on mice: see Figure 3(a) below. If this reaction-diffusion mechanism
is responsible for the laying down of the pattern at an early stage
of embryonic development the related embryonic surface has an equivalent a >> b and is thus quasi-one-dimensional. The melanin pattern
distribution (associated with a concentration here greater than the
steady state say) predicted is then a series of transverse stripes as
found experimentally: see Figure 3(a). The mechanism cannot realis-
tically produce longitudinal stripes since the one-dimensional modes
are too dominant. Thus the geometry at the time of laying down is
what precludes the possibility of longitudinal stripes which is in a
sense the same as saying the probability is negligible as supposed by
Mintz (1967). From her photographs, however, it seems that the
stripes are not all transverse which in turn implies that a and b
are perhaps more comparable in size at the time of laying down: see
also the critical discussion by McLaren (1976). Figure 3(b) is
reminiscent of Figure 2(b).

Consider now the the tapering geometry illustrated in Figure 4, the
surface of which is the reaction-diffusion domain. In terms of the

radial azimuthal and axial coordinates r, θ and z the eigensolutions equivalent to (23) are, typically

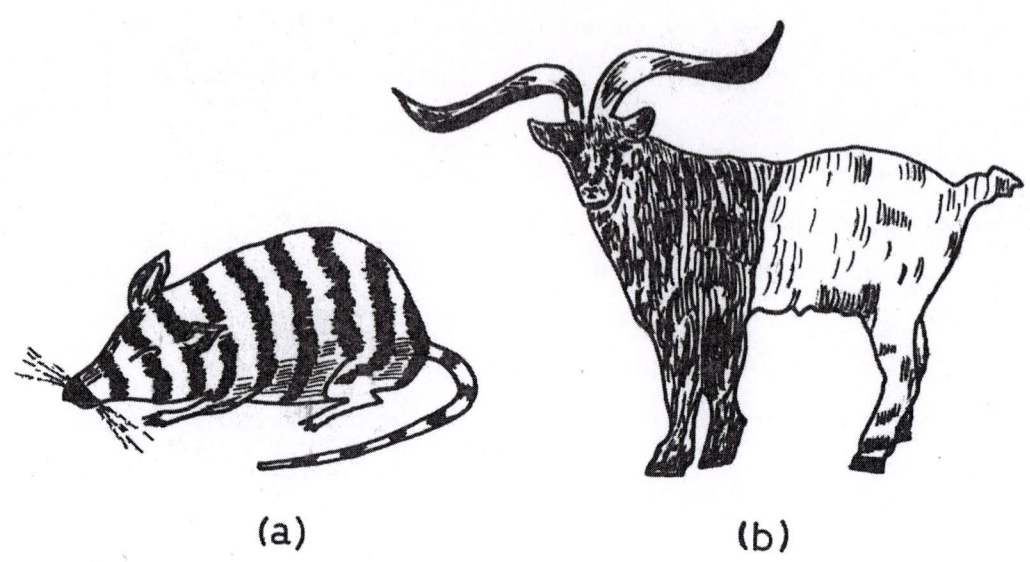

<u>Figure 3</u>

Simple melanistic patterns; (a) Chimaeric mouse, after Mintz (1967), (b) Valais goat after Heráň (1976).

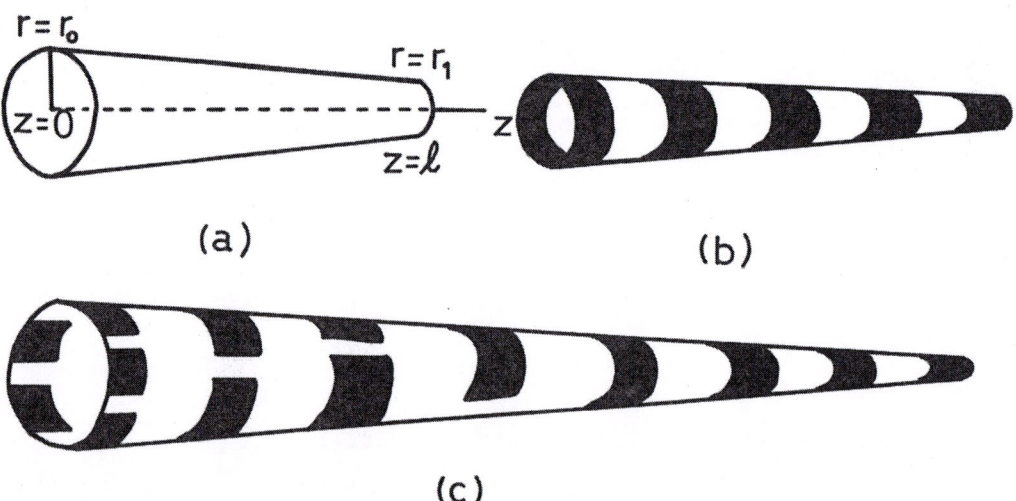

<u>Figure 4</u>

Cylindrical surface reaction-diffusion domain: (a) geometrical facts, (b) $r_0 < r < r_1$ with r_1 small, (c) r_1 small and r_0 large enough for two-dimensional effects near $z = 0$.

$$e^{\lambda_{mn} t} \cos n\theta \, \cos \frac{m\pi}{\ell} z \qquad\qquad (26)$$

where now the integers m, n for unstable modes satisfy (23).

If over the length of the cylinder r is small enough so that n^2/r^2 with $n \geq 1$ is too large to lie within the unstable range (23) then the only unstable eigensolutions have $n = 0$ and any m allowed by (23). From (26) then, this is simply the one-dimensional case illustrated in Figure 4(b) and is comparable to the plane case of Figure 2(e).

Suppose now that r_0 is not sufficiently small for $1/r_0^2$ to lie outside the range (23) but $1/r_1^2$ is. Then near $z = 0$ the inequality can yield modal pairs m, n with $m \geq 1$ and $n \geq 1$ while near $z = \ell$, $n = 0$, $m \geq 1$. Thus there can be a smooth transition from a definite two-dimensional structure near the thick end to a quasi-one-dimensional stripe pattern towards the thin end as illustrated in Figure 4(c). For the full nonlinear system the regular striping near $z = \ell$ is predicted by linear theory. We use these results below in Section 5.

Finally, let us consider the time scale for establishing such spatial patterns on a comparative domain scale basis. From equations (4) with (5) the size scale parameter γ appears only as a factor of the reaction rates in both equations for s and a. So if we redefine the time t by γt and all lengths L by $\sqrt{\gamma} L$, that is $\frac{1}{\gamma} \nabla^2$ by ∇^2, the system we get is exactly the original one with the effective $\gamma = 1$. If, for a given domain size, the pattern formation time is T say, then for a geometry of similar shape but 10 times larger (that is $\sqrt{\gamma} = 10$) the system to analyse is the same except that the corresponding time of formation is of the order of $100T$ (that is γT).

Consider now the effect of this increased time on the eigenfunction pairs m and n , in (20) for example, which give unstable eigensolutions because the corresponding $\lambda_{mn} > 0$. If the domain is large then for a fixed γ the dimensions a and b are large (or alternatively a and b are fixed and γ is large). This implies that at least one of m or n satisfying (20) must be large which in turn implies a large number of spatial structures. These patterns take a much longer time to develop than those for smaller integer pairs. It is likely that only a finite time is available for pattern formation and so the mechanism may in fact not have time to develop the ultimate picture and quasi-homogeneity could result. An alternative explanation, which is effectively the same is that structure only appears because of boundary influence (which determines the eigensolutions). In very large domains these are far from most of the reaction-diffusion domain and so their influence is too weak to effect a pattern in the time available.

In summary then if a domain is too small (a and b in Figure 2 are too small) no spatial structuring is possible while if the domain is too large the available time is not sufficient for the pattern to develop. In either extreme the ultimate picture obtained is homogeneity. Although very speculative, if a reaction-diffusion mechanism is responsible for the pre-pattern in aminal markings it could give certain order of magnitude times for the period of laying down. It also suggests a tentative explanation for the homogeneity of coat colour of large animals with long gestation periods and very small ones with short gestation periods.

5. APPLICATION OF PATTERN FORMATION MECHANISM TO
SPECIFIC GEOMETRIES AND ANIMALS

In this section we present some of the numerical results and
relate them to certain general features of animal markings. All the
results were obtained using a finite element numerical scheme on the
system (4) with (5) and zero flux of the concentrations s and a
across the boundary, that is boundary conditions (7). The initial
conditions used were random perturbations about the uniform steady
state $\tilde{s}, \tilde{a}$. The procedure was stopped when the heterogeneous
spatial structure at successive time steps satisfied a prescribed
convergence: 10^{-3} or less was used. In the figures the shaded
regions indicate areas where s > $\tilde{s}$ unless otherwise stated.
The numerical programme used was originally developed by Kernevez et
al. (1979) for the specific system (4) and (5).

The parameters for the system are α, ρ, K, s_0 and a_0 , which
determine the steady state $\tilde{s}, \tilde{a}$ and γ and β , which relate to the
diffusively driven unstable linear modes discussed above. There is
a wide range of parameter values which give rise to spatial structures
but we chose for illustrative purposes only 2 sets of α, ρ, K, s_0, a_0
and β and varied only the scale factor γ . Similar domains of
different size are easily compared by simply varying the scale parameter γ since domain size is directly proportional to $\sqrt{\gamma}$ as
mentioned before. In this way it is obviously not simply a judicious
choice of the several parameters which gives the varied patterns.
Even with such a restriction on parameters and initial conditions the
wealth of possible patterns for such a reaction-diffusion mechanism
is remarkable.

We consider first the typical markings found on animal tails
and legs which we represent by a tapering cylindrical geometry. For

visual and numerical convenience we considered the cylindrical surface as a tapered planar domain, in which b (the circumference)
varies with the length a . If the tail is sufficiently thin then
the equivalent b is small and essentially a one-dimensional situation obtains and diffusive instability gives rise to simple striping
along the length of the tail as predicted by linear theory with the
number being proportional to the length. Figure 5(a) is a typical
example: here $\gamma = 9$. As γ is increased, that is the domain is

larger, more of the two-dimensional influence is felt: see Figure 5(b).
Figure 5(c), with $\gamma = 25$, also has a much longer linear dimension
so as to illustrate the gradation from spots, a distinctly two-
dimensional behaviour, to stripes as the domain becomes thinner.

The general pattern is now clear. If the scale is increased even
further in the geometry of Figure 5(c) spots will be present further
down the tail while the converse holds for a decreased γ . If the
scale factor γ is small enough then only a uniform unpatterned
state is obtained.

Striped tailed animals are fairly common as on genets while
Figure 5(a) is a pattern from our mechanism. The number of stripes
in any species is not constant: in the genet for example, the author
has seen as few as 6 and as many as 13 black stripes. An immediate
consequence of the theory here is that the number is linearly
related to the tail length at the time of laying down of the stripe
pre-pattern. This does not necessarily mean that if the length of
adult tails differ then so does the number of stripes: it is the
length at the laying down which is critical. We envisage the genetic switch, which initiates the pattern formation, at a specific
time in the embryonic development. It is expected that the time of
switching and parameter values are inherited and so therefore are

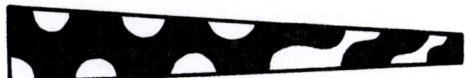

(a) $\gamma = 9$ (b) $\gamma = 15$

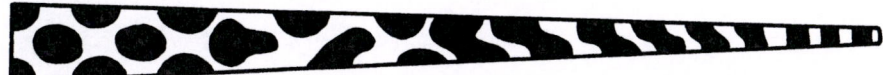

(c) $\gamma = 25$

Figure 5

    Results from numerical solution of equations (4) with (5) with
$\alpha = 1.5$, $K = 0.1$, $\rho = 18.5$, $s_0 = 92$, $a_0 = 64$ (steady state $\tilde{s} = 10$,
$\tilde{a} = 9$) and diffusion coefficient ratio $\beta = 10$: (a) Scale factor $\gamma = 9$,
dark regions $s > \tilde{s}$, (b) Scale factor $\gamma = 15$, dark regions $s > \tilde{s}$,
(c) Scale factor $\gamma = 25$, dark regions $s < \tilde{s}$.

the number of stripes unless the environment of the progenitors is altered. On the basis of extensive study on the external features of giraffe, particularly the neck markings, Dagg (1968) concluded that coat colour, area and shape of the spots are inherited. The theory we propose here is consistent with this.

We now relate our results to specific animals with the implication of course that the type of reaction-diffusion mechanism we have studied could be responsible for the melanin pattern observed in them. The interesting tail pattern in Figure 6(a) of a Chapman's zebra after Willoughby (1975) shows a striking resemblance to Figures 5(b) and 6(e). It also shows how the tail is a continuation of the dark spinal stripe: see also Figure 8 below which is related to the back marking. Figure 6(b) is a drawing of the tail of a post-natal genet: it should be compared with Figures 5(b) and 6(e) when rolled into a cylinder. Figures 6(c) and 6(d) are from photographs of a cheetah and jaguar and show, the former particularly, how the reducing diameter forces the spots to become stripes. The spot to stripe pattern is often seen towards the leg extremities: the same reasoning applies to these.

To consider body markings it would be useful to know the time of laying down of the pre-pattern so that the embryonic shape could be taken as a guide to domain geometry. This is in general not known: we briefly touch on this below in Section 6. In the giraffe Hall-Martin (1978) has mentioned that the pattern is laid down by about 100 days through the gestation period. By this time the animal has a shape recognisably similar to the grown species: it has it much earlier in fact as seen from 35-45 day giraffe embryos. For the zebra, the distinct body shape is only just emerging by the 5th week. We discuss certain aspects of zebra striping in more detail below. The

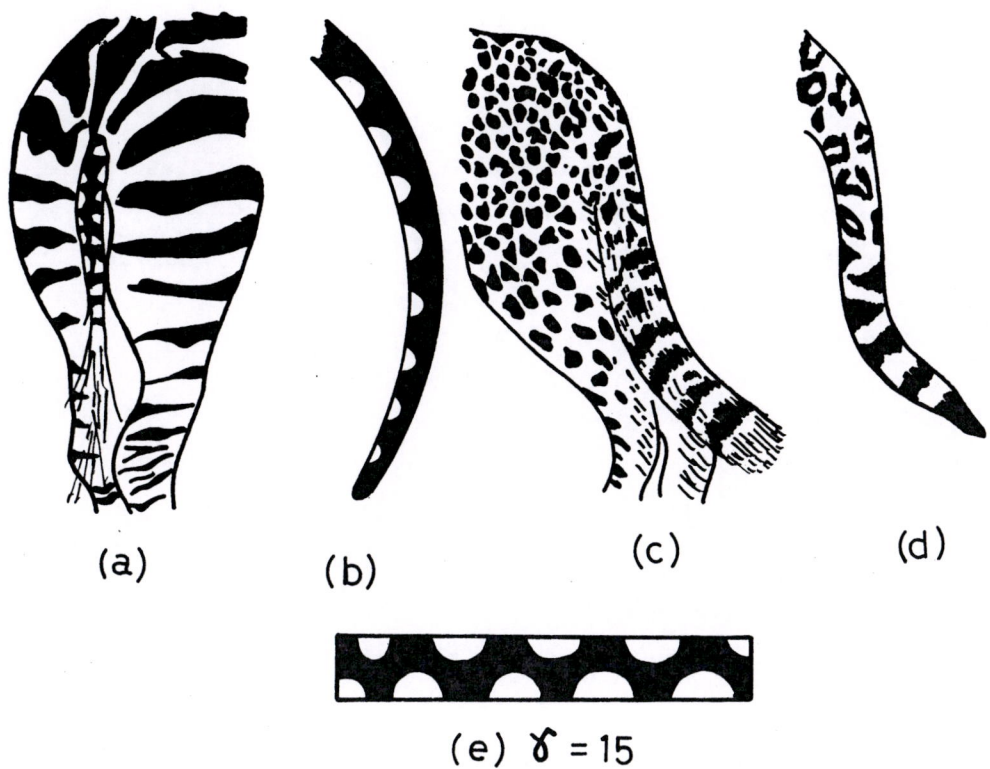

(a) (b) (c) (d)

(e) ♉ = 15

Figure 6

Various tail markings from (a) Zebra (Equus burchelli chapmani)
from Willoughby (1974), (b) Post-natal male genet (Genetta genetta),
Natural History Museum, London (66-6165): tail length 11 cm.,
(c) Cheetah (Acinonyx jubatus): (d) Jaguar (Panthera onca),
(e) Computed markings for rectangular domain (rolled out cylinder):
parameter values as in Figure 5.

leg and tail patterns in animals, from the point of view of our reaction-diffusion theory suggest that a 'reaction shape' qualitatively similar to the living animal has been reached by the time of pattern formation initiation. It seemed that it might be of interest therefore to consider a simple body surface shape as in Figure 7 to show the effect of scale on the patterns obtained.

Linear theory is of little practical use here except when the domain dimensions are small when a rough comparison with the rectangular domain in Figure 2 suffices. It should be emphasized here that we take this domain pattern only for illustration. The shape at the time of laying down the pre-pattern is as yet unknown.

For γ sufficiently small no pattern is obtained as in Figure 7(a). As the size (γ) increases the sequence of patterns quickly diverges from linear predictions based on Figure 2. The time required for establishing such patterns increased with increasing values of γ in keeping with the discussion in Section 4.

Considering the epidermal surface of the embryo as a planar domain the 'length' is larger than the 'width'. Thus modal patterns which appear for γ larger than in Figure 7(b) are stripes such as those found by Mintz (1967) in chimaeric mice. Figure 3(a) above is a sketch based on her results where she found 17 stripes: compare this with Figure 5(a). The pattern in Figure 7(b) is dramatically found in nature as shown in the sketch in Figure 3(b) of the domestic Valais goat after Heráň (1976).

From Figure 7 we see that as the domain size increases the larger body surface area becomes progressively more spotted but with the slender extremities like the legs and tail still retaining their striped pattern. This seems to be a common feature with many spotted

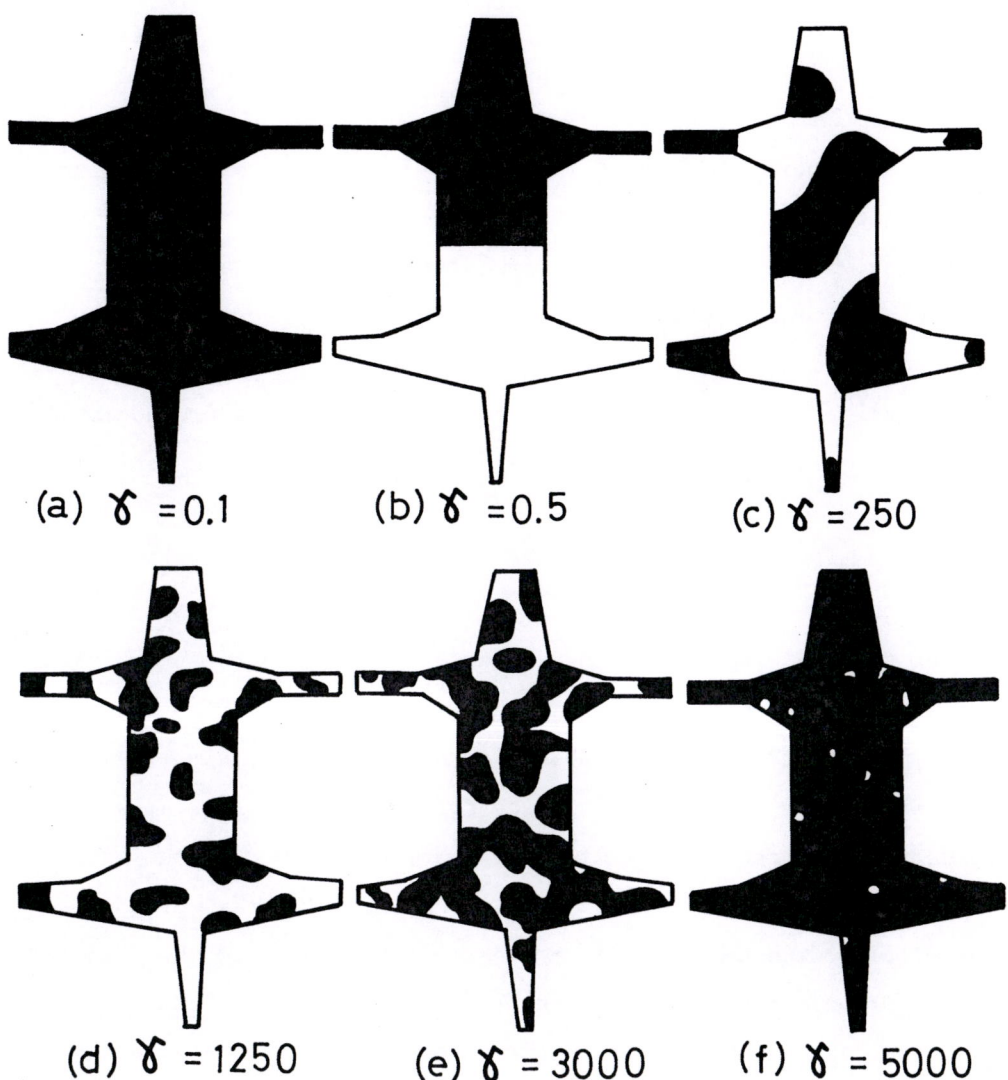

(a) $\gamma = 0.1$ (b) $\gamma = 0.5$ (c) $\gamma = 250$

(d) $\gamma = 1250$ (e) $\gamma = 3000$ (f) $\gamma = 5000$

Figure 7

Effect of body surface scale on pattern formed by the reaction-diffusion mechanism (4) with (5) for $\alpha = 1.5$, $K = 0.125$, $\rho = 13$, $s_0 = 103$, $a_0 = 77$ (steady state $\tilde{s} = 23$, $\tilde{a} = 24$) and $\beta = 7$. Domain dimension is proportional to $\sqrt{\gamma}$. Dark regions have $s \geq \tilde{s}$.

animals. With the giraffe the embryo is distinctly developed at the time of laying down and so a spotted coat including the tail and legs is as expected.

Consider now the zebra. Bard (1977) suggested that a regular stripe pattern laid down about 0.5 mm apart at a specific time would produce the observed number of stripes found on adult animals. We have seen above that the reaction-diffusion mechanism can produce a sequence of parallel stripes. Some of these become the distinctive caudal stripes due to differential foetal growth. The production of the traditional spinal stripe with the main stripes coming off at right angles to it is less obvious. Figure 8

however shows how this could be achieved from the pattern formation in Figure 8(a) by simple embryonic growth to Figure 8(b). Figure 8(c) is a typical back pattern in the tiger which exhibits similar striping. There is further supportive evidence for this in Figure 6(a) where the zebra tail pattern is similar to that in Figure 8(a) but which has undergone little radial growth as compared with that of the body. The spinal stripe in Figure 6(a) clearly continues onto the tail and is a simple earlier pattern of the back.

Consider now the pattern of scapular stripes at the foreleg-body junction in the zebra: a typical example is shown in Figure 9(a). This is the type of pattern that would be expected mathematically on the basis of two reaction-diffusion domains at approximately right angles to each other in each of which there are parallel stripes. The legs at the time of laying down of the pattern are such that only stripes are generated as in Figures 4(b) and 5(a), while the back, which is dimensionally larger, exhibits a pattern typically as in Figure 8(a) and (b). Figure 9(b) is what can be expected from the

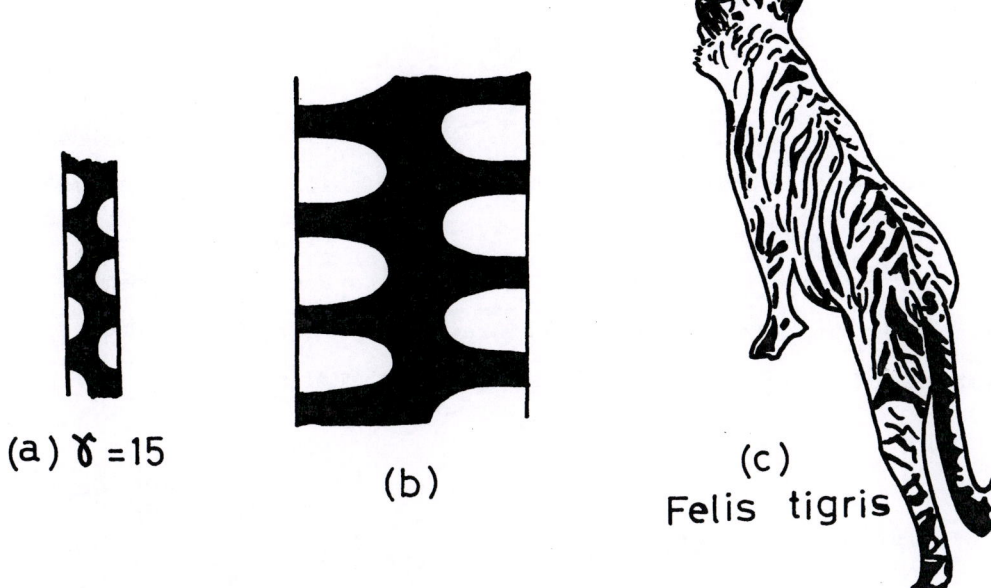

(a) $\gamma = 15$

(b)

(c)
Felis tigris

Figure 8

Possible back pattern formation for the zebra and tiger:
(a) Computed pattern from the reaction-diffusion mechanism (4) with
(5) and parameter values as in Figure 5, (b) Effect of lateral growth
on the pattern, (c) Typical tiger (Felis tigris) stripe pattern.

system (4) and (5).

The cases discussed here are only a few examples of the structural possibilities of just one reaction-diffusion mechanism of the
substrate inhibition type (4) and certainly do not exhaust the
possible patterns for geometries of interest. However they demonstrate certain general pattern features which are common to such
systems and are commonly observed in many marked animals.

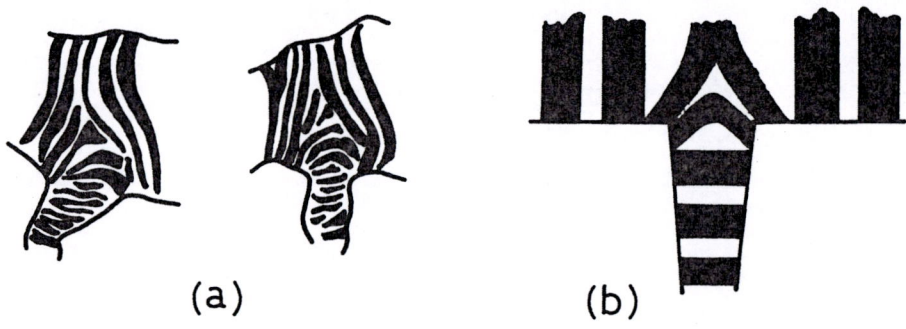

(a)   (b)

Figure 9

(a) Typical examples of scapular stripes on the foreleg of zebra,
after Briand Peterson (1972), (b) Expected mathematical pattern for
intersecting striped domains for the mechanism (2) and (3).

396

6. CONCLUSIONS

The main purpose of this paper is to present qualitative evidence
in support of a reaction-diffusion mechanism for the laying down of
the pre-patterns for animal markings. The specific mechanism we
consider is a substrate inhibition one which is a practical example
of what is a fairly common type found in practice. When such inhibition reaction systems are made diffusionally unstable by, for example,
a reduction in concentration of an inhibitor, spatial structures are
obtained in a time scale short compared with pure diffusion times.
The possible role of a reaction-diffusion switch to initiate and
terminate the pattern formation mechanism will be discussed elsewhere.

The role of geometry is shown to be important and the gradation
from spots to stripes is an immediate consequence of domain size
reduction as on tail and leg extremities. Since time of pattern formation is related to scale some tentative general conclusions can be
made as regards time of pre-pattern formation. The intimate relation
between geometry and size and the corresponding time scale required
for generating heterogeneous structure as opposed to homogeneity
gives a possible explanation for the uniformity in coat colour in
very small animals and very large ones.

The patterns discussed here only touch on the wealth of possibilities such simple two species reaction-diffusion systems can
exhibit. The genetic coding involvement is, in such a mechanism,
simply an elementary inhibitor-type switch.

If there is an all encompassing mechanism for pattern formation
in animal markings then a reaction-diffusion system seems to be a
serious candidate. It is efficient, simple and is capable of generating an infinite variety of possible structural patterns which
also exhibits a general behaviour which is closely related to geometry

and scale in a manner frequently observed in nature.

ACKNOWLEDGEMENTS

I would like to thank the many people who have been so helpful in providing information on specific animals, help with the numerical analysis, and for their general encouragement. In particular, I would like to mention Professor Anne Dagg, Dr. Hans Kruuk, Dr. Anthony Hall-Martin, Professor G.H. Findlay, Dr. N.F. Britton, Mr. Cinderey of the Whipsnade Zoological Gardens and, for the use of their finite numerical scheme, Professor J.-P. Kernevez and Drs. B. Bunow, M.C. Duban and G. Joly.

REFERENCES

Bagnara, J.T. and Hadley, M.E., *Chromatophores and Colour Change: The Comparative Physiology of Animal Pigmentation*, Prentice-Hall, New Jersey, 1973.

Bard, J.B.L., A unity underlying the different zebra striping patterns, J. Zool. Lond., 183, 527-539, 1977.

Dagg, A.I., External features of giraffe, Extrait de Mammalia, 32, No. 4, 657-669, 1968.

Fife, P., *Mathematical Aspects of Reacting and Diffusing Systems*, Lecture Notes in Biomathematics, Springer-Verlag, New York, 1979.

Findlay, G.H., Personal communication, 1978.

Fox, H.M. and Vevers, G., *The Nature of Animal Colours*, Sedgwick & Jackson, London, 1960.

Hall-Martin, A.J., Personal communication, 1978.

Heráň, I., *Animal Colouration:* The Nature and Purpose of Colours in Invertebrates, Hamlyn, London, 1976.

Kauffman, S., Shymko, R. and Trabert, K., Control of Sequential Compartment in *Drosophila*, Science, 199, 259-269, 1978.

Kernevez, J.P., Joly, G., Duban, M.C., Bunow, B., and Thomas, D., Hysterisis, oscillations, and pattern formation in realistic immobilized enzyme systems, J. Math. Biol., 7, 41-56, 1979.

Lewis, J., Slack, J.M.W., and Wolpert, L., Thresholds in Development, J. Theor. Biol., 65, 579-590, 1977.

McLaren, A., *Mammalian Chimaeras*, Cambridge University Press, Cambridge, 1976.

Meinhardt, H., and Gierer, A., Application of a Theory of Biological Pattern Formation based on Lateral Inhibition, J. Cell. Sci., 15, 321-346, 1974.

Mimura, M. and Murray, J.D., On a Diffusive Prey-Predator Model which Exhibits Patchiness, J. Theor. Biol., 75, 249-262, 1978a.

Mimura, M. and Murray, J.D., Spatial Structures in a Model Substrate-Inhibition Reaction Diffusion System, Z. Naturfosch. 33c, 580-586, 1978b.

Mintz, B., Gene Control of Mammalian Pigmentary Differentiation I. Clonal origin of melanocytes, Proc. Nat. Acad. Sci., Washington, 58, 344-351, 1967.

Mintz, B., Clonal Basis of Mammalian Differentiation, Symp. Soc. Exp. Biol., 345-370, 1971.

Murray, J.D., *Lectures on Nonlinear Differential Equation Models in Biology*, Clarendon Press, Oxford, 1977.

Nicolaus, R.A., *Melanins* (in Chem. Natural Products Series: ed. E. Lederer), Hermann, Paris, 1968.

Okubo, A., *Diffusion and Ecological Problems: Mathematical Models*, Springer-Verlag, Heidelberg , 1979.

Searle, A.G., *Comparative Genetics of Coat Colour in Mammals*, Academic Press, 1968.

Seelig, F.F., Chemical oscillations by substrate inhibition - a parametrically universal oscillator type in homogeneous catalysis by metal complex formation, Z. Naturfosch., 31a, 731-738, 1976.

Segel, L.A., Mathematical Models for Cellular Behaviour, in *A Study in Mathematical Biology*, (Ed. S. Levin), Math. Assoc. of America, 1976.

Thomas, D., Artificial enzyme membranes, transport, memory and oscillatory phenomena, Proc. Inst. Symp. on *Analysis and Control of Immobilized Enzyme Systems*, (Eds. D. Thomas and J.-P. Kernevez), May 1975, 115-150, 1976.

Turing, A.M., The Chemical Basis of Morphogenesis, Phil. Trans. Roy. Soc. (London) B, 237, 37-72, 1952.

Tyson, J.J., *The Belousov-Zhabotinskii reaction*, Lecture Notes in Biomathematics (Ed. S. Levin), Springer-Verlag, New York, 1976.

Willoughby, D.P., *The Empire of Equus*, Barnes and Co., New York, 1974.

Winfree, A.T., Rotating Chemical Reactions, Sci. Amer., 230, 82-95, 1974.

Winfree, A.T., Stably Rotating Patterns of Reaction and Diffusion, in Theoretical Chemistry, 4, 1-51, (Eds. H. Eyring and D. Henderson), Academic Press, N.Y., 1978.

Wolpert, L., Positional Information and the Spatial Pattern of Cellular Differentiation, J. Theor. Biol. 25, 1-47, 1969.

Wolpert, L. and Gingell, D., Striping and the Pattern of Melanocyte Cells in Chimaeric Mice, J. Theor. Biol., 29, 147-150, 1970.

CELL GROWTH AS AN AUTOCATALYTIC RELAXATION PROCESS

A. M. Liquori and A. Tripiciano

Istituto di Chimica Fisica, University of Rome

INTRODUCTION

One of the great merits of the extention of Thermodynamics to non-equilibrium systems achieved through the development of Irreversible Thermodynamics (1) lies in the close connection established between thermodynamic and kinetic aspects of chemical reactions.
        A chemical reaction may thus be considered as a "spontaneous" irreversible process driven toward equilibrium by its thermodynamic affinity, i. e., by the difference between the chemical potentials of the products and the reactants. In general, the relationship between the rate of a chemical reaction and its affinity is non linear. However, in two case it becomes linear: 1) the chemical reaction is not too far from equilibrium, or 2) the chemical reaction, even far from equilibrium, may be considered as a global reaction consisting of a large number of small steps, each of which is driven by an affinity small compared to RT, and a stationary regime is established. The latter condition implies that the rates of the chemical reactions become identical to the rate of the global reaction, so that any intermediate chemical species is consumed at the same rate it is produced. In both cases the relaxation equation which is obtained as solution of the linear differential equation displays a tipical behaviour. The extent of the reaction shows in fact a hyperbolic increase which tends to a constant equilibrium value.
        As a new approach to cell growth, this process might be considered as a complex global reaction consisting of a large number of chemical steps for which a stationary state may be assumed. However, a hyperbolic growth equation would be expected whereas growth curves show a characteristic sigmoidal behaviour. This means that growth should be considered as an "autocatalytic global reaction".
        It is then possible to treat growth as due to the combination of two global processes, a "slow process" and a "fast process". If it is assumed that a continuous transition from the slow process to the fast process takes place during the cell growth and the shift is regulated by the rate of the overall process, a sigmoidal relaxation equation may be obtained.
        As it will be shown the above equation fits very satisfactorily all the experimental growth curves thus far examined. It may be considered as a novel growth equation having a thermodynamic basis, and at the same time showing some advantages over previous equations (such as the logistic (2) and the Gompertz (3) equation). It only contains in fact two parameters (the relaxation times of the slow and fast processes) having a rather simple physical meaning.

RELAXATION TOWARD EQUILIBRIUM OF A GLOBAL REACTION UNDER STATIONARY STATE CONDITIONS

Let's consider a large set of q chemical reactions involving m molecular species. The rth reaction may be represented as

$$\nu_{r1} M_1 + \nu_{r2} M_2 + \cdots \underset{\longleftarrow}{\overset{\longrightarrow}{\quad}} \cdots \nu_{r\,m-1} M_{m-1} + \nu_{r\,m} M_m \qquad (1)$$

The whole set may be represented in compact form as

$$\sum_i \nu_{ri} M_i = 0 \qquad\qquad \begin{array}{l} r = 1,\ 2, \ldots,\ q \\ i = 1,\ 2, \ldots,\ m \end{array} \qquad (2)$$

ν_{ri} is the stoichiometric coefficient of the ith chemical species in the rth reaction and M_i is its molecular weight. The stoichiometric coefficients (to be taken positive or negative for the products and the reactants respectively) may therefore be considered as the elements of a large rectangular matrix.

The affinity of the rth reaction is

$$A_r = -\sum_i \nu_{ri} \mu_i \qquad (3)$$

where μ_i is the chemical potential of the ith species.

The rate of the rth reaction is

$$v_r = \dot{\xi}_r \qquad (4)$$

where ξ_r is the extent of the rth reaction.

For $A \ll RT$ a first order expansion of the rates as a function of the affinities is justified yelding the linear phenomenological equations (in matrix notation):

$$V = LA \qquad (5)$$

where the rth element of V is $\dot{\xi}_r$ and the rth element of A is A_r. L is a square matrix which , according to Onsager reciprocity relations, is symmetric, namely

$$L = L^T \qquad (6)$$

A similar first order expansion of the affinity as a function of the extents of the reactions holds yelding the linear equations

$$A = CX \qquad (7)$$

with

$$C = C^T \qquad (8)$$

The rth component of X is $\xi_r - \bar{\xi}_r$ where ξ_r is the extent of the rth reaction at time t and $\bar{\xi}_r$ its equilibrium value. Replacing (7) into (5) the following linear equations are obtained

$$V = FX \qquad (9)$$

F is a square symmetric matrix given by

$$F = LC \qquad (10)$$

Since it may be shown that the time derivative of the free energy is given by

$$-\dot{G} = V^T A = VA^T = V^T L^{-1} V = A^T LA \qquad (11)$$

it follows that

$$-\dot{G} = X^T H X \tag{12}$$

where

$$H = C^T L C \tag{13}$$

The quadratic form (12) may be reduced to a canonical form by a diagonalization of the matrix L and the matrix C which involves the diagonalization of F.
This may be achieved by finding the roots of the characteristic equations:

$$\left\| L - \lambda E \right\| = 0 \tag{14a}$$

$$\left\| C - \lambda E \right\| = 0 \tag{14b}$$

where E is the unit matrix.
Equation (9) therefore becomes

$$V' = T^{-1} X' \tag{15}$$

where T^{-1} is a diagonal matrix whose r^{th} element $-\tau_r^{-1}$ is the inverse of the rth relaxation time.

STATIONARY CONDITIONS

Let's now consider the ith species formed in the global reaction. Then

$$dn_i = \sum_r \gamma_{ir} \, d\xi'_r \tag{16}$$

$$d\xi'_g = \frac{dn_i}{\gamma_i} = \sum_r \frac{\gamma_{ir}}{\gamma_i} \, d\xi'_r \tag{17}$$

where ξ'_g is the extent of the global reaction, γ_{ir} is the stoichiometric coefficient of the ith species in the rth reaction and γ_i is the stoichiometric coefficient of the ith species in the global reaction. Equation (15) may now be inverted to

$$X' = T V' \tag{18}$$

Since

$$x'_g = \xi'_g - \bar{\xi}'_g = \sum_r \frac{\gamma_{ir}}{\gamma_i} (\xi'_r - \bar{\xi}'_r) \tag{19}$$

elements of the equation (18) may now be multiplied by $\frac{\gamma_{ir}}{\gamma_i}$ and summed. Accordingly to the condition of stationary state, i. e.

$$\dot{\xi}'_r = \dot{\xi}'_g \tag{20}$$

the following result is obtained

$$x'_g = \sum_r \frac{\nu_{ir}}{\gamma_i} x'_r = TrT \; \mathcal{F}'_g \qquad (21)$$

being $\sum \frac{\nu_{ir}}{\gamma_i} = 1$. TrT is the trace of the diagonal matrix T.
Equation (20) may now be inverted back into the equation

$$\mathcal{F}'_g = (TrT)^{-1} \; x'_g \qquad (22)$$

which may also be written as

$$\dot{\mathcal{F}}'_g = -\frac{1}{\tau}(\mathcal{F}'_g - \bar{\mathcal{F}}'_g) \qquad (23)$$

where

$$\frac{1}{\tau} = \frac{1}{\sum_r \tau} \qquad (24)$$

THE RELAXATION EQUATION OF THE GLOBAL REACTION

The linear differential equation (23) may be integrated to obtain

$$\mathcal{F}'_g(t) - \bar{\mathcal{F}}'_g = (\mathcal{F}'_g(0) - \bar{\mathcal{F}}'_g) \; \exp{-t/\tau} \qquad (25)$$

which for $\mathcal{F}'_g(0) = 0$ reduces to

$$\mathcal{F}'_g(t) = \bar{\mathcal{F}}'_g(1 - \exp{-t/\tau}) \qquad (26)$$

A reduced extent of the global reaction $y = \mathcal{F}'_g(t)/\bar{\mathcal{F}}'_g$ may be introduced which is given by

$$y = 1 - \exp{-t/\tau} \qquad (27)$$

It will be noticed that $y \rightarrow 0$ for $t \rightarrow 0$ and $y \rightarrow 1$ for $t \rightarrow \infty$. In other words y varies between 0 and 1 as the global reaction moves from the initial conditions to the equilibrium conditions.

THE OVERALL AUTOCATALYTIC GROWTH EQUATION

Equation (27) shows the asymptotic behaviour of cell growth but does not display the typical sigmoidal shape. The latter must in fact be due to autocatlysis.

Suppose in fact that the observable cell growth is the result of two simultaneous global reactions proceeding with relaxation times τ_1 and τ_2. The corresponding reduced extents of "slow growth" and "fast growth" will then be given by

$$y_1(t) = 1 - \exp{-t/\tau_1} \qquad (28a)$$

404

$$y_2(t) = 1 - \exp{-t/\tau_2} \tag{28b}$$

Autocatalysis may now be expressed through the equation

$$y(t) = y_1(t)(1 - y(t)) + y_2(t)y(t) \tag{29}$$

where $y(t)$ is the overall growth rate.

The above equation implies that at the beginning the reduced extent of growth is given by $y_1(t)$ (the slow rate) and during growth a continuous transition takes place from the slow growth, characterized by the reduced extent $y_1(t)$, to the fast growth, characterized by the reduced extent $y_2(t)$. The transition is regulated in time by the extent of the overall growth. In fact $y(t) \longrightarrow y_1(t)$ for $t \longrightarrow 0$ and $y(t) \longrightarrow y_2(t)$ for $t \longrightarrow \infty$ (at equilibrium).

Equation (26) may be rearranged and $y_1(t)$ and $y_2(t)$ may be replaced by (28a) and (28b). The resulting growth equation is

$$y(t) = \frac{1 - \exp{-t/\tau_1}}{1 - \exp{-t/\tau_1} + \exp{-t/\tau_2}} \tag{30}$$

The above equation displays the tipical sigmoidal shape of cell growth curves. This is shown in Fig. 1 where $y(t)$ is plotted against t. Two arbitrary values τ_1 and τ_2

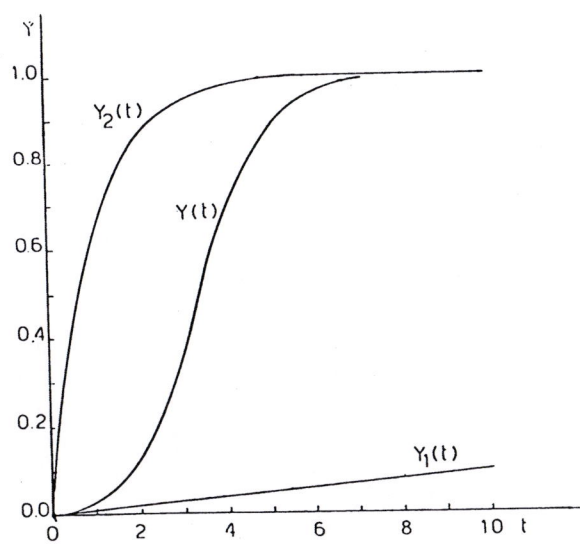

Figure 1. Plot of theoretical curves of $y_1(t)$, $y_2(t)$ and $y(t)$ according to Eq.(30). Arbitrary values of $\tau_1 = 100$ and $\tau_2 = 1$ were chosen.

have been used. In the same figure $y_1(t)$ and $y_2(t)$, corresponding to the reduced extents of slow and fast growth, are also plotted*.

The above result shows that cell growth may be considered as a spontaneous autocatalytic overall chemical process driven by the thermodynamic tendency of the system to decrease its free energy. The growth equation which has been derived may be used to analyze experimental growth curves and requires the determination of only two parameters τ_1 and τ_2, i. e. the relaxation time of slow and fast growth. Other growth processes (which may be simulated by chemical processes) common in economic or social sciences might be studied with the aid of equation (30).

Equation (30) fits very accurately the experimental growth data of several systems, such as bacteria, yeast, embryos. Furthermore, it has been used to analyze allometric growth curves, namely the growth curves of different parts of an organism.

Altough the fitting could be achieved using a computer, a simple metod was used which allows a rather straightforward fitting of a set of experimental data.

FITTING METHOD

The following function may be derived from Eq.(30):

$$\alpha(t) = \frac{y(t)}{1 - y(t)} = \frac{1 - x_1}{x_2} \tag{31}$$

where

$$x_1 = \exp{-t/\tau_1} \tag{32a}$$

$$x_2 = \exp{-t/\tau_2} \tag{32b}$$

Let's consider a pair of values $\alpha(t_n)$ and $\alpha(t_{2n})$ corresponding to double time values $(t_{2n} = 2t_n)$. Then

$$\alpha(t_n) = \frac{1 - x_1(t_n)}{x_2(t_n)} \tag{33a}$$

$$\alpha(t_{2n}) = \frac{1 - x_1^2(t_n)}{x_2^2(t_n)} = \frac{(1 - x_1(t_n))(1 + x_1(t_n))}{x_2^2(t_n)} \tag{33b}$$

$$\frac{\alpha(t_n)}{\alpha^2(t_n)} = \frac{1 + x_1(t_n)}{1 - x_1(t_n)} \tag{34}$$

Replacing (32a) and (32b) into (34) and solving for τ_1, the following result is obtained

$$\tau_1 = t_n \ln(1 + \frac{\alpha(2t_n)}{\alpha^2(t_n)} / \frac{\alpha(2t_n)}{\alpha^2(t_n)} - 1) \tag{35}$$

.Once τ_1 has been obtained from the above relation inserting the experimental values of $\alpha(t_n)$ and $\alpha(t_{2n})$, τ_2 may be obtained from equation (33a). When in fact the latter equation is solved for τ_2, the following result is obtained

$$\tau_2 = t_n \ln \frac{\alpha_2(t_n)}{1 - \exp{-t/\tau_1}} \qquad (36)$$

In order to fit a set of experimental growth data they were first plotted against $x = 1/t$ and the asymptotic value was found by extrapolation to $x \to 0$. A continuous curve was then drawn by interpolating the normalized experimental values (reduced extents of growth). Pairs of values were then selected corresponding to double time values ($t_{2n} = 2t_n$). The corresponding values of $\alpha(t_n)$ and $\alpha(t_{2n})$ were calculated from each pair and τ_1 and τ_2 were obtained according to (35) and (36). The average τ_1 and τ_2 values were then computed from a number of pairs and inserted into Eq. (30). The theoretical growth curve was thus calculated.

RESULTS

In Fig. 2 the fitting of the normalized experimental growth data with Eq.(30) of E. col in two different media are shown.

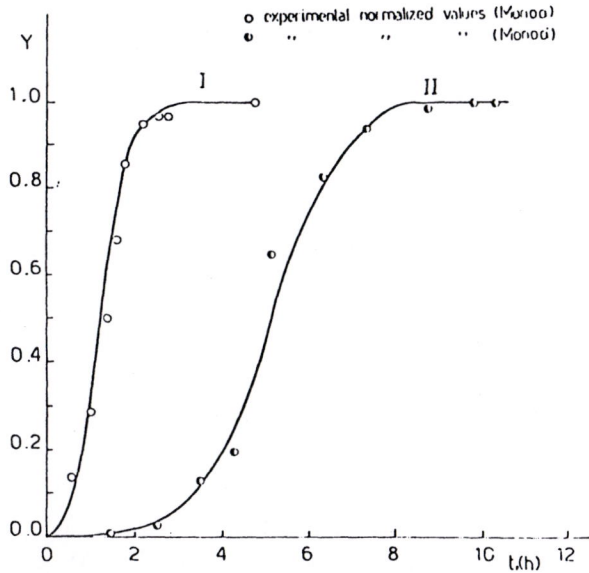

Figure 2.   Plot of the theoretical reduced extent of growth calculated according to Eq.(30) for two growth curves of E. coli in different media. τ_1= 22,733h and τ_2= 0,419h for curve I. τ_1= 1,075 10^3h and τ_2= 0,967h for curve II. The experimental reduced values have been obtained from tables reported in J. Monod Recherches sur la Croissance des Cultures Bacteriennes (4).

In Fig. 3 the fitting of the normalized experimental growth data of yeast with Eq.(30) is shown.

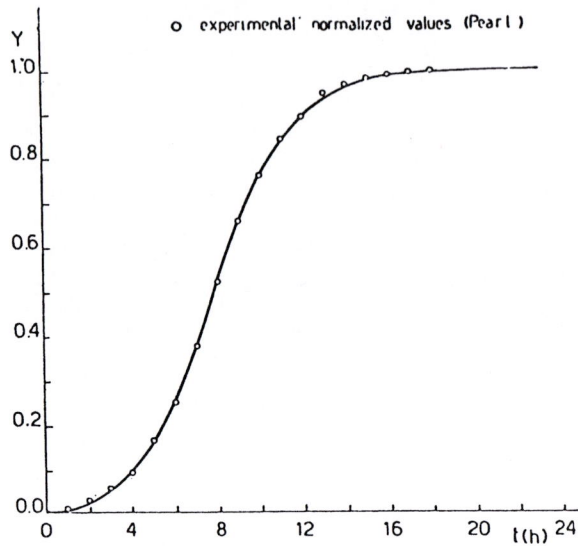

Figure 3. Plot of the theoretical reduced extent of growth calculated according to Eq. (30) for a growth curve of yeast. τ_1 = 0,1993 10^3h and τ_2 = 2,399 h. The experimental reduced values were obtained by a table in R. Pearl, Quart. Rev. Biol. 2, 532 (1927).

In Fig. 4 the fitting of the normalized experimental growth data of a chicken embryo is shown. In Fig. 5 the fitting of the normalized experimental growth data of the head and the trunk of a chicken embryo are shown. Finally, in Table I the values of τ_1 and τ_2 for the allometric growth curves of different parts of a chicken embryo are given.

DISCUSSION

From Figs. 2, 3, 4 and 5 it may it may be concluded that Eq.(30) fits rather accurately the experimental growth data of different grwth systems. It is therefore of practical utility in the analysis of cell growth. In the case of allometric growth curves it becomes possible to describe allometry as largely due to a difference in τ (the relaxation time of the "slow growth") for different parts of the same organism.

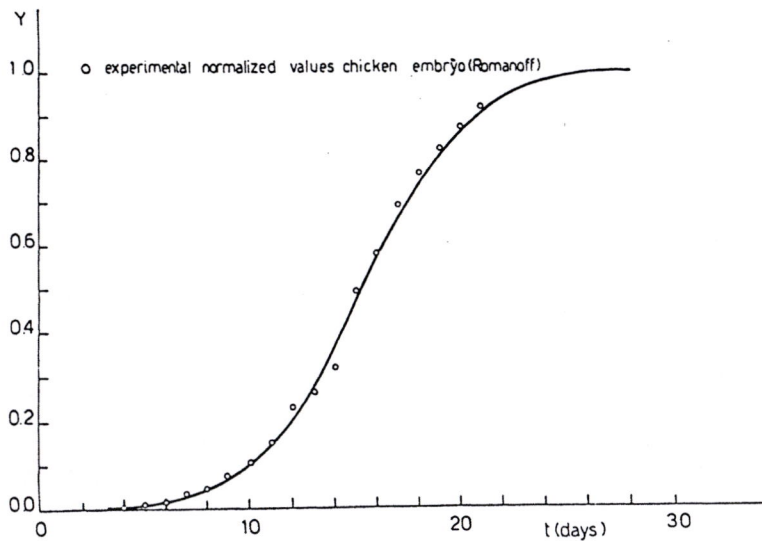

Figure 4. Plot of the theoretical reduced extent of growth calculated according to Eq. (30) for a growth curve of a chicken embryo. $\tau_1 = 2,648 \ 10^3$ days and $\tau_2 = 2,9629$ days. The experimental reduced values were obtained from a table in A. L. Romanoff, The Avian Embryo The MacMillian Co N. Y. 1960.

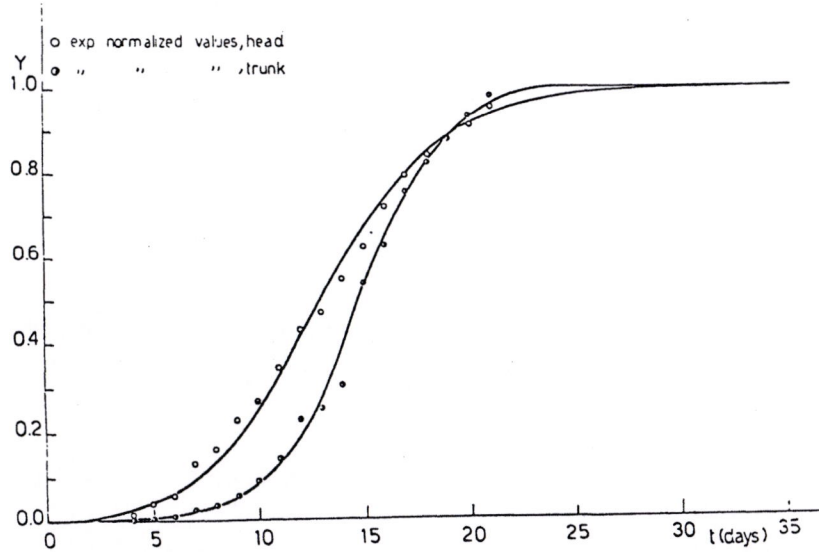

Figure 5. Plot of the theoretical reduced extents of growth calculated according to Eq. (30) for the growth curves of the head and the trunk of a chicken embryo. $\tau_1 = 0,5091 \ 10^3$ days, $\tau_2 = 3,5327$ days for head. $\tau_1 = 7,996 \ 10^3$ days and $\tau_2 = 2,3557$ days for trunk. The experimental reduced data were obtained from tables in A. L. Romanoff, The Avian Embryo The MacMillian Co. N. Y. 1960.

TABLE I

	$\tau_1 \; 10^3$ (days)	τ_2 (days)
Chicken embryo	2,648	2,9629
Head	0,5091	3,5327
Trunk	7,996	2,3557
Neck	11,169	2,2523
Hindlimb	59,223	1,8953
Forelimb	26,831	2,3508

REFERENCES

1) I. Prigogine, Introduzione alla Termodinamica dei Processi Irreversibili
        Leonardo E. S. ,Roma, 1971.
2) P. F. Verhulst, Corr. Math. PHys. 10, 113 (1838)
3) B. Gompertz, Phil. Trans. Roy. Soc. 513–585 (1825)
4) J. Monod, Recher ches sur la Croissance des Cultures Basteriennes 2^a ed. Paris
        (1958).

* Obviously the rate equation which may be obtained by deriving Eq.(30) with respect to time is not a linear differential equation.

VITO VOLTERRA AND CONTEMPORARY MATHEMATICAL BIOLOGY

A. Borsellino

Istituto de Cibernetica e Biofisica,
CNR, Camogli (Italy)
Istituto di Scienze Fisiche, Genova
(Italy)

Volterra and the Mathematical Biology

Let me recall briefly some aspects of the remarkable personality of
Vito Volterra.

Born in the year 1860 in Ancona, Volterra showed in his boyhood his
exceptional gifts for mathematical and physical thinking. At the age
of thirteen, after reading Verne's novel on the voyage from earth to
moon, he devised his own method to compute the trajectory under the gra-
vitational field of the earth and moon; the method was worth later development into a general procedure for solving differential equations.
He became a pupil of Dini at the Scuola Normale Superiore in Pisa and
published many important papers while still a student. He received his
degree in Physics at the age of 22 and was made full professor of Rational Mechanics at the same University only one year later, as a successor of Betti.

Volterra had many interests outside pure mathematics, ranging from
history to poetry, to music. When he was called to join in 1900 the University of Rome from Turin, he was invited to give the opening speech
of the academic year.

The title of his speech was: "On the Attempts to Apply Mathematics
to Biological and Social Sciences", a very indicative title when we
realize that the talk was given 25 years before Volterra's first contribution in the field of Mathematical Biology. The paper, reprinted
in 1906 in two other journals and later in his collected "Scientific
Essays" in 1920, makes still today a worthy reading[1]. In this paper
Volterra first of all recognized the existence of already well developed mathematical treatment in problems like blood circulation in elas-
tic vessels, locomotion mechanics, physiological thermodynamics, or
the great work of Helmholtz in sensory physiology. But these or similar
examples he considers as particular cases of ordinary mechanical or physical studies, for which no new ideas were involved or required. We
would include them today possibly in a list of biophysical problems.
Completely different, in Volterra's thought, are those problems which

he considered proper to Biology. After discussing some tentatives that
we would call today of morphotaxonomy or morphogenesis, Volterra indicates as really important to biology problems of genetics and evolution,
then just in the first exploratory steps for a mathematical development.
He describes quite in detail, showing more than reading knowledge of
the available literature, for example the new ideas and approaches advanced by Galton first and later developed by Pearson.

Without entering into more detail, I must emphasize that Volterra
was clearly bringing into focus just those very special and unique aspects that characterize biological objects, as they result from evolution. Accepting the reductionism of biology to physics does not avoid
or smooth the problems: they are of the same nature and scale as those
of the cosmological evolution of the Universe.

From his parallel discussion of mathematical economics in the same
talk, we can realize how large was Volterra's reading in fields different from his own specialization, a characteristic that he was able
to maintain also in later years. At the end of his talk Volterra expresses, with his usual warm eloquence, his great expectation that,
through a more extensive use of quantitative thinking and adequate
mathematics, these new approaches to the field of biology could be
developed and brought to the levels already reached by the classical
sciences of mechanics and physics. We can see today how much Volterra's
expectations have been fulfilled. This symposium is another demonstration that the mathematical developments wished by Volterra have been
largely brought to reality and multiplied in many directions.

Volterra was President of the Accademia dei Lincei in the years
1923 - 1926. He was also the founder of the Italian Society for the
Advancement of Science and of the National Council of Research. For
many years he was one of the most productive scientists and a very
influential personality in public life. When Fascism took power in
Italy, Volterra did not accept any compromise and preferred to leave
his public and academic activities.

I will not try to recall all the deep discoveries due to Volterra
in pure Mathematics, or his other important contributions. Instead I
will try to indicate some examples showing how Volterra's name and
mathematical inventions are present today in other fields of mathematical biology, quite different or apparently separated from that of
population dynamics.

Biology and Mathematical Models

The present status of what can be called mathematical biology shows
so many roads and different approaches that one finds great difficulties in trying to get a general view or indicate the main lines of development. One possibility is to start with a more or less exhaustive
list of "mathematical problems" originated and of relevant interest in
biology. One possible list can be found for example in a booklet by Fomin and Berkinblit[2]. Some of the examples, like the classical Hodgkin
and Huxley treatment of nervous excitation and nerve impulse propagation or the regulation of protein synthesis can be considered just direct, although complicated, applications of electrochemical or biochemical principles. Other problems, like those of neural networks, control,
memory, artificial intelligence, are discussed in the booklet as those
for which the appropriate models are still in question. A few of them
are already quite sophisticated in their mathematical treatment.

Let me spend a few moments to discuss the use of the word "model".
In using this word one often intends to assume an attitude of modesty,
implying that what is presented as a model is still not a "theory". The
model does not claim to fully describe the phenomenology that is treated;
it has some openly recognized limitation, and is "simpler than reality".
Sometimes a model is used only to deal with the more basic aspects, just
to see them more transparently without the clouding effect of irrelevant
complications[3]. However, I may note that Volterra never uses the word
model in this sense. When he uses the terms "mechanical model" or "geometrical model" they are referred as analogical or as "real" interpretations or descriptions of the discussed phenomenology.

From a methodological point of view, certainly no important distinction should be made between models and theories. Both are stages of the
treatment of empirical information, with the scope to encode it in an
efficient way, in the general aim to diminish or eliminate the large
informational redundancy that the data contain[4]. In scientific practice the only distinction that we usually apply is that a theory is a
mapping or encoding with a larger domain or a higher efficiency than
a model. When we treat the information acquired about biological objects, encoding it in the language of physics, we indulge in physical
reductionism. We must declare that Volterra was recognizing the need
for biology to develop its own code and language, whenever possible
with strong assistance from mathematics.

A very similar attitude is shared, as is well known, by different
lines of attack on biological problems that are discussed in the field

of theoretical biology. For example it is stressed, some times with strong emphasis, that biology typically has to deal with very complex systems, showing a high level of internal organization. Special aspects of such systems are studied by cybernetics, as initiated by Wiener. The possibility to reach high complexity and internal "order", and later to maintain it, is attributed to the fact that biological systems are open systems, not at thermodynamical equilibrium. Von Bertalanffy was the first to develop, to cover this phenomenon, a new "language", that of general system theory. In the last several years, Prigogine and his school have also strongly insisted that particularly the fluctuations in open systems, when far from equilibrium, can originate or maintain the high ordered complexity found in biological systems. While invited therefore to refuse the simple reductionism to the language of "ordinary" physics, as exemplified by macroscopic mechanics or equilibrium thermodynamics, we are not asked to abandon totally the language of physics but rather to enlarge it to make space for the new phenomenology. Cybernetics has been very useful to alert biologists that, when discussing for example homeostasis or reafference, they could profit from all the mathematical developments already in existence for similar problems as studied by engineers.

Volterra Systems and Volterra Series Expansion

One of Volterra's greatest mathematical creations was the theory of functionals. A functional, in the simplest case, is a quantity y depending on all the values taken by a function x in its interval of definition. An example is the length of a line.

Functional relations or functional equations are usually encountered as differential or integral equations. Volterra showed that the notion of continuity, differentiality and analyticity could be extended to functionals. Functionals can be linear or of first degree; in most cases they can be expressed as integrals, that is:

$$y(t) = \int K(t,t') x(t') dt'.$$

In circuit analysis, the kernel K is the response function h of the linear system, relating input x(t) to output y(t):

$$y(t) = \int h(t-t') x(t') dt'.$$

Volterra introduced funtionals of higher degree n, arriving at the power seriės:

$$y = \sum_{n=0}^{\infty} \int \cdots \int k_n(t_1, \cdots, t_n) x(t_1) \ldots x(t_n) dt_1 \ldots dt_n$$

as general expressions for analytical functionals.

Following N. Wiener, the general Volterra expanşion for functionals has been used in nonlinear circuit analysis. The effects of nonlinearity in communication systems, causing "distortion" or crosstalk interference, can be treated taking into consideration the first higher terms of the Volterra expansions. The various types of nonlinearity can be also classified by the higher order kernels k_n. Using sine waves as input and taking the Fourier transforms of the kernels k_n, one can define "Volterra transfer functions" of higher order. Passive time-invariant systems (starting with n=1) with finite memory are currently called "Volterra Systems" and a detailed classification of various types of nonlinearity has been undertaken[5].

Volterra expansion was also found useful in identification analysis of nonlinear systems. Starting with black-box assumptions, the system, when tested with known signals as the inputs, can reveal its significant k_n components, particularly through correlation analysis between output and input. This approach has been used particularly for biological system identification in sensory physiology and nervous networks[6] as in defining a strategy for the reconstruction of the neural interactions underlying patterns of behaviour[7].

Going to the single cell level, a neuron can be considered to operate as a black-box encoding a continuous signal as a train of spikes. Treating the neuron as a leaky integrator, the Volterra representation has been used[8] to obtain higher order (nonlinear) transfer functions B_n, as generalizations of the previous known linear approximation[9].

The problems so rapidly indicated are of great importance and the possibility to develop mathematical models of this type has great potentialities for behavior analysis, memory and in general nonlinear neural networks.

Limits to Growth. Neuronal Death and Plant Mortality

I mention two recent mathematical models that can be both traced to Volterra. The first refers to the future of human population as has

been analyzed by the Club of Rome group, in relation to the pollution
of the environment due to industrialization. Forrester world dynamics
and Meadows modeling of the growth limits are based on computer analysis, with functional dependences cast in tabulated form. One can show[10]
that their results can be well reproduced by using the integro-diffe-
rential equation introduced by Volterra in 1931:

$$\frac{dN}{dt} = \{\varepsilon - \gamma N - \int_0^t f(t-\tau)N(\tau)d\tau\}N$$

to treat the effects of intoxication due to the catabolic waste in the
environment of a bacterial population. The integral term represents the
accumulation of past pollution load. Assuming the present pollution as

$$P(t) = \int_0^{t-\theta} e^{-\delta(t-\theta-\tau)}N(\tau)d\tau$$

one obtains for the population-pollution competition the equations:

$$\begin{cases} \dot{P}(t) = -\delta P(t) + N(t-\theta) \\ \dot{N}(t) = \{\varepsilon - \gamma N(t) - \alpha P(t)\}N(t) \end{cases}$$

where the coefficient $\alpha = \alpha(P)$ characterizes how pollution affects the
population changes. Additional nonlinearities are introduced assuming
a quadratic dependence of α on P, while life time of pollutants δ^{-1} is
supposed also dependent on the total load. Suppression of population
growth by limited carrying capacity or by pollution, as well as cyclic
interplay of pollution and population can be seen in a more transparent
way by using this analytical model. For example a longer delay enhances
the population crisis in a very dramatic way. How realistic the model
is and which lesson it is teaching, only the future will reveal.

The last model to which I will refer regards the embryonic development of the nervous system, this has some relation to the previous
example. At the end of the proliferation phase, a peak in the number
of neuronal cells in a certain region of the embryo is reached, the
peak being followed by a high mortality phase. The cell number at the
final value gives mortality frequently as high as 50 % and in a few
systems up to 80 - 90 %. The phenomenon appears to be naturally occurring, with a well-defined timing, so that it is considered not a for-
tuitous accident of development, but as having a definite role in the
making of the nervous system.

One type of explanation calls for a system-matching mechanism. It
is assumed that cells compete for a limited number of available synaptic
fields. To survive the cells have to receive retrograde signals or sub-

stances from those cells with which they must extablish contacts; mortality is determined by the finite carrying capacity of such an environment. The cell competition, as the phenomenon was already called by Ramon y Cajal, can be relaxed or forced by experimentally increasing or reducing the synaptic targets. A model for the retinal ganglion cells in the chick embryo has been discussed by G. Rager[11]. Mathematically one can write the Volterra equations for two cell populations, the ganglion cells and their prey, the tectal cells that they must reach with their axonal arborization. In this case a retardation effect is introduced by the time required by the axons to grow inside the optical tract.

The cell mortality in embryonic neural development has a curious analogy with another case of high mortality that has been recently evidenced in even-aged monoculture of plants. Following a phase of bimodality in the statistical distribution of plant parameters (height, weight, etc.) the plant population shows a high mortality (50 %), settling finally again with a unimodal distribution.

The phenomenon is explained as a consequence of an interaction between the plants. In a pair of adjacent members of the population, one of the two by chance will be the more vigorous. This dominant member will grow faster and will damage the less vigorous one, shadowing it with its own higher and larger crown; analogous effects can come from inter-root competition. In these conditions the population will develop a bimodality, one peak contributed by the dominant plants, the other by the dominated ones. At the end the dominated members degenerate and, following a phase of high mortality, the population becomes unimodal again, with the surviving plants completing their growth.

Taking a random rectangular distribution for the vigour, Gates[12] has developed a mathematical model for the plant growth distribution and for the mortality rate.

On a similar line one can treat[13] the neural cell growth and the cell mortality during the embryonic development of the nervous system. In this case the vigour must be looked as a random variable expressing the result of many small independent factors affecting the growing cells in their microenvironment. In another view the vigour could be a measure of the success of one cell in reaching its target in a random sequence of attempts. This kind of models suggests that cells can compete between themselves during development. In this way a parallelism is established between phylogenesis and ontogenesis[14]. A competitive selection could ensure that the final nervous system is made only with selected cells, the surviving ones. In view of the non-renewable components of this system, the organism could get in this way an additional safety margin.

While the model gives some hints for understanding the phenomenon of neural death, there are still several aspects of it that are rather obscure and in need of further clarification. As usual, the nervous system offers the best examples of resistant complexity.

References

1. V. Volterra: Sui tentativi di applicazione delle matematiche alle scienze biologiche e sociali, Ann. R. Univ. Roma 1901-2, 3-28; Giorn. degli Econ., 23, 436-58, 1901; Rev. du Mois, Paris, I, 1-20, 1906; Arch. di Fisiologia, 3, 175-191, 1906; Saggi scientifici, Bologna, 1-33, 1920; Opere Matematiche, Roma, Vol. III, 14-29, 1957

2. S. Fomin, M. Berkiblit: Problèmes mathématiques en biologie, Moscow, 1975

3. J. Maynard Smith: Models in Ecology, Cambr. Univ. Press, London, 1974

4. A. Borsellino: L'informazione ed il progresso nella scienza in: "Il concetto di progresso nella scienza" (ed. E. Agazzi), 135-138, Milano, 1976

5. E. Bedrosian, S.O. Rice: The output properties of Volterra Systems (Nonlinear systems with Memory) driven by harmonic and gaussian inputs, Proc. IEEE, 59, 1688-1707, 1971

6. P.Z. Marmarelis, K.L. Naka: Identification of multi-input biological systems, IEEE Trans. Biom. Eng. 2, 88-101, 1974

7. T. Poggio, W. Reichardt: Visual control of orientation behaviour in the fly, p. II. Quart. Rev. of Biophys. 9, 377-438, 1976

8. T. Poggio, V. Torre: A Volterra representation for some neuron models, Biol. Cybernetics 27, 113-124, 1977

9. A. Borsellino, R.E. Poppele, C.A. Terzuolo: Transfer functions of the slowly adapting stretch receptor organ of Crustacea. Cold Spring Harbor Symp. Quant. Biol. 30, 581-586, 1965

10. A Borsellino, V. Torre: Limits to growth from Volterra theory of population, Kybernetik 16, 113-118, 1974

11. G. Rager: Systems-matching by degeneration, Exp. Brain Res. 33, 79-90, 1978

12. D.J. Gates: Bimodality in even-aged plant monocultures. J. Theor. Biol. 71, 525-540, 1978

13. A. Borsellino: Neuronal death in embryonic development. A model for selective cell competition and dominance. In: A multidisciplinary approach to brain development. (C. Di Benedetta, ed.), Elsevier, Amsterdam, 1980

14. R.J. Zilles: Ontogenesis of the visual system. Adv. Anat. Embryol. Cell Biol. 54, 9-138, 1978

_ecture Notes in Biomathematics

Vol. 26: M. B. Katz, Questions of Uniqueness and Resolution in Reconstruction fror Projections. IX, 175 pages. 1978.

Vol. 27: N. MacDonald, Time Lags in Biological Models. VII, 112 pages. 1978.

Vol. 28: P. C. Fife, Mathematical Aspects of Reacting and Diffusing Systems. IV, 185 pages. 1979.

Vol. 29: Kinetic Logic – A Boolean Approach to the Analysis of Complex Regulator Systems. Proceedings, 1977. Edited by R. Thomas. XIII, 507 pages. 1979.

Vol. 30: M. Eisen, Mathematical Models in Cell Biology and Cancer Chemotherapy. IX 431 pages. 1979.

Vol. 31: E. Akin, The Geometry of Population Genetics. IV, 205 pages. 1979.

Vol. 32: Systems Theory in Immunology. Proceedings, 1978. Edited by G. Bruni et a XI, 273 pages. 1979.

Vol. 33: Mathematical Modelling in Biology and Ecology. Proceedings, 1979. Edited by W. M. Getz. VIII, 355 pages. 1980.

Vol. 34: R. Collins, T. J. van der Werff, Mathematical Models of the Dynamics of the Human Eye. VII, 99 pages. 1980.

Vol. 35: U. an der Heiden, Analysis of Neural Networks. X, 159 pages. 1980.

Vol. 36: A. Wörz-Busekros, Algebras in Genetics. VI, 237 pages. 1980.

Vol. 37: T. Ohta, Evolution and Variation of Multigene Families. VIII, 131 pages. 1980.

Vol. 38: Biological Growth and Spread: Mathematical Theories and Applications. Pro ceedings, 1979. Edited by W. Jäger, H. Rost and P. Tautu. XI, 511 pages. 1980

Vol. 39: Vito Volterra Symposium on Mathematical Models in Biology. Proceedings, 1979 Edited by C. Barigozzi. VI, 417 pages. 1980.